Notice

The Doping Search Guide is an indicative guide that describes the status of pharmaceutical products or over the counter medicinal products and substances in relation to the World Anti-Doping Code List of Prohibited Substances and Methods which list can be found on the WADA website http://www.wada-ama.org.

Elsevier made reasonable effort to ensure the accuracy and completeness of the Doping Search Guide and Elsevier does not accept responsibility for any errors, omissions or inaccuracies that may arise.

No responsibility is assumed by Elsevier for any injury and/or damage to persons or property as a matter of products liability, negligence or otherwise, or from any use or operation of any methods, products, instructions or ideas contained in the material herein.

The Doping Search Guide is not intended to provide medical advice and independent verification of diagnoses and medication should be made.

TABLE OF CONTENT

Introduction 5

Searching Scientific Information 9
Introduction to EMTREE 11

Chapter 1 - EMTREE Terms per WADA category 15
Chapter 2 - EMTREE Terms and Synonyms 35
Chapter 3 - Index 219

INTRODUCTION

This guide refers to the 2004 WADA (World Anti-Doping Agency) List of Prohibited Substances and Methods. In addition to the introductory chapters, this book has three chapters containing lists of prohibited substances. In this introduction you will find instructions on how to use these lists, guidelines for searching biomedical databases and information about EMTREE, THE Life Science Thesaurus from Elsevier.

The WADA (World Anti-Doping Agency)

The World Anti-Doping Agency (WADA) seeks to foster a doping-free culture in sport. It combines the resources of sport and government to enhance, supplement and coordinate existing efforts to educate athletes about the harms of doping, reinforce the ideal of fair play and sanction those who cheat themselves and their sport.

WADA was established as an independent, non-governmental organization on November 10, 1999, as a result of provisions of the Lausanne Declaration on Doping in Sport. The Agency's headquarters are located in Montreal, Canada.

Key Activities are:

- Conducting unannounced out-of-competition doping control among elite athletes
- Monitoring acceptance of and compliance with the World Anti-Doping Code
- Funding scientific research to develop new detection methods
- Observing the doping-control and results-management programs of major events
- Educating athletes through the Athlete Outreach Program
- Providing anti-doping education to athletes, coaches and administrators
- Fostering the development of National Anti-Doping Organizations (NADO)

More information relating to the World Anti-Doping Code can be found on the WADA website: http://www.wada-ama.org/. This site contains all the official WADA publications and procedures (such as Therapeutic Use Exemptions) and is always the most up-to-date official resource.

HOW TO USE THIS BOOK

The first part of this book lists the prohibited substances subdivided according to the WADA groups.

S1. STIMULANTS
S2. NARCOTICS
S3. CANNABINOIDS
S4. ANABOLIC AGENTS
S5. PEPTIDE HORMONES
S6. BETA-2 AGONISTS
S7. AGENTS WITH ANTI-OESTROGENIC ACTIVITY
S8. MASKING AGENTS
S9. GLUCOCORTICOSTEROIDS
M1. ENHANCEMENT OF OXYGEN TRANSFER
P1. ALCOHOL
P2. BETA-BLOCKERS
P3. DIURETICS

The following WADA groups do not contain chemical compounds. So these have been omitted:

M2. PHARMACOLOGICAL, CHEMICAL AND PHYSICAL MANIPULATION
M3. GENE DOPING

The names of the substances are the EMTREE preferred terms. The selection of the terms has been made by matching the relevant EMTREE broader terms with the WADA categories. For instance: the substances listed under the WADA group S4. ANABOLIC AGENTS correspond to the EMTREE narrower terms listed under the broader terms: anabolic agent and androgen.

The number of terms selected from EMTREE for each WADA category exceeds the number of terms actually mentioned in the WADA list because it contains many other substances with similar chemical structures or similar pharmacological effects.

See the latest WADA instructions for detailed information about prohibition in-competition or in- and out-of-competition or exceptions depending on the administration route. This also applies for substances for which a medical notification is required in accordance with the International Standard for Therapeutic Use Exemptions (TUE).

The second part of the book lists the prohibited substances by their EMTREE preferred name together with all available information for each individual compound, in the following order:

EMTREE preferred term
WADA group
MeSH descriptor
CAS Registry number
Trade names and research codes
Short synonyms
Long synonyms

Example:

---

fadrozole

Wada group
S7. AGENTS WITH ANTI-OESTROGENIC ACTIVITY

MeSH descriptor
fadrozole

CAS Registry number
102676-31-3

Trade names and research codes
afema
arensin
cgs 16949
cgs16949
cgs 16949 a
cgs 16949a
cgs16949a

Short synonyms
fadrozole hydrochloride

Long synonyms
5 (4 cyanophenyl) 3,6,7,8 tetrahydro 5h imidazo [1,5 a]pyridine
4 (3,6,7,8 tetrahydro 5h imidazo[1,5 a]pyridin 5 yl) benzonitrile

Explanation:

MeSH descriptor (The Medical Subject Headings of the U.S. National Library of Medicine)
All MeSH descriptors are present in EMTREE, as synonyms or as preferred terms.
In this instance the EMTREE preferred term 'fadrozole' is also a MeSH descriptor.

CAS Registry number (Chemical Abstracts Registry number)
The CAS Registry number belonging to the EMTREE preferred term is listed here.
In some instances a CAS Registry number corresponding to a synonym is also listed here for ease of reference.

Trade names and research codes
Registered trade marks and codes referring to the manufacturer are listed here.

Short synonyms
Synonyms with not more than 30 characters not listed as trade names or research codes.
For instance short chemical names or (spelling) variants of the preferred term.

Long synonyms
Synonyms with more than 30 characters; for the most part these are (long) chemical synonyms.

The third part of the book is an alphabetical list of the entries listed in the second part i.e. it contains the EMTREE preferred terms and also all EMTREE short synonyms + trade names and research codes with their corresponding preferred term. The EMTREE preferred terms can be found between the lines, all other terms have no lines.

So this list is the index functioning as an easy entrance to find the information present in the other two chapters.

Example:

---

fadrozole

---

fadrozole hydrochloride
see: fadrozole

WARNING!

Terms in this book have been selected for EMTREE only if they were mentioned in at least a number of published scientific articles. This means that this guide does not per se cover every prohibited substance that exists. At the same time, certain substances that are covered in this guide are allowed under certain circumstances and/or for specific use.

If in doubt whether a specific substance is allowed or not, please seek the advice of an expert. Such experts are usually available at the National Doping Agencies. Contact information for those agencies is available at the WADA.

SEARCHING SCIENTIFIC INFORMATION

Nowadays many people have experience with Internet searching and search engines, most frequently with Google. Google is considered ideal for quick results that require little effort. But when there is a lot at stake and you need to find all of the relevant information, it is wise to take the time to prepare a search plan.

A search plan should consist of several elements, a description of your problem using relevant search terms, a selection of sources that are likely to contain the required information and a search strategy to retrieve the desired information.

Select search terms

Begin your search plan by creating an overview of your questions. This overview should describe your problem and consist of a word list, and a set of required information. Your problem or search question may have many components. What type of information are you seeking (i.e., facts, opinions, options)? What form will this information take (i.e., scientific articles, review articles, product information)? A word list typically consists of various key words organized in different groups; essential terms, narrower words, broader words, and related words.

Information Sources

Everyone has experience with high recall, usually when an Internet search engine provides you with thousands of ìhitsî for your search term(s). Preferably you want high precision, to find only the information that is highly relevant to your search question. The perfect match of content covered by a website and the search tools it provides depends on the situation. This might be a good opportunity to consider alternatives to your automatic choice of search engine. Here are some examples.

Scirus

According to Wired Magazine there is more than Google for searching the Internet, certainly if you're looking for scientific information on the Web. Many researchers instead turn to Scirus (www.scirus.com). Scirus is a science-specific search engine. Scirus searches over 167 million science-specific Web pages, enabling you to quickly pinpoint scientific, scholarly, technical and medical data on the Web. Scirus does cover the latest reports, peer-reviewed articles and journals that other search engines miss.

MEDLINE and PubMed

Some content is searchable on more than one website, such as MEDLINE that is searchable via Scirus but also via PubMed. MEDLINE is The National Library of Medicine's premier bibliographic database covering the fields of medicine, nursing, dentistry, veterinary medicine, the healthcare system, and the pre-clinical sciences, containing bibliographic citations and author abstracts from more than 4,300 biomedical journals. The file contains over 12 million citations dating from 1966 to the present.

PubMed, also from the National Library of Medicine, includes over 14 million citations for biomedical articles back to the 1950's. These citations are from MEDLINE and additional life science journals. PubMed includes links to many sites providing full text articles and other related resources. PubMed provides a range of tools for information searching.

EMBASE.com

EMBASE.com combines two high quality biomedical databases, EMBASE and Medline, in one website resulting in 16 million citations.
The coverage of EMBASE is different from Medline; it is more focussed towards drugs and pharmacology together with a less US centric journal policy.

EMBASE features comprehensive coverage of:

- Drug Research, Pharmacology, Pharmacy, Pharmacoeconomics, Pharmaceutics and Toxicology
- Human Medicine (Clinical and Experimental)
- Basic Biological Research
- Health Policy and Management
- Public, Occupational and Environmental Health
- Substance Dependence and Abuse
- Psychiatry
- Forensic Science
- Biomedical Engineering and Instrumentation

Therefore when there is a need to be complete, both databases should be included in your search strategy. EMTREE is applied in EMBASE.com as one consistent vocabulary that can be used to search both databases. EMBASE.com does have a good combination of content with a powerful though very easy to use interface. Note: it is not free.

Search Strategy

A Search Strategy usually has a multi-step approach to get the desired result list that is highly relevant and not too long. The specific implementation of a search strategy is dependent on the source and website of your choice. Therefore it is advisable to look at the help sections on the website. You can find valuable information there to complete your search strategy.

Field Searching

A bibliographic database consists of many records each organized in a similar manner. A record consists of various fields such as article title, journal title, abstract and many more. Field searching is a great tool because you can specify exactly where a key word should be found (e.g. in the field Drug Trade Name at EMBASE.com).

Boolean Logic

Boolean operators as AND, OR and NOT or equivalents such as + and – can be used in almost every search form to combine search terms. Consider using the less familiar proximity operators such as NEAR or ADJ (adjacent) as well. Do note that different search tools use different operators so look at the help files or search tips to find the proper operator.

Controlled Vocabulary

A Search Strategy benefits greatly from the presence of a thesaurus using controlled vocabulary. The indexing of the database will guarantee that every article on a topic represented by a thesaurus term is included in your search. Even when the term is quite broad, an explosion search will include all narrower terms in your search results without the need to include all these narrower terms in your search command. Often good suggestions for more terms or more precise terms can be found in some record from your initial search results.
The EMTREE chapter contains a detailed description of this controlled vocabulary.

INTRODUCTION TO EMTREE

EMTREE is Elsevier's Life Science Thesaurus. It is a hierarchically structured, controlled vocabulary, for Biomedicine and related Life Sciences.

EMTREE provides a consistent description of biomedical information:

- it offers indexers a comprehensive vocabulary to describe the content of biomedical data
- for database users, it facilitates comprehensive searching and high precision retrieval

EMTREE history

EMTREE evolved from the Master List of Medical Terms (MALIMET), originally created in 1963 to control and standardize the subject indexes of over 40 printed Excerpta Medica abstract journals. But MALIMET grew rapidly as new terms were proposed by the abstract journal editors, until by the end of the 80's it contained an unwieldy 250,000 preferred terms.

EMTREE was created in 1988 by pruning MALIMET to the most frequently indexed 25,000 terms, and imposing upon these terms a hierarchical structure based on that of MeSH, the thesaurus used by the U.S. National Library of Medicine for MEDLINE and PubMed. Over the past 16 years, EMTREE has been developed and broadened to its current size: a thesaurus comprising almost 48,000 preferred terms, which is actively maintained and updated with up to 1000 new terms every year.

EMTREE is integrated into Elsevier's Bibliographic Databases, EMBASE and EMBASE.com, and is an important part of the Elsevier Customized Bibliographic Services (EMSCOPES). EMTREE is also available in a three-volume print format.

EMTREE content

EMTREE comprises more than 48,000 preferred terms, most of which have one or more synonyms that are available as entry points for indexers and database users. The number of synonyms can be very large: for example the drug isoniazid has more than 200 synonyms, including many trade names and laboratory codes by which it is known. Overall EMTREE has almost 200,000 synonyms: an average of more than four synonyms for each preferred term.

For the user, this means that searching does not require advance knowledge of EMTREE's preferred terminology; any phrase describing the required concept is enough. Simply by looking up the phrase in the alphabetical index or (more generally) by checking any of its component words in the permuted index (of all EMTREE's words), users can identify the EMTREE keywords - preferred terms or synonyms - for the concepts they have in mind.

EMTREE structure

EMTREE preferred terms are not independent of each other, but are organised into a hierarchical structure with 15 branches, which we call facets:

A Anatomical concepts
B Organisms
C Physical diseases, disorders and abnormalities
D Chemicals and drugs
E Analytical, diagnostic and therapeutic techniques, equipment and parameters
F Psychological and psychiatric phenomena
G Biological phenomena and functions
H Chemical, physical and mathematical phenomena
I Society and environment
J Types of article or study
K Geographic names
L Groups by age and sex

M Named groups of persons
N Healthcare
O Biomedical disciplines, science and art

This structure is modeled on that of MeSH (see EMTREE History above). However, the distribution of terms differs from that of MeSH: EMTREE - with its focus on drug names - has more drugs and chemicals in facet D (ca. 24,000 in 2004) than MeSH has total terms (ca. 23,000 in 2004).

Each facet represents a single term type, as described by the facet name. Within each facet, terms are organised into a hierarchical tree (up to 12 levels deep). Individual terms may appear more than once in the hierarchy, i.e. EMTREE is polyhierarchical (explained below).

EMTREE's hierarchical tree - the facet structure - is defined by some 10,000 preferred terms, sometimes referred to in this context as nodes or explosion terms[1]. The image below is a representation of the nodes in facets A-E. The facet with the most nodes is Facet C (Physical diseases, disorders and abnormalities), followed by facet D (Chemicals and drugs):

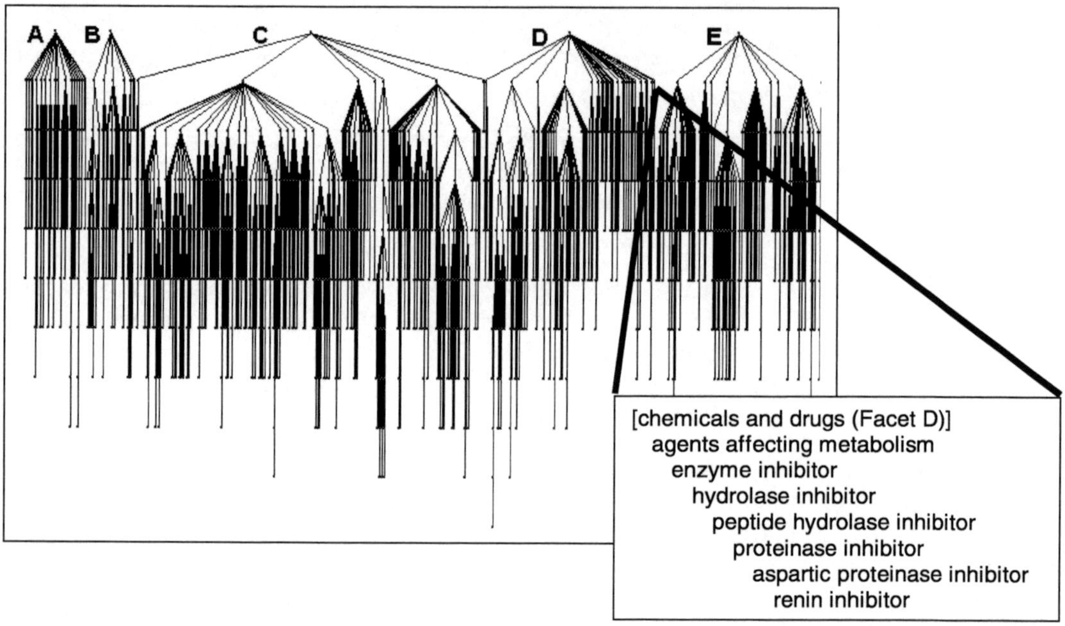

Terms at different levels in the hierarchy have a broader-narrower term relationship with each other, as shown in the inset, which represents part of facet D (e.g. hydrolase inhibitor is a narrower term of the higher level term enzyme inhibitor).

[1] In the printed EMTREE, explosion terms have codes which identify their place in the tree structure. This enables users to find the hierarchical location of terms which they have identified in the alphabetical index.

Several additional aspects of the facet structure merit special attention:

- Polyhierarchical structure: terms may be listed in several different parts of the hierarchy. For example, leukemia is listed both in the malignant neoplastic disease (cancer) tree and in the leukocyte disorder tree. If such multiply-listed terms are explosion terms (i.e. head a hierarchy of narrower terms), EMTREE displays the same hierarchy in all locations[2].

- Non-explosion terms: these are terms - 38,000 in all - which lack their own codes and which are associated as narrower terms with one or more explosion terms. In the inset, the explosion term renin inhibitor has 30 narrower non-explosion terms, including inhibitors such as ciprokiren and zankiren.

- Explosion searches: the tree structure allows users to do explosion searches to retrieve groups of hierarchically related terms in a single search. For example, an explosion search on proteinase inhibitor retrieves records indexed with either this term or any of its narrower terms, including aspartic proteinase inhibitor, renin inhibitor, as well as all narrower (non-explosion) terms of these terms (such as ciprokiren and zankiren).

If explosion searches are carried out using terms present in more than one place in the hierarchy (as in the case of leukemia, see above), then all narrower terms are retrieved.

[2] The only exception is subfacet D4 (natural product) which excludes synthetic substances from its hierarchy.

EMTREE Terms per WADA category

S1. STIMULANTS

adrafinil
adrenalin
☝ adrenalone
allylglycine
almitrine
almitrine dimesilate
amfepramone
amfonelic acid
4 amino 1 (6 bromo 2 pyridyl)piperidine
4 amino 1 (6 chloro 2 pyridyl)piperidine
aminorex
amiphenazole
amphetamine
amphetamine derivative
amphetaminil
anorexigenic agent
apomorphine
apraclonidine
bamethan
bemegride
1 (1,3 benzodioxol 5 yl) n methyl 2 butanamine
benzphetamine
brimonidine
brolamfetamine
bromantan
brucine
buphenine
tert butylbicycloorthobenzoate
tert butylbicyclophosphorothioate
cafedrine plus theodrenaline
☝ caffeine
☝ caffeine benzoate
☝ caffeine citrate
carphedon
central stimulant agent
chloramphetamine
4 chloromethamphetamine
chlorphentermine
citicoline
clobenzorex
clorprenaline
clortermine
cocaine
convulsant agent
cropropamide
crotetamide
5 (2 cyclohexylideneethyl) 5 ethylbarbituric acid
cyclopentamine
deanol
dexamphetamine
dexfenfluramine
dexmethylphenidate
dexnorfenfluramine
dexoxadrol
2,6 dichloro 4 dimethylaminoamphetamine
dimefline
dimetamfetamine
2,5 dimethoxy 4 methylamphetamine
n (3,5 dimethoxyphenethyl) 5 methoxy 2 (phenylethynyl)amphetamine
5 (1,3 dimethylbutyl) 5 ethylbarbituric acid
dimetofrine
☝ diphenylpyraline plus phenylpropanolamine
dipivefrine
dobutamine
☝ dopamine
dopexamine
doxapram
ephedrine
etafedrine
etamivan
ethimizole
n ethyl 3,4 methylenedioxyamphetamine
5 ethyl 5 (3 methyl 2 butenyl)barbituric acid
4 ethyl 6,7 dimethoxy beta carboline 3 carboxylic acid methyl ester
n ethylamphetamine
etilefrine
etilefrine pivalate
fencamfamin
fenetylline
fenfluramine
fenoldopam
fenoldopam 7,8 bis(n ethylcarbamate)
fenoldopam mesilate
fenproporex
flurothyl
fominoben
formetorex
furfenorex
furfurylamphetamine
gepefrine
gepefrine tartrate
heptaminol
homococaine
n hydroxy 3,4 methylenedioxyamphetamine
hydroxyamphetamine
n hydroxyamphetamine
ibogaine
4 iodo 2,5 dimethoxyamphetamine
4 iodoamphetamine
iofetamine
lefetamine
levofacetoperane
lobeline
mazindol
meclofenoxate
mefenorex
mefexamide
mephentermine
metaraminol
methamphetamine
methcathinone
4 methoxyamphetamine
2 methoxymethamphetamine
3 methoxymethamphetamine
4 methoxymethamphetamine
methoxyphenamine
4 methylaminorex
4 methylamphetamine
3,4 methylenedioxyamphetamine
3,4 methylenedioxyamphetamine derivative
3,4 methylenedioxymethamphetamine
methylephedrine
methylphenidate
midodrine
modafinil
morazone
nikethamide
noradrenalin
norcocaine

☝ *probably not prohibited*

norfenfluramine
norpseudoephedrine
oxilofrine
oxyfedrine
pemoline
pemoline magnesium
pentetrazole
phendimetrazine
phendimetrazine embonate
phendimetrazine tartrate
phenmetrazine
phentermine
phentermine resin
☝ phenylpropanolamine
pholedrine
picamilon
picrotoxin
☝ pipradol
prenylamine
prethcamide
prolintane
propylhexedrine
psychostimulant agent
pyrovalerone
racephedrine
selegiline
strychnine
sydnocarb
sydnofen
tetrabenazine
tetramethylsuccinimide
theodrenaline
xamoterol
xamoterol hydrogen fumarate

☝ *probably not prohibited*

S2. NARCOTICS

buprenorphine
dextromethorphan plus morphine
dextromoramide
diamorphine
hydromorphone
levomethadone
methadone
morphine
morphine 6 acetate
morphine sulfate
nicomorphine
oxycodone
oxymorphone
pentazocine
percocet
percodan
pethidine

S3. CANNABINOIDS

ajulemic acid
anandamide
2 arachidonoylglycerol
cannabichromene
cannabidiol
cannabidiol derivative
cannabidiol dimethyl ether
cannabidiol methyl ether
cannabielsoin
cannabigerol
cannabinoid
cannabinoid derivative
cannabinol
cannabinol derivative
cannabis
cannabis derivative
deacetyllevonantradol
dexanabinol
dextronantradol
2,3 dihydro 5 methyl 3 (morpholinomethyl) 6 (1 naphthoyl)pyrrolo[1,2,3 de][1,4]benzoxazine
4 (1,1 dimethylheptyl) 1',2',3',4',5',6' hexahydro 2,3' dihydroxy 6' (3 hydroxypropyl)biphenyl
5 (1,1 dimethylheptyl) 2 (3 hydroxy 7 hydroxymethyldecahydro 1 naphthyl)phenol
dronabinol
3' hydroxy delta9 tetrahydrocannabinol
11 hydroxydronabinol
levonantradol
methanandamide
nantradol
palmidrol
tetrahydrocannabinol
delta8 tetrahydrocannabinol
delta9(11) tetrahydrocannabinol
tetrahydrocannabinol derivative
delta8 tetrahydrocannabinol derivative
tetrahydrocannabinolic acid

S4. ANABOLIC AGENTS

adrenosterone
amafolone
ambroxol plus clenbuterol
anabolic agent
androgen
androst 1 ene 3,17 dione
androsta 4,16 dien 3 one
5alpha androstan 3 one
androstanediol
3beta androstanediol
androstanedione
androstanolone
5beta androstanolone
androstanolone bromoacetate
androstanolone derivative
androstanolone propionate
4 androstenediol
androstenediol
androstenediol derivative
androstenedione
androstenedione derivative
androsterone
androsterone derivative
atromid
benorterone
bolandiol
bolasterone
boldenone
boldenone undecenoate
boldione
calusterone
4 chloro 17beta hydroxy 17 methylandrosta 1,4 dien 3 one
clenbuterol
clostebol
clostebol acetate
danazol
deoxycorticosterone phenpropionate plus nandrolone phenpropionate
dexatopic
drostanolone
drostanolone propionate
epiandrosterone
estr 4 ene 3,17 dione
estratest
ethinylestradiol plus methyltestosterone
2beta ethoxy 3alpha hydroxy 11alpha isopentylamino 5alpha androstane 17beta carboxylic acid methyl ester
13beta ethyl 17beta hydroxygon 4 en 3 one
ethylestrenol
etiocholanone
fluoxymesterone
formebolone
furazabol
gestrinone
11beta hydroxyandrostenedione
19 hydroxyandrostenedione
4 hydroxytestosterone
mepitiostane
mestanolone
mesterolone
metandienone
metenolone
metenolone acetate
metenolone enantate
methandriol
methandriol dipropionate
methyldienolone
methyltestosterone
metribolone
mibolerone
nandrolone
nandrolone 4 hexyloxyhydrocinnamate
nandrolone cyclohexylpropionate
nandrolone decanoate
nandrolone derivative
nandrolone furylpropionate
nandrolone laurate
nandrolone phenpropionate
nandrolone undecanoate
norboletone
norclostebol
norclostebol acetate
norethandrolone
oxabolone
oxabolone cipionate
oxandrolone
19 oxoandrostenedione
11 oxotestosterone
oxymesterone
oxymetholone
prasterone
prasterone acetate
prasterone sulfate
quinbolone
stanozolol
stenbolone
stenbolone acetate
testololactone
1 testosterone
testosterone
testosterone 4 butylcyclohexanecarboxylate
testosterone cipionate
testosterone derivative
testosterone enantate
testosterone enantate benziloylhydrazone
testosterone ester
testosterone ether
testosterone phenylpropionate
testosterone propionate
testosterone undecanoate
tetrahydrogestrinone
tibolone
trenbolone
17alpha trenbolone
trenbolone acetate
trestolone
zearalanone
zearalenone
zeranol
zilpaterol

S5. PEPTIDE HORMONES

adenohypophysis hormone
aldosterone
alsactide
1 [2 (2 amino 2 methylpropionylamino) 3 (1h indol 3 yl)propionyl] 3 benzyl 3 piperidinecarboxylic acid ethyl ester
3 amino 3 methyl n [2,3,4,5 tetrahydro 2 oxo 1 [[2' (1h tetrazol 5 yl) 1,1' biphenyl 4 yl]methyl] 1h 1 benzazepin 3 yl]butanamide
2 amino 4 (methylsulfonyl)butyrylglutamylhistidylphenylalanyl dextro lysylphenylalanine
asialochorionic gonadotropin
biosynthetic human proinsulin
biphasic insulin
bovine insulin
buserelin
buserelin acetate
chorionic gonadotropin
chorionic gonadotropin alpha subunit
chorionic gonadotropin beta subunit
corticotropin
corticotropin[1-10]
corticotropin[11-24]
corticotropin[1-17]
corticotropin[1-39]
corticotropin[18-39]
corticotropin[4-10]
corticotropin[7-10]
corticotropin[7-16]
corticotropin derivative
corticotropin releasing factor
corticotropin releasing factor[9-41]
corticotropin releasing factor derivative
deglycochorionic gonadotropin
deoxycorticosterone
deoxycorticosterone acetate
deoxycorticosterone phenpropionate plus nandrolone phenpropionate
deoxycorticosterone pivalate
deslorelin
ebiratide
ebiratide acetate
erythropoietin
folligen
follitropin
follitropin beta subunit
follitropin derivative
follitropin receptor binding inhibitor
follitropin releasing factor
giractide
gonadorelin
gonadorelin[1-9][6 dextro alanine]
gonadorelin[1-9] ethylamide[6 dextro alanine]
gonadorelin[1-9] ethylamide[6 dextro tryptophan]
gonadorelin[6 dextro [3 (2 naphthyl)alanine] 10 azaglycine]
gonadorelin[6 dextro lysine] 2 pyrrolinodoxorubicin
gonadorelin[6 dextro lysine] doxorubicin
gonadorelin[6 medphalan]
gonadorelin acetate
gonadorelin agonist
gonadorelin associated peptide
gonadorelin associated peptide derivative
gonadorelin derivative
gonadotropin
gonadotropin derivative
goserelin
growth hormone
growth hormone derivative
growth hormone releasing factor
growth hormone releasing factor[1-29]
growth hormone releasing factor derivative
hexarelin
histidyl dextro tryptophylalanyltryptophyl dextro phenylalanyllysinamide
histrelin
human growth hormone
human insulin
human menopausal gonadotropin
3 (2 hydroxypropylamino) 3 methyl n [2,3,4,5 tetrahydro 2 oxo 1 [[2' (1h tetrazol 5 yl) 1,1' biphenyl 4 yl]methyl] 1h 1 benzazepin 3 yl]butanamide
hypothalamus releasing factor
ibutamoren
immunocortin
immunoreactive insulin
insulin
insulin aspart
insulin[B28 lysine B29 proline]
insulin deoctapeptide
insulin derivative
insulin detemir
insulin glargine
insulin glulisine
insulin zinc suspension
ipamorelin
isophane insulin
leuprorelin
luteinizing hormone
luteinizing hormone beta subunit
luteinizing hormone derivative
lutrelin
methallibure
monocomponent insulin
nafarelin
nafarelin acetate
neutral insulin
novel erythropoiesis stimulating protein
ovurelin
pig insulin
pralmorelin
preproinsulin
proinsulin
recombinant chorionic gonadotropin
recombinant erythropoietin
recombinant follitropin
recombinant growth hormone
recombinant human insulin
recombinant luteinizing hormone
recombinant somatomedin B
recombinant somatomedin C
relefact
sauvagine
seric gonadotropin
sermorelin
somatomedin
somatomedin A
somatomedin B
somatomedin C
somatrem
synthetic insulin

probably not prohibited

tabimorelin
☝ tetracosactide
☝ tetracosactide zinc phosphate
triptorelin
urofollitropin

☝ *probably not prohibited*

S6. BETA-2 AGONISTS

alifedrine
ambroxol plus clenbuterol
6 amino alpha [[(1 methyl 3 phenylpropyl)amino]methyl] 3 pyridinemethanol
bambuterol
bamethan
alpha [[[3 (1 benzimidazolyl) 1,1 dimethylpropyl]amino]methyl] 2 fluoro 4 hydroxybenzyl alcohol
beta 1 adrenergic receptor stimulating agent
beta 2 adrenergic receptor stimulating agent
beta 3 adrenergic receptor stimulating agent
beta adrenergic receptor stimulating agent
4 [3 [bis(beta hydroxyphenethyl)amino]butyl]benzamide
bitolterol
bitolterol mesilate
broxaterol
budesonide plus formoterol
carbuterol
3 chloro n (1,2,3,4 tetrahydro 7 hydroxy 2 naphthyl)phenylethanolamine
3 chloro n (7 ethoxycarbonylmethoxy 1,2,3,4 tetrahydro 2 naphthyl)phenylethanolamine
[[7 [[2 (3 chlorophenyl) 2 hydroxyethyl]amino] 5,6,7,8 tetrahydro 2 naphthyl]oxy]acetic acid ethyl ester
5 [2 [[2 (3 chlorophenyl) 2 hydroxyethyl]amino]propyl] 1,3 benzodioxole 2,2 dicarboxylic acid
4 [2 [[2 (3 chlorophenyl) 2 hydroxyethyl]amino]propyl]phenoxyacetic acid
4 [2 [[2 (3 chlorophenyl) 2 hydroxyethyl]amino]propyl]phenoxyacetic acid methyl ester
cicloprolol
cimaterol
clenbuterol
clorprenaline
combivent
cromoglycate disodium plus reproterol
cyclohexyl[4 [2 [2 hydroxy 3 (4 hydroxyphenoxy)propylamino]ethyl]phenoxymethyl]phosphinic acid
denopamine
dichlorisoprenaline
1 (3,4 dihydroxyphenoxy) 3 (3,4 dimethoxyphenethylamino) 2 propanol
3 (3,4 dihydroxyphenyl) 2 [3 (4 fluorophenyl)propylamino] 3 hydroxypropionic acid pyrrolidine amide
6 [2 (3,4 dihydroxyphenyl) 2 hydroxyethylamino] n [4 (trifluoromethyl)phenyl]heptanamide
ditec
dopexamine
doxaminol
epanolol
epinine
etafedrine
etanterol
etilefrine
etilefrine pivalate
fenoterol
fenoterol plus ipratropium bromide
flerobuterol
fluticasone propionate plus salmeterol
formoterol
formoterol fumarate
gepefrine
gepefrine tartrate
hexoprenaline
4 [2 [(2 hydroxy 2 phenylethyl)amino]ethoxy]phenylacetic acid
4 [2 [(2 hydroxy 2 phenylethyl)amino]propyl]benzoic acid
4 [2 [(2 hydroxy 2 phenylethyl)amino]propyl]benzoic acid methyl ester
4 [2 [(2 hydroxy 2 phenylethyl)amino]propyl]benzoic acid methyl ester hydrogen maleate
n [2 [2 hydroxy 3 [4 (2 isobutoxyethoxy)phenoxy]propylamino]ethyl] 4 morpholinecarboxamide
n [4 [2 [[2 hydroxy 3 (4 hydroxyphenoxy)propyl]amino]ethyl]phenyl]benzenesulfonamide
4 [2 [(2 hydroxy 3 phenoxypropyl)amino]ethoxy] n (2 methoxyethyl)phenoxyacetamide
4 [2 [(2 hydroxy 3 phenoxypropyl)amino]ethoxy]phenoxyacetic acid
8 hydroxy 5 [1 hydroxy 2 [n [2 (4 methoxyphenyl) 1 methylethyl]amino]ethyl]carbostyril
4 hydroxy 7 [2 [2 [3 (2 phenylethoxy)propylsulfonyl]ethylamino]ethyl] benzothiazol 2(3h) one
hydroxyamphetamine
hydroxybenzylisoprenaline
3 hydroxydenopamine
4 hydroxy n [2 [2 hydroxy 3 [4 [2 (isobutoxy)ethoxy]phenoxy]propylamino]ethyl] 1 piperidinecarboxamide
ibopamine
ibuterol
imoxiterol
isoetarine
isoprenaline
isoxsuprine
levalbuterol
mabuterol
methoxamine
methoxyphenamine
naminterol
noradrenalin
noradrenalin bitartrate
orciprenaline
oxyfedrine
picumeterol
pirbuterol
pirbuterol acetate
prenalterol
procaterol
quinprenaline
ractopamine
reproterol
rimiterol
ritodrine
salbutamol
salbutamol sulfate
salmefamol
salmeterol

salmeterol xinafoate
soterenol
tazolol
terbutaline
terbutaline sulfate
n (1,2,3,4 tetrahydro 7 hydroxy 2
naphthyl)phenylethanolamine
trecadrine
tretoquinol
tretoquinol derivative
n (3,4,5 trimethoxyphenethyl)noradrenalin
tulobuterol
xamoterol
xamoterol hydrogen fumarate
zilpaterol
zinterol

S7. AGENTS WITH ANTI-OESTROGENIC ACTIVITY

acefluranol
aminoglutethimide
aminoglutethimide derivative
aminoglutethimide phosphate
7alpha (4 aminophenylthio)androstenedione
anastrozole
androsta 1,4,6 triene 3,17 dione
androsta 4,6,8(9) triene 3,17 dione
anordiol
antiestrogen
aromatase inhibitor
arzoxifene
atamestane
bazedoxifene
1 [4 [n,n bis(2 chloroethyl)carbamoyloxy]phenyl] 1 (4 hydroxyphenyl) 2 phenyl 1 butene
2,3 bis(2 fluoro 4 hydroxyphenyl) 2,3 dimethylbutane
2,3 bis(2 fluoro 4 hydroxyphenyl) 2,3 dimethylbutane derivative
2,3 bis(4 hydroxyphenyl) 2,3 dimethylbutane
bis(4 hydroxyphenyl)cyclohexylidenemethane
4 [n (4 bromobenzyl) n (1,2,4 triazol 4 yl)amino]benzonitrile
n butyl 11 (16alpha chloro 3,17beta dihydroxyestra 1,3,5(10) trien 7alpha yl) n methylundecanamide
n butyl 11 (3,17beta dihydroxyestra 1,3,5(10) trien 7alpha yl) n methylundecanamide
centchroman
8 chloro 3 methylnaringenin
8 chloro 5 (4 chlorophenyl) 5h indeno[1,2 d]pyrimidine
clomifene
clomifene citrate
cyclofenil
1,1 dichloro 2,3 diphenylcyclopropane
1 (4,4' dicyanobenzhydryl)imidazole
4 (2 diethylaminoethoxy) alpha' ethyl alpha (4 hydroxyphenyl) 4' methoxystilbene
11 [4 (2 dimethylaminoethoxy)phenyl]estradiol
dimethylstilbestrol
droloxifene
enclomifene
enclomifene citrate
☝ epimestrol
ethamoxytriphetol
exemestane
fadrozole
finrozole
formestane
fulvestrant
6 hydroxy 2 (4 hydroxyphenyl) 3 [4 [2 (1 pyrrolidinyl)ethoxy]benzoyl]benzo[b]thiophene
3 (4 hydroxyphenyl) 4 methyl 2 [4 [2 (1 piperidinyl)ethoxy]phenyl] 2h 1 benzopyran 7 ol
hydroxytamoxifen
4 hydroxytamoxifen
4 hydroxytoremifene
idoxifene
lasofoxifene
letrozole
liarozole
liarozole fumarate
mepitiostane
4 [4 methyl 2 [4 [2 (1 piperidinyl)ethoxy]phenyl] 7 pivaloyloxy 2h 1 benzopyran 3 ylphenyl] pivalate
3 methylnaringenin
minamestane
miproxifene phosphate
nafoxidine
nitromifene
nortamoxifen
ospemifene
panomifene
11 [4 [[5 [(4,4,5,5,5 pentafluoropentyl)sulfonyl]pentyl]oxy]phenyl]estradiol
pipendoxifene
2 [4 (2 piperidinoethoxy)phenyl] 3 phenyl 2h 1 benzopyran
10 propargylestr 4 ene 3,17 dione
pyridoglutethimide
raloxifene
tamoxifen
tamoxifen aziridine
tamoxifen citrate
tamoxifen derivative
tesmilifene
testolactone
3 [4 (1,2,3,4 tetrahydro 6 methoxy 2 phenyl 1 naphthyl)phenoxy] 1,2 propanediol
toremifene
1,3,8 trichloro 6 methyldibenzofuran
trioxifene
trioxifene mesilate
1,1,2 triphenylethylene derivative
vorozole
zindoxifene
zuclomifene
zuclomifene citrate

☝ *probably not prohibited*

S8. MASKING AGENTS

acetazolamide
actovegin
aldactazine
altizide
amiloride
amiloride plus cyclopenthiazide
amiloride plus hydrochlorothiazide
2 amino 4 (bicyclo[2.2.1]hept 2 ylamino) n (n isopropylcarbamoyl) 5 pyrimidinesulfonamide
2 [4 (3 aminomethyl 4 hydroxybenzoyl) 2,3 dichlorophenoxy]acetic acid ethyl ester
2 aminomethyl 4 tert butyl 6 iodophenol
ammonium acetate
4 anilino 2 methylthiopyrido[2,3 d]pyrimidine
artificial blood
atenolol plus chlortalidone
azosemide
bemetizide
bemitradine
benazepril plus hydrochlorothiazide
bendroflumethiazide
bendroflumethiazide plus nadolol
benzthiazide
benzthiazide plus triamterene
besulpamide
bisoprolol fumarate plus hydrochlorothiazide
blood derivative
blood extract
blood substitute
briserin
brocrinat
bumetanide
butizide
butizide plus spironolactone
canrenoate potassium
canrenoic acid
canrenone
canrenone derivative
captopril plus hydrochlorothiazide
chlormerodrin
8 chloro 1 [alpha (2 dimethylaminoethyl)benzyl] 6 phenyl 4h 1,2,4 triazolo[4,3 a][1,4]benzodiazepine
8 chloro 3 (2 fluorophenyl) 5,6 dihydrofuro[3,2 f][1,2]benzisoxazole 6 carboxylate potassium
[[5 chloro 3 (2 methylphenyl) 4 oxo 4h benzopyran 7 yl]oxy]acetic acid
chlorothiazide
chlorothiazide derivative
chlortalidone
chlortalidone plus metoprolol
chlortalidone plus reserpine
cilazapril plus hydrochlorothiazide
clopamide
cyclopenthiazide
cyclopenthiazide plus guanethidine
cyclopenthiazide plus oxprenolol
cycloteriam
cyclothiazide
dextran
dextran 40
dextran 60
dextran 70
3,5 diamino 6 chloro n [1 [n [2 [2 hydroxy 3 (1 naphthoxy)propylamino]ethyl]carbamoyl] 1 methylethyl]pyrazine 2 carboxamide
6,7 dichloro 2,3 dihydro 5 (n,n dimethylsulfamoyl)coumarilic acid
diclofenamide
dihydralazine plus hydrochlorothiazide plus reserpine
2,4 dihydro 6,8 dinitro 1,2,4 triazolo[3,4 c][1,4]benzoxazin 1 one
6,7 dihydrocanrenone
diucomb
diuretic agent
☝ drospirenone
☝ drospirenone plus estradiol
☝ drospirenone plus ethinylestradiol
enalapril plus hydrochlorothiazide
epinine
epitestosterone
epitizide
eplerenone
etacrynic acid
ethiazide
ethoxzolamide
etozolin
fenquizone
2 [2 (4 fluorophenoxy)ethyl]phenol
[2 [2 (4 fluorophenoxy)ethyl]phenyl] sulfate
fresh frozen plasma
frumil
furosemide
furosemide plus triamterene
gelatinol
gelatin succinate
guanethidine plus hydrochlorothiazide
hemodialysis fluid
hetastarch
hydralazine plus hydrochlorothiazide
hydralazine plus hydrochlorothiazide plus reserpine
hydrochlorothiazide
hydrochlorothiazide plus irbesartan
hydrochlorothiazide plus lisinopril
hydrochlorothiazide plus losartan
hydrochlorothiazide plus metoprolol
hydrochlorothiazide plus metoprolol tartrate
hydrochlorothiazide plus propranolol
hydrochlorothiazide plus quinapril
hydrochlorothiazide plus telmisartan
hydrochlorothiazide plus triamterene
hydrochlorothiazide plus valsartan
hydroflumethiazide
17 hydroxy 15beta,16beta methylene 7alpha methylthio 3 oxo 17alpha pregna 1,4 diene 21 carboxylic acid gamma lactone
ibopamine
indacrinone
indapamide
isosorbide
kadiur
loop diuretic agent
mannitol
mefruside
mersalyl
mespirenone
methazolamide
methyclothiazide
15beta,16beta methylenemexrenone
metolazone

☝ *probably not prohibited*

metyrapone
mexrenoate potassium
mexrenoic acid
mexrenone
muzolimine
niravoline
osmotic diuretic agent
oxprenoate potassium
oxyamal
oxypolygelatin
ozolinone
perhexiline
perhexiline maleate
piretanide
plasma substitute
plasmion
polygeline
polymerized hemoglobin
polythiazide
potassium sparing diuretic agent
probenecid
7alpha propylspironolactone
pyridoxylhemoglobin
pyridoxylpolyhemoglobin
quinethazone
rheodextran
sali aldopur
skf 105494
sorbitol
spironolactone
spiroxasone
tensigradyl
thiazide diuretic agent
thrombocyte concentrate
tiamizide
tienilic acid
tienoxolol
torasemide
torrat
trasitensin
traxanox
trepress
triamterene
triamterene plus xipamide
trichlormethiazide
triniton
tripamide
trometamol
trometamol edetate
ultroser g
veratide
viskaldix
xipamide

S9. GLUCOCORTICOSTEROIDS

alclometasone
alclometasone dipropionate
amcinonide
baycuten
beclometasone
beclometasone dipropionate
betamethasone
betamethasone acetate
betamethasone acetate plus betamethasone sodium phosphate
betamethasone benzoate
betamethasone derivative
betamethasone dipropionate
betamethasone sodium phosphate
betamethasone sodium phosphate plus neomycin
betamethasone valerate
budesonide
budesonide plus formoterol
celestamine
chloroprednisone
ciclesonide
ciprocinonide
clioquinol plus dexamethasone
clioquinol plus flumetasone pivalate
clobetasol
clobetasol butyrate
clobetasol propionate
clobetasone
clobetasone butyrate
clocortolone
clocortolone pivalate
cloprednol
cortisone
cortisone acetate
cortisone derivative
cortisporin
cortivazol
crotamiton plus hydrocortisone
daktacort
deflazacort
desonide
desoximetasone
dexamethasone
dexamethasone 17,21 dipropionate
dexamethasone 17 valerate
dexamethasone 21 mesilate
dexamethasone acetate
dexamethasone derivative
dexamethasone isonicotinate
dexamethasone plus tobramycin
dexamethasone sodium phosphate
dexatopic
diflorasone
diflorasone diacetate
diflucortolone
diflucortolone valerate
6alpha,9alpha difluoro 11beta,17alpha dihydroxy 16beta methyl 17beta methylthiocarbonylandrosta 1,4 dien 3 one 17 acetate
6alpha,9alpha difluoro 11beta,17alpha dihydroxy 16beta methyl 17beta methylthiocarbonylandrosta 1,4 dien 3 one 17 propionate
difluprednate
20 dihydroprednisolonic acid methyl ester
11beta,17beta dihydroxy 17 (1 propynyl)androsta 1,4,6 trien 3 one
11beta,17beta dihydroxy 6 methyl 17alpha (1 propynyl)androsta 1,4,6 trien 3 one
domoprednate
drocinonide
dutimelan
epihydrocortisone
fluclorolone
fluclorolone acetonide
fludrocortisone
fludrocortisone acetate
fludroxycortide
flumetasone
flumetasone acetate
flumetasone pivalate
flumetasone pivalate plus salicylic acid
flumetasone pivalate plus triclosan
flumoxonide
flunisolide
flunisolide acetate
fluocinolone
fluocinolone acetonide
fluocinonide
fluocortin
fluocortin butyl
fluocortolone
fluocortolone caproate
fluocortolone pivalate
fluorometholone
fluprednidene
fluprednidene acetate
fluprednisolone
fluticasone
fluticasone propionate
fluticasone propionate plus salmeterol
formocortal
glucocorticoid
halcinonide
halometasone
halopredone
halopredone acetate
hydrallostane
hydrocortisone
hydrocortisone 17 butyrate 21 propionate
hydrocortisone acetate
hydrocortisone butyrate
hydrocortisone derivative
hydrocortisone plus urea
hydrocortisone sodium phosphate
hydrocortisone sodium succinate
hydrocortisone valerate
18 hydroxyhydrocortisone
6beta hydroxyhydrocortisone
16alpha hydroxyprednisolone
isoflupredone
isoflupredone acetate
lorinden a
lorinden t
loteprednol etabonate
lotricomb
mazipredone
medrysone
meprednisone
methylprednisolone
16beta methylprednisolone
methylprednisolone aceponate

Terms per WADA category

probably not prohibited

methylprednisolone acetate
methylprednisolone sodium succinate
methylprednisolone suleptanate
mometasone furoate
mycolog
nicocortonide
nivacortol
oropivalone
18 oxohydrocortisone
paramethasone
paramethasone acetate
prednicarbate
prednisolone
prednisolone 21 phosphate
prednisolone 3 sulfobenzoate
prednisolone acetate
prednisolone derivative
prednisolone hemisuccinate
prednisolone pivalate
prednisolone sodium phosphate
prednisolone sodium succinate
prednisolone sodium tetrahydrophthalate
prednisone
prednisone acetate
prednival acetate
prednylidene
pregnenolone
pregnenolone derivative
pregnenolone sulfate
procinonide
rimexolone
sofradex
terracortril
tetrahydrocortisol
tetrahydrocortisone
ticabesone
ticabesone propionate
timobesone
timobesone acetate
tipredane
tixocortol
tixocortol pivalate
triamcinolone
triamcinolone acetate
triamcinolone acetonide
triamcinolone diacetate
triamcinolone hexacetonide
11beta,17alpha,21 trihydroxy 3,20 dioxopregna 1,4 diene 16alpha carboxylic acid methyl ester
ulobetasol propionate
uniderm

M1. ENHANCEMENT OF OXYGEN TRANSFER

actovegin
artificial blood
bis(perfluorohexyl)ethylene
blood derivative
blood extract
blood substitute
carboxyhemoglobin
continuous erythropoiesis receptor activator
deoxyhemoglobin
diaspirin crosslinked hemoglobin
efaproxiral
erythrocruorin
erythropoietin
fluosol
fluosol da
fresh frozen plasma
glycosylated hemoglobin
hemoglobin
hemoglobin A
hemoglobin A1c
hemoglobin A2
hemoglobin alpha chain
hemoglobin beta chain
hemoglobin C
hemoglobin chain
hemoglobin delta chain
hemoglobin derivative
hemoglobin E
hemoglobin F
hemoglobin gamma chain
hemoglobin H
hemoglobin J
hemoglobin M
hemoglobin S
hemoglobin variant
leghemoglobin
methemoglobin
novel erythropoiesis stimulating protein
oxyhemoglobin
perfluorobutyltetrahydrofuran
perfluorodecalin
perfluorooctyl bromide
perfluoroperhydrofluoranthene
perfluorotributylamine
perfluorotripropylamine
plasma substitute
plasmion
polymerized hemoglobin
pyridoxylhemoglobin
pyridoxylpolyhemoglobin
recombinant erythropoietin
recombinant hemoglobin
sulfhemoglobin
thrombocyte concentrate

P1. ALCOHOL

alcohol

P2. BETA-BLOCKERS

acebutolol
acebutolol plus nifedipine
adimolol
afurolol
alprenolol
alprenolol derivative
amosulalol
arotinolol
atenolol
atenolol plus chlortalidone
atenolol plus nifedipine
befunolol
bendroflumethiazide plus nadolol
beta 1 adrenergic receptor blocking agent
beta 2 adrenergic receptor blocking agent
beta 3 adrenergic receptor blocking agent
beta adrenergic receptor blocking agent
betaxolol
bevantolol
bfe 55
bisoprolol
bisoprolol fumarate
bisoprolol fumarate plus hydrochlorothiazide
bopindolol
bornaprolol
brefonalol
8 bromoacetamido 1 [2 hydroxy 3 (4 indolyloxy)propylamino] para menthane
bromoacetylalprenololmenthane
bucindolol
bucumolol
bufetolol
bufuralol
bunitrolol
bunolol
bupranolol
butofilolol
butoxamine
4 (3 tert butylamino 2 hydroxypropoxy) 2 benzimidazolone
1 tert butylamino 3 (2 chlorophenoxy) 2 propanol
1 tert butylamino 3 (2 methyl 4 indolyloxy) 2 propanol
1 tert butylamino 3 (3 methyl 2 nitrophenoxy) 2 propanol
9 (1 tert butylamino 3 hydroxy 2 propyloxyimino)fluorene
carazolol
n [1 carboxy 5 [4 (2 hydroxy 3 isopropylaminopropoxy)indole 2 carboxamido]pentyl]alanylproline
carteolol
carvedilol
celiprolol
cetamolol
chlortalidone plus metoprolol
cloranolol
cyanoiodopindolol
1 (2 cyanophenoxy) 3 [2 (3 phenylureido)ethylamino] 2 propanol
cyanopindolol
4 cyclohexylamino 1 (1 naphthyloxy) 2 butanol
cyclopenthiazide plus oxprenolol
n [2 [3 [4 [2 (2 cyclopropylmethoxyethoxy)ethyl]phenoxy] 2 hydroxypropylamino]ethyl] 4 hydroxy 1 piperidinecarboxamide
6 [4 [3 [[3 [4 [2 (cyclopropylmethoxy)ethyl]phenoxy] 2 hydroxypropyl]amino]propionamido]phenyl] 4,5 dihydro 5 methyl 3(2h) pyridazinone
deacetylmetipranolol
diacetolol
3,5 diamino 6 chloro n [1 [n [2 [2 hydroxy 3 (1 naphthoxy)propylamino]ethyl]carbamoyl] 1 methylethyl]pyrazine 2 carboxamide
1 (2,4 dichlorophenoxy) 3 [2 (3,4 dimethoxyphenyl)ethylamino] 2 propanol
dihydralazine plus oxprenolol
dihydroalprenolol
dilevalol
epanolol
esmolol
1 (2 ethylphenoxy) 3 (1,2,3,4 tetrahydro 1 naphthylamino) 2 propanol oxalate
exaprolol
falintolol
falintolol oxalate
felodipine plus metoprolol
flestolol
flusoxolol
hydrochlorothiazide plus metoprolol
hydrochlorothiazide plus metoprolol tartrate
hydrochlorothiazide plus propranolol
4 [2 hydroxy 3 [(1 methyl 3 phenylpropyl)amino]propoxy]benzeneacetamid e
5 [2 [[2 hydroxy 3 [4 (1 methyl 4 trifluoromethyl 2 imidazolyl)phenoxy]propyl]amino]ethoxy]salic ylamide
n [2 [2 hydroxy 3 [4 (2 isobutoxyethoxy)phenoxy]propylamino]ethyl] 4 morpholinecarboxamide
4 (2 hydroxy 3 isopropylaminopropoxy)carbanilic acid propyl ester
3 [4 (2 hydroxy 3 isopropylaminopropoxy)phenyl]propionic acid
hydroxybenzylpindolol
8 hydroxycarteolol
alpha hydroxymetoprolol
indenolol
iodopindolol
iprocrolol
isamoltane
2 isopropylamino 1 (4 tolyl)propanol
3 isopropylamino 1 (7 methyl 4 indanyloxy) 2 butanol
1 isopropylamino 3 [4 (2 methoxyethoxy)phenoxy] 2 propanol
isoxaprolol
labetalol
landiolol
levobunolol
levomoprolol
medroxalol
mepindolol
mercuderamide
4' methylthiopropranolol
metipranolol
metoprolol
metoprolol fumarate

metoprolol succinate
metoprolol tartrate
moprolol
nadolol
1 (1 naphthyloxy) 3 [6 [2 (2 pyridyl)ethoxy]hexylamino] 2 propanol
nebivolol
nifenalol
nipradilol
oxprenolol
pafenolol
pamatolol
penbutolol
pindolol
pindolol derivative
practolol
primidolol
prizidilol
procinolol
pronetalol
propranolol
propranolol derivative
proxodolol
ridazolol
salcardolol
sandoz 204545
soquinolol
soquinolol mucate
sotalol
spirendolol
talinolol
tertatolol
tienoxolol
tilisolol
timolol
timolol maleate
tolamolol
toliprolol
trasitensin
trepress
tribendilol
viskaldix
xibenolol

P3. DIURETICS

acetazolamide
aldactazine
altizide
amiloride
amiloride plus cyclopenthiazide
amiloride plus hydrochlorothiazide
2 amino 4 (bicyclo[2.2.1]hept 2 ylamino) n (n isopropylcarbamoyl) 5 pyrimidinesulfonamide
2 [4 (3 aminomethyl 4 hydroxybenzoyl) 2,3 dichlorophenoxy]acetic acid ethyl ester
2 aminomethyl 4 tert butyl 6 iodophenol
ammonium acetate
4 anilino 2 methylthiopyrido[2,3 d]pyrimidine
atenolol plus chlortalidone
azosemide
bemetizide
bemitradine
benazepril plus hydrochlorothiazide
bendroflumethiazide
bendroflumethiazide plus nadolol
benzthiazide
benzthiazide plus triamterene
besulpamide
bisoprolol fumarate plus hydrochlorothiazide
briserin
brocrinat
bumetanide
butizide
butizide plus spironolactone
canrenoate potassium
canrenoic acid
canrenone
canrenone derivative
captopril plus hydrochlorothiazide
chlormerodrin
8 chloro 1 [alpha (2 dimethylaminoethyl)benzyl] 6 phenyl 4h 1,2,4 triazolo[4,3 a][1,4]benzodiazepine
8 chloro 3 (2 fluorophenyl) 5,6 dihydrofuro[3,2 f][1,2]benzisoxazole 6 carboxylate potassium
[[5 chloro 3 (2 methylphenyl) 4 oxo 4h benzopyran 7 yl]oxy]acetic acid
chlorothiazide
chlorothiazide derivative
chlortalidone
chlortalidone plus metoprolol
chlortalidone plus reserpine
cilazapril plus hydrochlorothiazide
clopamide
cyclopenthiazide
cyclopenthiazide plus guanethidine
cyclopenthiazide plus oxprenolol
cycloteriam
cyclothiazide
3,5 diamino 6 chloro n [1 [n [2 [2 hydroxy 3 (1 naphthoxy)propylamino]ethyl]carbamoyl] 1 methylethyl]pyrazine 2 carboxamide
6,7 dichloro 2,3 dihydro 5 (n,n dimethylsulfamoyl)coumarilic acid
diclofenamide
dihydralazine plus hydrochlorothiazide plus reserpine
2,4 dihydro 6,8 dinitro 1,2,4 triazolo[3,4 c][1,4]benzoxazin 1 one
6,7 dihydrocanrenone
diucomb
diuretic agent
☝ drospirenone
☝ drospirenone plus estradiol
☝ drospirenone plus ethinylestradiol
enalapril plus hydrochlorothiazide
epinine
epitizide
eplerenone
etacrynic acid
ethiazide
ethoxzolamide
etozolin
fenquizone
2 [2 (4 fluorophenoxy)ethyl]phenol
[2 [2 (4 fluorophenoxy)ethyl]phenyl] sulfate
frumil
furosemide
furosemide plus triamterene
guanethidine plus hydrochlorothiazide
hydralazine plus hydrochlorothiazide
hydralazine plus hydrochlorothiazide plus reserpine
hydrochlorothiazide
hydrochlorothiazide plus irbesartan
hydrochlorothiazide plus lisinopril
hydrochlorothiazide plus losartan
hydrochlorothiazide plus metoprolol
hydrochlorothiazide plus metoprolol tartrate
hydrochlorothiazide plus propranolol
hydrochlorothiazide plus quinapril
hydrochlorothiazide plus telmisartan
hydrochlorothiazide plus triamterene
hydrochlorothiazide plus valsartan
hydroflumethiazide
17 hydroxy 15beta,16beta methylene 7alpha methylthio 3 oxo 17alpha pregna 1,4 diene 21 carboxylic acid gamma lactone
ibopamine
indacrinone
indapamide
isosorbide
kadiur
loop diuretic agent
mannitol
mefruside
mersalyl
mespirenone
methazolamide
methyclothiazide
15beta,16beta methylenemexrenone
metolazone
mexrenoate potassium
mexrenoic acid
mexrenone
muzolimine
niravoline
osmotic diuretic agent
oxprenoate potassium
ozolinone
perhexiline
perhexiline maleate
piretanide
polythiazide
potassium sparing diuretic agent
7alpha propylspironolactone
quinethazone
sali aldopur
skf 105494

☝ *probably not prohibited*

sorbitol
spironolactone
spiroxasone
tensigradyl
thiazide diuretic agent
tiamizide
tienilic acid
tienoxolol
torasemide
torrat
trasitensin
traxanox
trepress
triamterene
triamterene plus xipamide
trichlormethiazide
triniton
tripamide
trometamol
trometamol edetate
veratide
viskaldix
xipamide

EMTREE Terms and Synonyms

acebutolol

WADA group
P2. BETA-BLOCKERS

MeSH descriptor
acebutolol

CAS Registry number
34381-68-5
37517-30-9

Trade names and research codes
bay c 7705
bay c7705
espesil
il 17803a
il17803a
m and b 17803 a
m and b 17803a
prent
sectral

Short synonyms
acebutolol hydrochloride
neptall

Long synonyms
1 (2 acetyl 4 butyramidophenoxy) 2 hydroxy 3 isopropylaminopropane
1 (2 acetyl 4 n butyramidophenoxy) 2 hydroxy 3 isopropylaminopropane hydrochloride
n [3 acetyl 4 [2 hydroxy 3 [(methylethyl)amino]propoxy]phenyl]butanamide

acebutolol plus nifedipine

WADA group
P2. BETA-BLOCKERS

Trade names and research codes
bay l 5240
bay l5240
tredalat

acefluranol

WADA group
S7. AGENTS WITH ANTI-OESTROGENIC ACTIVITY

CAS Registry number
80595-73-9

Trade names and research codes
bx 591
bx591

acetazolamide

WADA group
S8. MASKING AGENTS
P3. DIURETICS

MeSH descriptor
acetazolamide

CAS Registry number
1424-27-7
59-66-5

Trade names and research codes
compound 6063
dazamide
diacarb
diamox
diuramide
fonurit
glaupax
storzolamide

Short synonyms
acetamox
acetazolam
acetazolamid
acetazol amide
acetazolamide sodium
acetazolamine
acetazoleamide
acetozolamide
acetozolamine
azetazolamide
cidamex
dehydratin
diluran
diomax
diuriwas wassermann barcelona
diutazol
edemox
eumicton
glaucomide
natrionex
nephramid
novozolamide
ulcosilvanil
ulcosylvanil

Long synonyms
5 acetamido 1,3,4 thiadiazole 2 sulfonamide
5 acetamido 2 sulfamoyl 1,3,4 thiadiazole
2 acetylamino 1,3,4 thiadiazole 5 sulfonamide
carbonic anhydrase inhibitor no 6063

actovegin

WADA group
S8. MASKING AGENTS
M1. ENHANCEMENT OF OXYGEN TRANSFER

CAS Registry number
63748-11-8

Trade names and research codes
actovegin
mf 125

Short synonyms
actovegin forte

adenohypophysis hormone

WADA group
S5. PEPTIDE HORMONES

MeSH descriptor
pituitary hormones, anterior

Short synonyms
pituitary hormones, anterior

adimolol

WADA group
P2. BETA-BLOCKERS

CAS Registry number
75708-29-1
78459-19-5

Short synonyms
adimolol hydrochloride hydrate
men 935

Long synonyms
1 [3 [[2 hydroxy 3 (1 naphthoxy)propyl]amino] 3,3 dimethylpropyl] 2 benzimidazolinone
1 [3 [[2 hydroxy 3 (1 naphthyloxy)propyl]amino] 3 methylbutyl] 2 benzimidazolinone
1 [3 [[3 (1 naphthoxy) 2 hydroxypropyl]amino] 3,3 dimethylpropyl] 2 benzimidazolinone

adrafinil

WADA group
S1. STIMULANTS

CAS Registry number
63547-13-7

Trade names and research codes
crl 40028
crl40028
olmifon
psl 14 537
psl 14537
psl14 537
psl14537

Long synonyms
benzhydrylsulfinylacetohydroxamic acid
[(diphenylmethyl)sulfinyl]acetohydroxamic acid
2 [(diphenylmethyl)sulfinyl]acetohydroxamic acid

adrenalin

WADA group
S1. STIMULANTS

MeSH descriptor
epinephrine

CAS Registry number
51-43-4
55-31-2
6912-68-1

Trade names and research codes
glaucon
simplene

Short synonyms
adnephrin
adnephrine
adrenalin chloride
adrenaline
adrenaline chloride
adrenaline hydrochloride
adrenalin hydrochloride
adrenamine
adrenapax
adrenazin
adrenine
adrin
adrine
advaradin
asthmahaler
balmadren
biorenine
bosmin
bronitin mist
bronkaid mist
chelafrin
d adrenalin
dextro adrenalin
dl adrenalin
drenamist
dylephrin
dyspne inhal
epiglaufrin
epimephrine
epinefrina
epinephran
epinephrin
epinephrine
epinephrine chloride
epinephrine hydrochloride
epipen
epirenamine
epirenan
exadrin
glaucosan
glin epin
glycirenan
haemostatin
hemisine
hemostasin
hemisine
hemostasin
hemostatin
hypernephrin
isopto epinal
l adrenalin
l adrenaline
l epinephrine
levo adrenalin
levoadrenalin
levo adrenaline
levoadrenaline
levo adrenalin hydrochloride
levo epinephrine
levoepinephrine
levorenin
levorenine
methylaminoethanolcatechol
methylarterenol
mucidrina
myosthenine
nephridine
nieraline
paranephrin
primatene mist
racemic adrenalin
renaglandin
renaleptine
renalina
renaline
renoform
renostypticin
renostyptin
scurenaline
soladren
sphygmogenin
styptirenal
supracapsulin
supranephrane
supranephrin
supranol
suprarenaline
suprel
surenine
surrenine
susphrine
sympathin i
takamina
tonogen
trenamist
vasoconstrictine

Terms and Synonyms

vasodrine
vasotonin
vasotonin forte seron

Long synonyms
3,4 dihydroxy alpha [(methylamino)methyl]benzyl alcohol
3,4 dihydroxy 1 [1 hydroxy 2 (methylamino)ethyl]benzene
1 (3,4 dihydroxyphenyl) 2 (methylamino)ethanol

☝ adrenalone

WADA group
S1. STIMULANTS

CAS Registry number
99-45-6

Trade names and research codes
haemodan
kephrin
kephrine
stryphnon
stryphnone
stypnon
stypnone

Short synonyms
adrenalon
adrenone
methylaminoacetopyrocatechol
4 methylaminoacetopyrocatechol

Long synonyms
3,4 dihydroxy alpha methylaminoacetophenone
3',4 dihydroxy 2 (methylamino)acetophenone
3',4 dihydroxy 2 methylaminoacetophenone
3',4' dihydroxy 2 methylaminoacetophenone

adrenosterone

WADA group
S4. ANABOLIC AGENTS

CAS Registry number
37-82-1
382-45-6

Short synonyms
androst 4 ene 3,11,17 trione
4 androstene 3,11,17 trione
androstenetrione
11 oxoandrost 4 enedione
11 oxo delta 4 androstenedione
reichstein substance g

afurolol

WADA group
P2. BETA-BLOCKERS

CAS Registry number
65776-67-2

Long synonyms
7 (3 tert butylamino 2 hydroxypropoxy)phthalide
1 tert butylamino 3 phthalid 7 yloxy 2 propanol

ajulemic acid

WADA group
S3. CANNABINOIDS

CAS Registry number
137945-48-3

Trade names and research codes
ct 3
ct3
ip 751
ip751

Long synonyms
1',1' dimethylheptyl delta8 tetrahydrocannabinol 11 oic acid

alclometasone

WADA group
S9. GLUCOCORTICOSTEROIDS

CAS Registry number
67452-97-5

Trade names and research codes
aclosone

Short synonyms
alclomethasone

Long synonyms
7alpha chloro 11beta,17,21 trihydroxy 16alpha methylpregna 1,4 diene 3,20 dione
7alpha chloro 16alpha methylprednisolone
prednisolone,7alpha chloro 16alpha methyl
pregna 1,4 diene 11beta,17,21 triol 3,20 dione,7alpha chloro 16alpha methyl

alclometasone dipropionate

WADA group
S9. GLUCOCORTICOSTEROIDS

CAS Registry number
66734-13-2

Trade names and research codes
almeta
delonal
logoderm
modrasone
sch 22219
vaderm

Short synonyms
aclovate
alclomethasone dipropionate
s 3460

Long synonyms
alclometasone 17,21 dipropionate
7alpha chloro 11beta,17,21 trihydroxy 16alpha methylpregna 1,4 diene 3,20 dione 17,21 dipropionate
7alpha chloro 11beta hydroxy 16alpha methyl 17,21 bis(1 oxopropoxy)pregna 1,4 diene 3,20 dione
7alpha chloro 16alpha methylprednisolone 17,21 dipropionate
prednisolone 17,21 dipropionate,7alpha chloro 16alpha methyl

alcohol

WADA group
P1. ALCOHOL

MeSH descriptor
ethanol

Terms and Synonyms

☝ *probably not prohibited*

CAS Registry number
64-17-5

Short synonyms
alcohol concentration
alcohol, ethyl
alcohol vapor
ethanol
ethanol solution
ethyl alcohol
ethylalcohol

aldactazine

WADA group
S8. MASKING AGENTS
P3. DIURETICS

CAS Registry number
76270-06-9

Trade names and research codes
aldactazide
aldactazine
spirozide

Short synonyms
althiazide with spironolactone
altizide plus spironolactone
pinactizine
practazin
prinactizide
spiroctazide
spironolactone plus altizide

aldosterone

WADA group
S5. PEPTIDE HORMONES

MeSH descriptor
aldosterone

CAS Registry number
52-39-1
6251-69-0

Trade names and research codes
aldocorten
electrocortin
elektrocortin

Short synonyms
aldosteron
d aldosterone
dextro aldosterone
l aldosterone
levo aldosterone
18 oxocorticosterone

Long synonyms
11beta,21 dihydroxy 3,20 dioxopregn 4 en 18 al(11,18)lactol
3,20 dioxo 11beta,18 oxido 4 pregnene 18,21 diol

alifedrine

WADA group
S6. BETA-2 AGONISTS

CAS Registry number
72913-80-5
78756-61-3

Trade names and research codes
d 13 625
d 13625
d13 625
d13625

Short synonyms
alifedrine hydrochloride

Long synonyms
1 cyclohexyl 3 (2 hydroxy 1 methyl 2 phenylethylamino) 1 propanone

allylglycine

WADA group
S1. STIMULANTS

MeSH descriptor
allylglycine

CAS Registry number
1069-48-3

Short synonyms
allylglycin
2 amino 4 pentenoic acid

almitrine

WADA group
S1. STIMULANTS

MeSH descriptor
almitrine

CAS Registry number
27469-53-0

Long synonyms
2,4 bis(allylamino) 6 [4 [bis(4 fluorophenyl)methyl]piperazin 1 yl] s triazine
2,4 bis(allylamino) 6 [4 [bis(4 fluorophenyl)methyl] 1 piperazinyl] 1,3,5 triazine
1 [4,6 bis(allylamino) s triazin 2 yl] 4 (4,4' difluorobenzhydryl)piperazine
1 (4,6 diallylamino 2 triazinyl) 4 (4,4' difluorobenzhydryl)piperazine
n,n' diallyl 6 [4 (4,4' difluorobenzhydryl)piperazin 1 yl] 1,3,5 triazine 2,4 diyldiamine

almitrine dimesilate

WADA group
S1. STIMULANTS

CAS Registry number
29608-49-9

Trade names and research codes
s 2620
s2620
se 2620
se2620
servier 2620
vectarion

Short synonyms
almitrine bismesilate
almitrine bismesylate
almitrine dimesylate
almitrine dimethanesulfonate

probably not prohibited

alprenolol

WADA group
P2. BETA-BLOCKERS

MeSH descriptor
alprenolol

CAS Registry number
13655-52-2
13707-88-5
39405-98-6
58615-82-0

Trade names and research codes
aptin
aptin durules
aptine
astra
betacard
gubernal

Short synonyms
alloprenalol
alpheprol
alprendol
alprenol
alprenolol hydrochloride
alprenolol isomer
apliobal
aprenolol
aptia
aptol
aptol duriles
betapin
ciba 39.889 ba
h 56-23
h 56-26
h 56 28
h 56-28
l alprenolol
levo dextro alprenolol

Long synonyms
1 (2 allylphenoxy) 3 isopropylamine 2 propanol hydrochloride
1 (2 allylphenoxy) 3 isopropylamino 2 propanol
1 (2 allylphenoxy) 3 isopropylamino 2 propanol hydrochloride
1 (2 allylphenoxy) 3 isopropylaminopropan 2 ol
1 (2 allylphenoxy) 3 isopropylaminopropanol
1 (2 allylphenoxy) 3 isopropylaminopropanol hydrochloride
dl 1 (ortho allylphenoxy) 3 isopropylamino 2 propanol hydrochloride
1 isopropylamino 2 hydroxy 3 (ortho allylphenoxy)propane
1 isopropylamino 2 hydroxy 3 (ortho allylphenoxy)propane hydrochloride
1 (o allyl phenoxy) 3 iso propyl amino 2 propanol
1 (o allylphenoxy) 3 isopropyl amino 2 propanol
1 (o allylphenoxy) 3 isopropylamino 2 propanol
1 (ortho allylphenoxy) 3 isopropyl amino 2 propanol
1 (ortho allylphenoxy) 3 isopropylamino 2 propanol
1 [1 (ortho allylphenoxy) 3 isopropylamino 2 propanol]
1 (ortho allylphenoxy) 3 isopropylamino 2 propanol hydrochloride
1 (ortho allylphenoxy) 3 isopropylaminopropan 2 ol

alprenolol derivative

WADA group
P2. BETA-BLOCKERS

alsactide

WADA group
S5. PEPTIDE HORMONES

CAS Registry number
34765-96-3

Trade names and research codes
hoe 433
synchrodyn 1-17
synchrodyn[1-17]

Short synonyms
alisactide

Long synonyms
1 beta alanine 17 [2,6 diamino n (4 aminobutyl)hexanamide] alpha 1-17 corticotrophin
corticotropin[1-17][1 alanine 4 amino n butylamide 17 lysine]

altizide

WADA group
S8. MASKING AGENTS
P3. DIURETICS

CAS Registry number
5588-16-9

Short synonyms
althiazide
p 1779

Long synonyms
3 [(allylthio)methyl] 6 chloro 3,4 dihydro 2h 1,2,4 benzothiadiazine 7 sulfonamide 1,1 dioxide
3 allylthiomethyl 6 chloro 3,4 dihydro 2h 1,2,4 benzothiadiazine 7 sulfonamide 1,1 dioxide

amafolone

WADA group
S4. ANABOLIC AGENTS

CAS Registry number
50588-47-1
51740-76-2

Trade names and research codes
org 6001

Long synonyms
3alpha amino 2beta hydroxy 17 oxo 5alpha androstane
3alpha amino 2beta hydroxy 5alpha androstan 17 one
3alpha amino 2beta hydroxy 5alpha androstan 17 one hydrochloride
3alpha amino 5alpha androstan 2beta ol 17 one
androstan 2beta ol 17 one,3alpha amino

ambroxol plus clenbuterol

WADA group
S4. ANABOLIC AGENTS
S6. BETA-2 AGONISTS

Trade names and research codes
chf 023
chf023
mucosolvan compositum
spasmo mucosolvan

Terms and Synonyms

Short synonyms
clenbuterol plus ambroxol

amcinonide

WADA group
S9. GLUCOCORTICOSTEROIDS

CAS Registry number
51022-69-6

Trade names and research codes
amciderm
amicla
cl 34699
cl34699
cyclocort
penticort
visderm

Short synonyms
visderm h

Long synonyms
triamcinolone cyclic 16,17 acetal with cyclopentanone, 21 acetate

amfepramone

WADA group
S1. STIMULANTS

MeSH descriptor
diethylpropion

CAS Registry number
134-80-5
90-84-6

Trade names and research codes
moderatan
regenon
tenuate
tenuate dospan
tepanil

Short synonyms
adiposon
alipid
amphepramon
anorex
anorexil
apisate
1 benzoyltriethylamine
derfon
diepropon
diethylaminopropiophenone
2 diethylaminopropiophenone
diethyl propion
diethylpropion
diethylpropione
diethylpropione hydrochloride
diethylpropion hydrochloride
dobesin
dualid
magrene
moludar
obesitex
phepranon
regenon retard
t 712
tylinal

Long synonyms
alpha benzoyltriethylamine hydrochloride
alpha diethylaminopropiophenone
alpha diethylaminopropiophenone hydrochloride

amfonelic acid

WADA group
S1. STIMULANTS

CAS Registry number
15180-02-6
82800-74-6

Short synonyms
amfolenic acid
amphonelic acid
nsc 100638
win 25978

Long synonyms
7 benzyl 1 ethyl 1,4 dihydro 4 oxo 1,8 naphthyridine 3 carboxylic acid

amiloride

WADA group
S8. MASKING AGENTS
P3. DIURETICS

MeSH descriptor
amiloride

CAS Registry number
2016-88-8
2609-46-3

Trade names and research codes
arumil
midamor

Short synonyms
amiclaran
amilorid
amiloride chloride
amiloride hcl
amiloride hydrochlorhydrate
amiloridehydrochlorhydrate
amiloride hydrochloride
amiloride hydroxychloride
amiloridine
amipramidine
amyloride
berkamil
colectril
guanamprazine
mk 870
modamide

Long synonyms
3,5 diamino 6 chloropyrazinoylguanidine
3,5 diamino 6 chloropyrazinoylguanidine hydrochloride
n amidino 3,5 diamino 6 chloropyrazinamide
n amidino 3,5 diamino 6 chloropyrazinamide hydrochloride

amiloride plus cyclopenthiazide

WADA group
S8. MASKING AGENTS
P3. DIURETICS

Trade names and research codes
navispare

Long synonyms
cyclopenthiazide plus amiloride

amiloride plus hydrochlorothiazide

WADA group
S8. MASKING AGENTS
P3. DIURETICS

CAS Registry number
57017-78-4

Trade names and research codes
aquaretic
diursan
durarese
moduret
moduretic
rhefluin
rhefluin mite

Short synonyms
co amilozide

Long synonyms
amiloride with hydrochlorothiazide
hydrochlorothiazide plus amiloride
hydrochlorothiazide with amiloride

4 amino 1 (6 bromo 2 pyridyl)piperidine

WADA group
S1. STIMULANTS

CAS Registry number
98644-22-5

Trade names and research codes
cm 57373
cm57373

4 amino 1 (6 chloro 2 pyridyl)piperidine

WADA group
S1. STIMULANTS

Trade names and research codes
cm 57227
cm57227
sr 57227
sr57227
sr 57227a
sr57227a

Long synonyms
1 (6 chloro 2 pyridyl) 4 piperidinamine
1 (6 chloro 2 pyridyl)piperidin 4 amine

1 [2 (2 amino 2 methylpropionylamino) 3 (1h indol 3 yl)propionyl] 3 benzyl 3 piperidinecarboxylic acid ethyl ester

WADA group
S5. PEPTIDE HORMONES

CAS Registry number
170842-48-5

Trade names and research codes
1 163540

Long synonyms
3 benzyl 1 (2 methylalanyl dextro tryptophyl) 3 piperidinecarboxylic acid ethyl ester
1 (2 methylalanyl dextro tryptophyl) 3 phenylmethyl 3 piperidinecarboxylic acid ethyl ester

3 amino 3 methyl n [2,3,4,5 tetrahydro 2 oxo 1 [[2' (1h tetrazol 5 yl) 1,1' biphenyl 4 yl]methyl] 1h 1 benzazepin 3 yl]butanamide

WADA group
S5. PEPTIDE HORMONES

CAS Registry number
145455-23-8

Trade names and research codes
1 692428
1 692429

2 amino 4 (bicyclo[2.2.1]hept 2 ylamino) n (n isopropylcarbamoyl) 5 pyrimidinesulfonamide

WADA group
S8. MASKING AGENTS
P3. DIURETICS

CAS Registry number
124788-46-1

Trade names and research codes
ay 31906
ay31906

2 amino 4 (methylsulfonyl)butyrylglutamylhistidylphenylalanyl dextro lysylphenylalanine

WADA group
S5. PEPTIDE HORMONES

CAS Registry number
50913-82-1

Trade names and research codes
org 2766

Long synonyms
s,s dioxymethionylglutamylhistidylphenylalanyl dextro lysylphenylalanine

6 amino alpha [[(1 methyl 3 phenylpropyl)amino]methyl] 3 pyridinemethanol

WADA group
S6. BETA-2 AGONISTS

CAS Registry number
103583-08-0

Trade names and research codes
1 644969

aminoglutethimide

WADA group
S7. AGENTS WITH ANTI-OESTROGENIC ACTIVITY

Terms and Synonyms

MeSH descriptor
aminoglutethimide

CAS Registry number
125-84-8

Trade names and research codes
ba 16038
ba16038
cytadren
cytadren ag
elipten
eliptin
orimeten
orimetene
rodazol

Short synonyms
amino glutethimide
aminogluthimide
nd 1966

Long synonyms
3 (4 aminophenyl) 3 ethyl 2,6 piperidinedione
3 (4 aminophenyl) 3 ethylpiperidine 2,6 dione
3 ethyl 3 (para aminophenyl) 2,6 dioxopiperidine
2 (para aminophenyl) 2 ethylglutarimide
3 (para aminophenyl) 3 ethyl 2,6 piperidinedione

aminoglutethimide derivative

WADA group
S7. AGENTS WITH ANTI-OESTROGENIC ACTIVITY

Long synonyms
3 (4 aminophenyl) 3 ethyl 2,6 piperidinedione derivative

aminoglutethimide phosphate

WADA group
S7. AGENTS WITH ANTI-OESTROGENIC ACTIVITY

CAS Registry number
13256-45-6
23734-88-5
32066-27-6

Short synonyms
amino glutethimide phosphate

Long synonyms
2 (4 aminophenyl) 2 ethylglutarimide phosphate

2 [4 (3 aminomethyl 4 hydroxybenzoyl) 2,3 dichlorophenoxy]acetic acid ethyl ester

WADA group
S8. MASKING AGENTS
P3. DIURETICS

CAS Registry number
78235-72-0

Trade names and research codes
a 49816
a49816

2 aminomethyl 4 tert butyl 6 iodophenol

WADA group
S8. MASKING AGENTS
P3. DIURETICS

CAS Registry number
58456-91-0

Trade names and research codes
mk 447

Long synonyms
2 (aminomethyl) 4 (1,1 dimethylethyl) 6 iodophenol
2 aminomethyl 4 (1,1 dimethylethyl) 6 iodophenol
2 aminomethyl 4 (tert butyl) 6 iodophenol
2 aminomethyl 6 iodo 4 (1,1 dimethylethyl)phenol
phenol,2 aminomethyl 4 tert butyl 6 iodo
3 tert butyl 6 hydroxy 5 iodobenzylamine

7alpha (4 aminophenylthio)androstenedione

WADA group
S7. AGENTS WITH ANTI-OESTROGENIC ACTIVITY

Trade names and research codes
um 583

Long synonyms
7alpha (4' amino)phenylthioandrost 4 ene 3,17 dione
7alpha (4' amino)phenylthioandrostenedione
androstenedione,7alpha (4' amino)phenylthio

aminorex

WADA group
S1. STIMULANTS

MeSH descriptor
aminorex

CAS Registry number
13425-22-4
2207-50-3

Short synonyms
2 amino 5 phenyl 2 oxazoline
2 amino 5 phenyloxazoline
aminorex fumarate
aminorexfumarate
aminorexum
aminoxafen
aminoxaphen
apiquel
mcn 742
menocil
nsc 66952

Long synonyms
2 amino 5 phenyl 2 oxazoline fumarate

amiphenazole

WADA group
S1. STIMULANTS

CAS Registry number
490-55-1

Trade names and research codes
daftazol
daptazile

daptazole
dha 245
dha245
dizol
fenamizol

Short synonyms
amiphenazol
2,4 diamino 5 phenylthiazole
phenamizole
5 phenyl 2,4 thiazolediamine

ammonium acetate

WADA group
S8. MASKING AGENTS
P3. DIURETICS

CAS Registry number
631-61-8

Short synonyms
acetate,ammonium

amosulalol

WADA group
P2. BETA-BLOCKERS

CAS Registry number
70958-86-0
85320-68-9
93633-92-2

Trade names and research codes
howgan
lowgan
ym 09538

Short synonyms
amosulalol hydrochloride
amsolulol
ym 9538

Long synonyms
5 [1 hydroxy 2 [2 (2 methoxyphenoxy)ethylamino]ethyl] 2 methylbenzenesulfonamide
5 [1 hydroxy 2 [[2 (2 methoxyphenoxy)ethyl]amino]ethyl] 2 methylbenzenesulfonamide

amphetamine

WADA group
S1. STIMULANTS

MeSH descriptor
amphetamine

CAS Registry number
1200-47-1
139-10-6
156-34-3
2706-50-5
300-62-9
51-62-7
60-13-9
60-15-1

Trade names and research codes
adderall
adderall xr
benzedrine
obetrol
phenamin
zedrin

Short synonyms
actedron
actemin
adipan
aktedrin
aktedron
alentol
allodene
alpha amphetamine
alpha methylphenethylamine
alpha methylphenylethylamine
amfetamine
2 amino 1 phenylpropane
amphamed
amphamine
amphetaime
amphetamin
amphetamine base phosphate
amphetamine base sulfate
amphetamine hydrochloride
amphetamine phosphate
amphetamine sulfate
amphetaminyl
amphethamine
amphezamin
anara
astedin
badrin
benzafinyl
benzebar
benzolone
benzpropamin
benzpropamine
beta aminopropylbenzene
betafen
beta phenyl isopropylamine
beta phenylisopropylamine
bluzedrin
centramine
delta amphetamine
desoxynorephedrin
dextro levo amphetamine
dextrolevo amphetamine
diethamine
diethanine
dipan
d l amphetamine
elastonin
elastonon
euphobine
euphodine
euphodyn
fabedrine
fenara
fenedrin
ibiozedrine
isoamin
isoamine
isoamyn
isoamyne
isomyn
l amphetamine
levamfetamine
levamphetamine
levedrine
levo amphetamine
levoamphetamine
levo amphetamine sulphate
linampheta
mecodrin
mimetina
monetamin
monophos
noclon

Terms and Synonyms

norephedrane
norphedrane
novydrine
obesin andromacro
oktedrin
oraldrina
ortedrine
percomon
pharmamedrine
pharmedrine
phenedrine
phenoprominum
phenpromin
1 phenyl 2 aminopropane
1 phenyl 2 propanamine
phenylaminopropane
(phenylisopropyl) amine
(phenylisopropyl)amine
phenyl isopropylamine
profamina
profetamine
propisamine
psychedrin
psychedrine
psychoton
racemic desoxy nor ephedrine
racemic desoxy norephedrine
racephen
raphetamine
rhinalator
sedolin
simpamina
simpamine
simpatedrin
simpatedrine
stimulan
sympametin
sympamine
sympatedrine
theptine
vapedrine
zedrine

Long synonyms
dextro levo 2 methylphenethylamine
dextro levo 2 methylphenetylamine
dextro levo alpha methylphenethylamine

amphetamine derivative

WADA group
S1. STIMULANTS

MeSH descriptor
amphetamines

Short synonyms
amphetamines

Long synonyms
2 amino 1 phenylpropane derivative
1 phenyl 2 aminopropane derivative
2 phenylisopropylamine derivative

amphetaminil

WADA group
S1. STIMULANTS

CAS Registry number
17590-01-1

Short synonyms
amfetaminil
an 1
aponeuron

Long synonyms
(alpha methylphenethyl)aminophenylacetonitrile
alpha phenyl alpha n (alpha phenylisopropyl)aminoacetonitrile
amphetamine,n (alpha cyanobenzyl)
2 [(1 methyl 2 phenylethyl)amino] 2 phenylacetonitrile
n (alpha cyanobenzyl)amphetamine
2 phenyl 2 (phenylisopropylamino)acetonitrile

anabolic agent

WADA group
S4. ANABOLIC AGENTS

MeSH descriptor
anabolic steroids

Short synonyms
anabolic agents
anabolic drug
anabolic hormone
anabolic steroid
anabolic steroid agent
anabolic steroids
anabolizing agent
anabolizing cream
anabolizing drug
anabolizing treatment
steroid,anabolic

anandamide

WADA group
S3. CANNABINOIDS

CAS Registry number
94421-68-8

Short synonyms
arachidonoylethanolamide
arachidonylethanolamide

anastrozole

WADA group
S7. AGENTS WITH ANTI-OESTROGENIC ACTIVITY

CAS Registry number
120511-73-1

Trade names and research codes
arimidex
ici d1033
icid1033
zd 1033
zd1033

Short synonyms
anastrazole

Long synonyms
2,2' [5 (1h 1,2,4 triazol 1 ylmethyl) 1,3 phenylene]bis(2 methylpropionitrile)

androgen

WADA group
S4. ANABOLIC AGENTS

MeSH descriptor
androgens, synthetic
androgens

Short synonyms
androgenic agent
androgenic hormone
androgenic steroid
androgens
androgens, synthetic
androgen sulfate

androst 1 ene 3,17 dione

WADA group
S4. ANABOLIC AGENTS

Short synonyms
1 androstene 3,17 dione
delta 1 androstene 3,17 dione
delta1 androstene 3,17 dione

Long synonyms
5alpha androst 1 ene 3,17 dione

androsta 1,4,6 triene 3,17 dione

WADA group
S7. AGENTS WITH ANTI-OESTROGENIC ACTIVITY

CAS Registry number
633-35-2

Short synonyms
1,4,6 androstatrien 3,17 dione

Long synonyms
1,4,6 androstatriene 3,17 dione

androsta 4,16 dien 3 one

WADA group
S4. ANABOLIC AGENTS

CAS Registry number
4-7-4075

Short synonyms
4,16 androstadien 3 one
androstadienone
delta4,16 androstadien 3 one

androsta 4,6,8(9) triene 3,17 dione

WADA group
S7. AGENTS WITH ANTI-OESTROGENIC ACTIVITY

CAS Registry number
115930-43-3

Trade names and research codes
fce 24918
fce24918

5alpha androstan 3 one

WADA group
S4. ANABOLIC AGENTS

Short synonyms
androstanolone,17 deoxy
17 deoxyandrostanolone
17 deoxydihydrotestosterone

Long synonyms
17 deoxy 5alpha dihydrotestosterone

androstanediol

WADA group
S4. ANABOLIC AGENTS

MeSH descriptor
androstane-3,17-diol

CAS Registry number
1852-53-5
25126-76-5
67332-38-1

Short synonyms
adiol
3alpha,17beta androstanediol
3alpha androstanediol
5 alpha androstanediol
5alpha androstanediol
androstandiol
androstane-3,17-diol
androstane 3alpha,17beta diol
dihydroandrosteron
hombreol

Long synonyms
3alpha,17beta dihydroxy 5alpha androstane
3alpha,17beta dihydroxyandrostanediol
5alpha androstan 3,17 beta diol
5 alpha androstan 3 alpha,17 beta diol
5alpha androstan 3alpha,17beta diol
5alpha androstane 3,17beta diol
5alpha androstane 3alpha 17beta diol
5alpha androstane 3alpha,17beta diol

3beta androstanediol

WADA group
S4. ANABOLIC AGENTS

Trade names and research codes
xenabol

Short synonyms
5alpha,3beta androstanediol
androstan 3beta,17beta diol
androstane 3beta,17beta diol
3beta,5alpha androstanediol
3beta diol
drostanediol

Long synonyms
5 alpha androstan 3beta,17 beta diol
5alpha androstan 3beta,17beta diol
5alpha androstane 3beta,17beta diol
3beta,17beta dihydroxy 5alpha androstane
3beta,17beta dihydroxyandrostane

androstanedione

WADA group
S4. ANABOLIC AGENTS

Short synonyms
5 alpha androstanedione
5alpha androstanedione
androstandione

androstanolone

WADA group
S4. ANABOLIC AGENTS

MeSH descriptor
stanolone

CAS Registry number
521-18-6

Trade names and research codes
andractim

Short synonyms
5alpha androstanolone
5alpha dihydrotestosterone
anaboleen
anabolex
anabol tablinen
anaprotin
androlone
androstan 17beta ol 3 one
5 androstan 17 beta ol 3 one
5 androstan 17beta ol 3 one
5 androstan 3 one 17b ol
17beta hydroxyandrostan 3 one
cristerona
cristerone mb
dihydrotestosterone
5 dihydrotestosterone
lg 152
neodrol
pesomax
proteina
protona
stanaprol
stanolone
stanoprol
stanorone

Long synonyms
5alpha androstan 17beta ol 3 one
5alpha androstane 17beta ol 3 one
5alpha androstane 3 one 17beta ol
5 alpha androstanolone 17 beta ol 3 one
17 beta hydroxy 5 alpha androstan 3 one
17beta hydroxy 5 alpha androstan 3 one
17beta hydroxy 5alpha androstan 3 one
17beta hydroxy 5alpha androstane 3 one

5beta androstanolone

WADA group
S4. ANABOLIC AGENTS

Short synonyms
5 beta dihydrotestosterone
5beta dihydrotestosterone
etiocholan 17beta ol 3 one

Long synonyms
5 beta androstan 17 beta ol 3 one
5 beta androstan 17beta ol 3 one
5beta androstan 17beta ol 3 one
17beta hydroxy 5beta androstan 3 one
17beta hydroxy etiocholan 3 one

androstanolone bromoacetate

WADA group
S4. ANABOLIC AGENTS

CAS Registry number
66656-21-1

Short synonyms
androstanolone 17 bromoacetate

Long synonyms
5alpha androstan 17beta ol 3 one 17 bromoacetate
5alpha androstan 3 one 17beta bromoacetate
5alpha dihydrotestosterone bromoacetate
17beta bromoacetoxy 5alpha androstan 3 one
17beta bromoacetoxy 5alpha dihydrotestosterone
17beta hydroxy 5alpha androstan 3 one 17 bromoacetate
dihydrotestosterone bromoacetate

androstanolone derivative

WADA group
S4. ANABOLIC AGENTS

Short synonyms
dihydrotestosterone derivative
stanolone derivative

Long synonyms
5alpha androstan 17beta ol 3 one derivative
5alpha dihydrotestosterone derivative
17beta hydroxy 5alpha androstan 3 one protein complex
17beta hydroxyandrostan 3 one derivative

androstanolone propionate

WADA group
S4. ANABOLIC AGENTS

CAS Registry number
855-22-1

Short synonyms
dihydrotestosterone propionate
stanolone propionate

Long synonyms
5alpha dihydrotestosterone propionate
androst 4 en 5alpha,17beta diol 3 one propionate

4 androstenediol

WADA group
S4. ANABOLIC AGENTS

CAS Registry number
1156-92-9

Short synonyms
4 androsten 3beta,17beta diol
androst 4 enediol
delta 4 androstenediol
delta4 androstenediol

Long synonyms
4 androstene 3beta,17beta diol
androst 4 ene 3beta,17beta diol

androstenediol

WADA group
S4. ANABOLIC AGENTS

MeSH descriptor
androst-5-ene-3 beta,17 beta-diol

CAS Registry number
28652-91-7
521-17-5

Short synonyms
androst 5 en 3beta,17beta diol
androst 5 ene 3,17beta diol
5 androsten 3beta,17beta diol
5 androstene 3,17beta diol
5 androstene 3beta,17beta diol
androstene diol
5 androstenediol
17 beta androstenediol
delta 5 androstenediol
delta5 androstenediol

Long synonyms
androst 5 ene 3 beta,17 beta diol
androst-5-ene-3 beta,17 beta-diol
3beta,17beta dihydroxyandrost 5 ene
delta 5 androstene 3beta,17beta diol
delta5 androstene 3beta,17beta diol

androstenediol derivative

WADA group
S4. ANABOLIC AGENTS

MeSH descriptor
androstenediols

Short synonyms
5 androstenediol derivative
androstenediols

Long synonyms
androst 5 ene 3beta,17beta diol derivative
5 androstene 3,17 diol derivative
5 androstene 3beta,17alpha diol derivative
5 androstene 3 beta,17 alpha diol derivatives
5 androstene 3beta,17beta diol derivative
5 androstene 3 beta,17 beta diol derivatives

androstenedione

WADA group
S4. ANABOLIC AGENTS

MeSH descriptor
androstenedione

CAS Registry number
26264-53-9
63-05-8

Short synonyms
5alpha androstenedione
androst 4 en 3,17 dione
androst 4 ene 3,17 dione
4 androsten 3,17 dione
androstendione
androstene 3,17 dione
4 androstene 3,17 dione
androstene dione
4 androstenedione
androtex
d 4 androstenedione
delta 4 androsten 3,17 dione
delta 4 androstene 3,17 dione
delta 4 androstenedione
delta4 androstenedione
u4 3,17 androstenedione
u4 androsten 3,17 dione
u4 androstene 3,17 dione
u4 androstenedione

androstenedione derivative

WADA group
S4. ANABOLIC AGENTS

Long synonyms
androst 4 ene 3,17 dione derivative
delta4 androstene 3,17 dione dioxime derivative

androsterone

WADA group
S4. ANABOLIC AGENTS

MeSH descriptor
androsterone

CAS Registry number
53-41-8

Short synonyms
5alpha androsterone
3alpha hydroxy 17 androstanone
androstan 3alpha ol 17 one
androsteron

Long synonyms
5alpha androstan 3alpha ol 17 one
5alpha androstane 3alpha ol 17 one
3alpha hydroxy 5alpha androstan 17 one
3 alpha hydroxyandrostan 17 one
3alpha hydroxyetioallocholan 17 one
3 epihydroxyetioallocholan 17 one

androsterone derivative

WADA group
S4. ANABOLIC AGENTS

4 anilino 2 methylthiopyrido[2,3 d]pyrimidine

WADA group
S8. MASKING AGENTS
P3. DIURETICS

CAS Registry number
72564-74-0

Trade names and research codes
md 39 am

anordiol

WADA group
S7. AGENTS WITH ANTI-OESTROGENIC ACTIVITY

CAS Registry number
1045-29-0

Trade names and research codes
af 45
af45

Long synonyms
2alpha,17alpha diethynyl a nor 5alpha androstane 2beta,17beta diol

anorexigenic agent

WADA group
S1. STIMULANTS

MeSH descriptor
appetite depressants

Short synonyms
agent,anorexiant
anorectic agent
anorectic drug
anorexant agent
anorexiant
anorexiant agent
anorexiant drug
anorexic agent
anorexic drug
anorexigen
anorexigenic compound
anorexigenic drug
antiappetite agent
appetite depressant agent
appetite depressants
appetite inhibitor
appetite reducer
appetite reducing drug
appetite restrainer
appetite suppressant
appetite suppressing agent

antiestrogen

WADA group
S7. AGENTS WITH ANTI-OESTROGENIC ACTIVITY

MeSH descriptor
estradiol antagonists
estrogen antagonists

Short synonyms
anti estrogen
antiestrogen agent
antiestrogenic agent
estradiol antagonists
estrogen antagonist
estrogen antagonists
estrogen suppression

apraclonidine

WADA group
S1. STIMULANTS

CAS Registry number
66711-21-5

Trade names and research codes
alo 2145
alo2145
iopidine
lapidine

Short synonyms
4 aminoclonidine
aplonidine
aplonidine hydrochloride
clonidine,4 amino
para aminoclonidine

Long synonyms
2 (4 amino 2,6 dichlorophenyl)iminoimidazolidine
2 (4 amino 2,6 dichlorophenylimino)imidazolidine

apomorphine

WADA group
S1. STIMULANTS

MeSH descriptor
apomorphine

CAS Registry number
314-19-2
58-00-4

Trade names and research codes
apokinon
ixense
taluvian
uprima

Short synonyms
apomorfine
apomorphine hydrochloride
apormorphine

2 arachidonoylglycerol

WADA group
S3. CANNABINOIDS

Short synonyms
2 arachidonylglycerol
glycerol 2 arachidonate

aromatase inhibitor

WADA group
S7. AGENTS WITH ANTI-OESTROGENIC ACTIVITY

Short synonyms
estrogen synthetase inhibitor
steroid aromatase inhibitor

arotinolol

WADA group
P2. BETA-BLOCKERS

CAS Registry number
68377-91-3
68377-92-4

Trade names and research codes
almarl
s 596

Short synonyms
arotinolol hydrochloride

Long synonyms
2 [(3 butylamino 2 hydroxypropyl)thio] 4 (5 carbamoyl 2 thienyl)thiazole
2 (3 tert butylamino 2 hydroxypropylthio) 4 (5 carbamoyl 2 thienyl)thiazole
5 [2 (3 tert butylamino 2 hydroxypropylthio) 4 thiazolyl] 2 thiophenecarboxamide
2 [2 [(3 tert butylamino 2 hydroxypropyl)thio] 4 thiazolyl] 5 thiophenecarboxamide

Terms and Synonyms

☝ *probably not prohibited*

artificial blood

WADA group
S8. MASKING AGENTS
M1. ENHANCEMENT OF OXYGEN TRANSFER

Short synonyms
blood,artificial

arzoxifene

WADA group
S7. AGENTS WITH ANTI-OESTROGENIC ACTIVITY

CAS Registry number
182133-25-1
182133-27-3

Trade names and research codes
ly 353381
ly353381

Short synonyms
arzoxifene hydrochloride

Long synonyms
6 hydroxy 2 (4 methoxyphenyl) 3 [4 [2 (1 piperidinyl)ethoxy]phenoxy]benzo[b]thiophene
2 (4 methoxyphenyl) 3 [4 [2 (piperidin 1 yl)ethoxy]phenoxy]benzo[b]thiophen 6 ol

asialochorionic gonadotropin

WADA group
S5. PEPTIDE HORMONES

Short synonyms
asialo chorionic gonadotropin
asialochorionogonadotropin
asialo hCG
desialo hcg

Long synonyms
desialylated human chorionic gonadotropin

atamestane

WADA group
S7. AGENTS WITH ANTI-OESTROGENIC ACTIVITY

CAS Registry number
96301-34-7

Trade names and research codes
sh 489

Long synonyms
androsta 1,4 diene 3,17 dione,1 methyl
1 methyl 1,4 androstadiene 3,17 dione
1 methylandrosta 1,4 diene 3,17 dione

atenolol

WADA group
P2. BETA-BLOCKERS

MeSH descriptor
atenolol

CAS Registry number
29122-68-7

Trade names and research codes
atenol
blokium
ici 66,082
ici 66082
neotenol
normiten
ormidol
tenoblock
tenolol
tenormin

Short synonyms
tenormin mite
tensinor

Long synonyms
1 (4 carbamoylmethylphenoxy) 3 isopropylamino 2 propanol
4 (2 hydroxy 3 isopropylaminopropoxy) phenylacetamide

atenolol plus chlortalidone

WADA group
S8. MASKING AGENTS
P2. BETA-BLOCKERS
P3. DIURETICS

CAS Registry number
73677-19-7

Trade names and research codes
blokium diu
teneretic
tenoretic

Short synonyms
atenigron
chlortalidone plus atenolol
co tenidone
diube
tenorectic
tenoret
tenoretic ge
tenoretic mite

atenolol plus nifedipine

WADA group
P2. BETA-BLOCKERS

Trade names and research codes
bay r 1999
bay r1999
beta adalat
beta adalate
niften
tenif
tenordate

Short synonyms
nifedipine plus atenolol

atromid

WADA group
S4. ANABOLIC AGENTS

CAS Registry number
8075-95-4

Trade names and research codes
atromid

Short synonyms
androsterone plus clofibrate
clofibrate plus androsterone

azosemide

WADA group
S8. MASKING AGENTS
P3. DIURETICS

CAS Registry number
27589-33-9

Trade names and research codes
luret
ple 1053
sk 110

Long synonyms
2 chloro 5 (1h tetrazol 5 yl) 4 [(2 thienylmethyl)amino]benzenesulfonamide
2 chloro 5 (1h tetrazol 5 yl) n4 (2 thenyl)sulfanilamide
5 [4 chloro 5 sulfamoyl 2 (2 thenylamino)phenyl]tetrazole

bambuterol

WADA group
S6. BETA-2 AGONISTS

CAS Registry number
81732-65-2

Trade names and research codes
bambec

Long synonyms
5 (2 tert butylamino 1 hydroxyethyl)resorcinol bis(n,n dimethylcarbamate)

bamethan

WADA group
S1. STIMULANTS
S6. BETA-2 AGONISTS

CAS Registry number
3692-39-5
3703-79-5
5716-20-1

Short synonyms
bamethane
bamethane sulfate
bamethan succinate
bamethan sulfate
bupatol
butedrin
butedrine
butyl norsynephrine
butyloctopamine
butylsympathol
butylsympatol
sim pelate
vasculat
vasculate
vasculit

Long synonyms
alpha butylaminomethyl para hydroxybenzylalcohol
2 butylamino 1 (para hydroxyphenylethanol)
1 (4' hydroxyphenyl) 1 hydroxy 2 butylaminoethane sulfonate
1 (4 hydroxyphenyl) 2 butylaminoethanol

baycuten

WADA group
S9. GLUCOCORTICOSTEROIDS

Trade names and research codes
baycuten
bay f 4797
bay f4797

Long synonyms
azidamfenicol plus clotrimazole and dexamethasone
azidamfenicol with clotrimazole and dexamethasone

bazedoxifene

WADA group
S7. AGENTS WITH ANTI-OESTROGENIC ACTIVITY

CAS Registry number
198481-32-2
198481-33-3

Trade names and research codes
tse 424
tse424
way 140424
way140424

Short synonyms
bazedoxifene acetate

Long synonyms
5 hydroxy 2 (4 hydroxyphenyl) 3 methyl 1 [4 [2 (perhydro 1 azepinyl)ethoxy]benzyl]indole
2 (4 hydroxyphenyl) 3 methyl 1 [4 [2 (perhydroazepin 1 yl)ethoxy]benzyl] 1h indol 5 ol acetate

beclometasone

WADA group
S9. GLUCOCORTICOSTEROIDS

MeSH descriptor
beclomethasone

CAS Registry number
4419-39-0

Short synonyms
beclomethasone

Long synonyms
9alpha chloro 16beta methylprednisolone
9 chloro 11beta,17,21 trihydroxy 16beta methylpregna 1,4 diene 3,20 dione
prednisolone,9alpha chloro 16beta methyl
pregna 1,4 diene 11beta,17,21 triol 3,20 dione,9 chloro 16beta methyl

beclometasone dipropionate

WADA group
S9. GLUCOCORTICOSTEROIDS

CAS Registry number
8-9-5534

Trade names and research codes
alanase
aldecin
aldecina
aldecine
atomide

beclate
beclazone
becloasma
becloforte
beclojet
beclomet
beclorhinol
beclosol
beclotaide
becloturmant
becloturmat
beclovent
becodisk
becodisks
beconase
beconase aq
beconasol
becotide
clenil
qvar
respocort
rhinivict
sanasthmax
sanasthmyl
vancenase
vancenase aq
vanceril
viarox

Short synonyms
beclamet
beclomethasone dipropionate
beclomethazone dipropionate
propaderm
propaderm forte
sch 18020w
viarex

Long synonyms
beclomethasone 17,21 dipropionate
9 chloro 11beta,17,21 trihydroxy 16beta methylpregna 1,4 diene 3,20 dione dipropionate

befunolol

WADA group
P2. BETA-BLOCKERS

CAS Registry number
39543-79-8
39552-01-7

Trade names and research codes
bentos
bentos ophtadose
bfe 60
bfe60
glauconex

Short synonyms
befnolol
benfuran
bentox
glaukonex

Long synonyms
2 acetyl 7 (2 hydroxy 3 isopropylaminopropoxy)benzofuran
1 (2 acetylbenzofuran 7 yloxy) 3 isopropylamino 2 propanol
7 (2 hydroxy 3 isopropylaminopropoxy) 2 benzofuranyl methyl ketone

bemegride

WADA group
S1. STIMULANTS

MeSH descriptor
bemegride

CAS Registry number
64-65-3

Trade names and research codes
megimide

Short synonyms
ab 01
bemequide
bemigride
3 ethyl 3 methylglutarimide
eukraton
malysol
methetharimide
mikedimide
np 13

Long synonyms
beta ethyl beta methylglutarimide
4 ethyl 4 methyl 2,6 piperidinedione

bemetizide

WADA group
S8. MASKING AGENTS
P3. DIURETICS

CAS Registry number
1824-52-8

Long synonyms
6 chloro 3,4 dihydro 3 (alpha methylbenzyl) 2h 1,2,4 benzothiadiazine 7 sulfonamide 1,1 dioxide
6 chloro 3,4 dihydro 3 (alpha methylbenzyl) 7 sulfamoyl 2h 1,2 4 benzothiadiazine 1,1 dioxide

bemitradine

WADA group
S8. MASKING AGENTS
P3. DIURETICS

CAS Registry number
88133-11-3

Trade names and research codes
sc 33643

Long synonyms
5 amino 8 (2 ethoxyethyl) 7 phenyl 1,2,4 triazolo[2,3 c]pyrimidine
8 (2 ethoxyethyl) 7 phenyl 1,2,4 triazolo[1,5 c]pyrimidin 5 amine
8 (2 ethoxyethyl) 7 phenyl[1,2,4]triazolo[1,5 c]pyrimidin 5 amine

benazepril plus hydrochlorothiazide

WADA group
S8. MASKING AGENTS
P3. DIURETICS

Trade names and research codes
cibadrex
lotensin HCT

Terms and Synonyms

Long synonyms
hydrochlorothiazide plus benazepril

bendroflumethiazide

WADA group
S8. MASKING AGENTS
P3. DIURETICS

MeSH descriptor
bendroflumethiazide

CAS Registry number
73-48-3

Trade names and research codes
aprinox
be 724 a
be 724a
be724a
ft 81
ft81
naturetin
neo naclex
neonaclex k
pluryl
sinesalin

Short synonyms
bendrofluazide
bendrofluazide k
benzhydroflumethiazide
benzydroflumethiazide
benzyl hydroflumethiazide
benzylhydroflumethiazide
berkozide
bristuron
centonuron
centyl
naturetin k
naturine
neo nadex k
neonadex k
pluryle
repicin
salures
salures k

Long synonyms
3 benzyl 3,4 dihydro 7 sulfamoyl 6 trifluoromethyl 1,2,4 benzothiadiazine 1,1 dioxide

bendroflumethiazide plus nadolol

WADA group
S8. MASKING AGENTS
P2. BETA-BLOCKERS
P3. DIURETICS

Trade names and research codes
corgaretic
corgaretic n
corgaretic s
corzide

Long synonyms
nadolol plus bendroflumethiazide

benorterone

WADA group
S4. ANABOLIC AGENTS

CAS Registry number
3-10-3570

Trade names and research codes
skf 7692

Short synonyms
17 methyl b nortestosterone

Long synonyms
17 alpha methyl beta nortestosterone
17alpha methyl beta nortestosterone
17alpha methyl betanortestosterone
17alpha methyl b nortestosterone
17beta hydroxy 17 methyl b norandrost 4 en 3 one
testosterone,17alpha methyl b nor

alpha [[[3 (1 benzimidazolyl) 1,1 dimethylpropyl]amino]methyl] 2 fluoro 4 hydroxybenzyl alcohol

WADA group
S6. BETA-2 AGONISTS

CAS Registry number
73865-18-6

Trade names and research codes
som 1122

1 (1,3 benzodioxol 5 yl) n methyl 2 butanamine

WADA group
S1. STIMULANTS

CAS Registry number
103818-46-8

Long synonyms
1 (1,3 benzodioxol 5 yl) n methyl 2 butylamine
5 (2 methylaminobutyl) 1,3 benzodioxole
n methyl 1 (1,3 benzodioxol 5 yl) 2 butanamine

benzphetamine

WADA group
S1. STIMULANTS

MeSH descriptor
benzphetamine

CAS Registry number
156-08-1
5411-22-3

Trade names and research codes
didrex

Short synonyms
benzfetamine
benzphetamine hydrochloride
benzylmetamphetamine
dextro benzphetamine
l benzphetamine
levo benzphetamine
n benzylmethamphetamine
n benzyl n methylamphetamine

Long synonyms
n benzyl n,alpha dimethylphenethylamine
n benzyl n methyl 1 phenyl 2 propanamine
1 phenyl 2 (n methyl n benzylamino)propane

benzthiazide

WADA group
S8. MASKING AGENTS
P3. DIURETICS

CAS Registry number
91-33-8

Trade names and research codes
aquatag
dytide n
exna
fovane
marazide
p 1393
p1393

Short synonyms
benzothiazide
benzylthiomethylchlorothiazide
exosalt
naclex robins
proaqua

Long synonyms
3 benzylthiomethyl 6 chloro 7 sulfamoyl 2h 1,2,4 benzothiadiazine 1,1 dioxide

benzthiazide plus triamterene

WADA group
S8. MASKING AGENTS
P3. DIURETICS

Trade names and research codes
diteriam
dytid
dytide

Short synonyms
triamterene plus benzthiazide

besulpamide

WADA group
S8. MASKING AGENTS
P3. DIURETICS

CAS Registry number
90992-25-9

Long synonyms
1 (4 chloro 3 sulfamoylbenzamido) 2,4,6 trimethylpyridinium hydroxide

beta 1 adrenergic receptor blocking agent

WADA group
P2. BETA-BLOCKERS

Short synonyms
beta 1 adrenergic antagonist
beta 1 adrenergic blocker
beta 1 adrenoceptor blocker

Long synonyms
beta 1 adrenergic blocking agent
beta 1 adrenergic receptor blocker

beta 1 adrenergic receptor stimulating agent

WADA group
S6. BETA-2 AGONISTS

Short synonyms
beta 1 adrenergic agonist
beta 1 adrenergic stimulant

beta 2 adrenergic receptor blocking agent

WADA group
P2. BETA-BLOCKERS

Short synonyms
beta 2 adrenergic antagonist
beta 2 adrenergic blocker

Long synonyms
beta 2 adrenergic blocking agent
beta 2 adrenergic receptor blocker

beta 2 adrenergic receptor stimulating agent

WADA group
S6. BETA-2 AGONISTS

Short synonyms
beta 2 adrenergic agent
beta 2 adrenergic agonist
beta 2 adrenergic stimulant

Long synonyms
beta 2 adrenergic receptor agonist
beta2 adrenergic receptor stimulating agent

beta 3 adrenergic receptor blocking agent

WADA group
P2. BETA-BLOCKERS

Short synonyms
beta 3 adrenergic antagonist
beta 3 adrenergic blocker
beta 3 adrenoceptor antagonist

Long synonyms
beta 3 adrenergic blocking agent
beta 3 adrenergic receptor antagonist
beta 3 adrenergic receptor blocker

beta 3 adrenergic receptor stimulating agent

WADA group
S6. BETA-2 AGONISTS

Short synonyms
beta 3 adrenergic agonist
beta 3 adrenoceptor agonist

Long synonyms
beta 3 adrenergic receptor agonist

beta adrenergic receptor blocking agent

WADA group
P2. BETA-BLOCKERS

MeSH descriptor
adrenergic beta-antagonists

Short synonyms
adrenergic beta-antagonists
beta adrenergic antagonist
beta adrenergic blocker
beta adrenergic blockers
beta adrenergic blocking agent
beta adrenergic blocking drug
beta adrenoceptor antagonist
beta adrenolytic
beta adrenolytic agent
beta antagonist
beta antiadrenergic agent
beta blocker
beta blocking adrenergic agent
beta blocking agent
beta blocking drug
beta receptor blocker
beta receptor blocking agent
beta sympathicolytic agent
beta sympathicolytics
beta sympatholytic agent
betasympatholytic agent

Long synonyms
beta adrenergic receptor antagonist
beta adrenergic receptor blocker
beta adrenoceptor blocking agent
beta adrenoceptor blocking drug
beta receptor adrenergic blocking agent

beta adrenergic receptor stimulating agent

WADA group
S6. BETA-2 AGONISTS

MeSH descriptor
adrenergic beta-agonists

Short synonyms
adrenergic beta-agonists
beta adrenergic agent
beta adrenergic agonist
beta adrenergic drug
beta adrenergic receptor agent
beta adrenergic stimulant
beta adrenergic stimulator
beta adrenoceptor agonist
beta agonist
beta mimetic agent
beta stimulating drug
beta sympathetic agent
beta sympathicomimetic
beta sympathicomimetic agent
beta sympathomimetic agent
beta sympathomimetic drug

Long synonyms
beta adrenergic receptor agonist
beta adrenergic receptor stimulant
beta adrenergic receptor stimulant agent
beta adrenergic stimulating agent
beta adrenoceptor stimulating agent

betamethasone

WADA group
S9. GLUCOCORTICOSTEROIDS

MeSH descriptor
betamethasone

CAS Registry number
378-44-9

Trade names and research codes
betnelan
betnesol v
betsolan
betsolon
celestan
celestan v
celestene
celestone
rinderon

Short synonyms
betacortril
betadexamethasone
betametasone
betamethasolone
beta methason
betamethason
beta methasone
betamethasone alcohol
betamethasonium
betamethasonum
betamethazone
betnasol
betnesol h
betnovate a
betsopart
celestan depot
celestona
celeston chronodose
cidoten
flubenisolone
methasone
nsc 39470
rg 833
sch 4831

Long synonyms
9alpha fluoro 11beta,17,21 trihydroxy 16beta methylpregna 1,4diene 3,20 dione
9alpha fluoro 11beta,17alpha,21 trihydroxy 16beta methylpregna 1,4 diene 3,20 dione
9alpha fluoro 16beta methyl 1,4 pregnadiene 3,20 dione 11beta,17alpha,21triol
9alpha fluoro 16beta methylprednisolone
betamethasone 17,21 (methylorthobenzoate)
betamethasone 17alpha,21 orthobenzoate
16beta methyl 9alpha fluoro delta 1 hydrocortisone
16beta methyl 9alpha fluoroprednisolone
prednisolone,9alpha fluoro 16beta methyl
pregna 1,4 diene 11beta,17alpha,21 triol 3,20 dione,9alpha fluoro 16beta methyl
pregna 1,4 diene 3,20 dione 11,17,21 triol, 9 alpha fluoro 16beta methyl

betamethasone acetate

WADA group
S9. GLUCOCORTICOSTEROIDS

CAS Registry number
987-24-6

Short synonyms
betamethasone 21 acetate

betamethasone acetate plus betamethasone sodium phosphate

WADA group
S9. GLUCOCORTICOSTEROIDS

CAS Registry number
2-8-8064

Trade names and research codes
celestone soluspan

Long synonyms
betamethasone sodium phosphate plus betamethasone acetate

betamethasone benzoate

WADA group
S9. GLUCOCORTICOSTEROIDS

CAS Registry number
22298-29-9

Trade names and research codes
euvaderm
fluobate
flurobate

Short synonyms
beben
benisone
betamethasone 17 benzoate
beta methazone 17 benzoate
fluorobate
ms 1112
uticort

betamethasone derivative

WADA group
S9. GLUCOCORTICOSTEROIDS

betamethasone dipropionate

WADA group
S9. GLUCOCORTICOSTEROIDS

CAS Registry number
5593-20-4

Trade names and research codes
alphatrex
diproderm
diprolene
diprophos
diprosalic
diprosis
diprosone
lotrisone
rinderon dp

Short synonyms
beloderm
betametasone dipropionate
diprocel
sch 11460

Long synonyms
betamethasone 17,21 dipropionate

betamethasone sodium phosphate

WADA group
S9. GLUCOCORTICOSTEROIDS

CAS Registry number
151-73-5
360-63-4

Trade names and research codes
bentelan
betnesol
diprospan
durabetason
rinderon a

Short synonyms
beta corlan
betamethasone 21 phosphate
beta methasone phosphate
betamethasone phosphate
betnesol inj
etnesol
solucelestan

Long synonyms
betamethasone 21 disodium phosphate
beta methasone disodium phosphate
betamethasone di sodium phosphate
betamethasone disodium phosphate
9 fluoro 11 beta, 17,21 trihydroxy 16 beta methylpregna 1,4 diene 3,20 dione 21(disodium phosphate)

betamethasone sodium phosphate plus neomycin

WADA group
S9. GLUCOCORTICOSTEROIDS

Trade names and research codes
betnesol n

Long synonyms
neomycin plus betamethasone sodium phosphate

betamethasone valerate

WADA group
S9. GLUCOCORTICOSTEROIDS

MeSH descriptor
betamethasone 17-valerate

CAS Registry number
2152-44-5
57654-97-4

Trade names and research codes
bemetson
betacort
betatrex
beta val
betneval
betnovat
betnovate
celestoderm
ectosone
goldline
metaderm
rinderon v
valisone
valnac

Short synonyms
betaderm
beta metasone 17 valerate
betametasone 17 valerate
betamethason 17 valerate
beta methasone 17 valerate
betamethasone 17 valerate
betamethasone 17-valerate
beta methasone valerate
betamethasone valerianate
betamethazone 17 valerate
betamethazone valerate
betaval
betnelan v
betnovate c
bextasol
celestoderm v
celestona c
celestone valerate
delmit
ecoval 70
retenema
tokuderm

Long synonyms
betamethasone 17 valerate ester

betaxolol

WADA group
P2. BETA-BLOCKERS

MeSH descriptor
betaxolol

CAS Registry number
63659-18-7
72424-72-7

Trade names and research codes
betaxon
betoptic
betoptima
kerlon
kerlone

Short synonyms
alo 1401 02
betaxolol hydrochloride
sl 75212

Long synonyms
[4 (2 cyclopropylmethoxyethyl) 3 isopropylaminophenoxy]propan 2 ol
1 [4 (2 cyclopropylmethoxyethyl)phenoxy] 3 isopropylamino 2 propanol

bevantolol

WADA group
P2. BETA-BLOCKERS

CAS Registry number
59170-23-9

Trade names and research codes
benatol
calvan
ci 755
ci755
ci 775
ci775
cl 775
cl775
nc 1400
nc1400
ranestol
vantol

Short synonyms
bevantolol hydrochloride

Long synonyms
1 [(3,4 dimethoxyphenethyl)amino] 3 (3 methylphenoxy) 2 propanol

bfe 55

WADA group
P2. BETA-BLOCKERS

CAS Registry number
21151-91-7

Trade names and research codes
bfe 55
bfe55

biosynthetic human proinsulin

WADA group
S5. PEPTIDE HORMONES

Short synonyms
human proinsulin,biosynthetic
proinsulin,human biosynthetic

biphasic insulin

WADA group
S5. PEPTIDE HORMONES

CAS Registry number
8063-29-4

Trade names and research codes
rapitard
rapitard mc

Short synonyms
biphasic insulin injection
insulin novo rapitard
rapitard insulin

1 [4 [n,n bis(2 chloroethyl)carbamoyloxy]phenyl] 1 (4 hydroxyphenyl) 2 phenyl 1 butene

WADA group
S7. AGENTS WITH ANTI-OESTROGENIC ACTIVITY

2,3 bis(2 fluoro 4 hydroxyphenyl) 2,3 dimethylbutane

WADA group
S7. AGENTS WITH ANTI-OESTROGENIC ACTIVITY

Trade names and research codes
d 18954
d18954

2,3 bis(2 fluoro 4 hydroxyphenyl) 2,3 dimethylbutane derivative

WADA group
S7. AGENTS WITH ANTI-OESTROGENIC ACTIVITY

2,3 bis(4 hydroxyphenyl) 2,3 dimethylbutane

WADA group
S7. AGENTS WITH ANTI-OESTROGENIC ACTIVITY

CAS Registry number
74385-27-6

Short synonyms
tetramethylhes
tetramethylhexestrol

Long synonyms
1,2 bis(4 hydroxyphenyl) 1,1,2,2 tetramethylethane
1,1,2,2 tetramethyl 1,2 bis(4 hydroxyphenyl)ethane

bis(4 hydroxyphenyl)cyclohexylidenemethane

WADA group
S7. AGENTS WITH ANTI-OESTROGENIC ACTIVITY

CAS Registry number
5189-40-2

Trade names and research codes
f 6060
f6060

Short synonyms
cyclofenil diphenol

Long synonyms
bis(para hydroxyphenyl) cyclohexylidenemethane
bis(para hydroxyphenyl)cyclohexylidenemethane
cyclohexylidenebis(para hydroxyphenyl)methane

4 [3 [bis(beta hydroxyphenethyl)amino]butyl]benzamide

WADA group
S6. BETA-2 AGONISTS

CAS Registry number
90505-66-1

Trade names and research codes
ro 16 8714
ro 16-8714

Long synonyms
4 [3 [bis(2 hydroxy 2 phenylethyl)amino]butyl]benzamide

bisoprolol

WADA group
P2. BETA-BLOCKERS

MeSH descriptor
bisoprolol

CAS Registry number
66722-44-9

Trade names and research codes
detensiel
soprol

Long synonyms
1 [[alpha (2 isopropoxyethoxy) para tolyl]oxy] 3 isopropylamino 2 propanol
1 [4 [(2 isopropoxyethoxy)methyl]phenoxy] 3 isopropylamino 2 propanol

bisoprolol fumarate

WADA group
P2. BETA-BLOCKERS

CAS Registry number
104344-23-2

Trade names and research codes
bisobloc
bisocor
cl 297939
cl297939
concor
emconcor
emcor
emd 33512
emd33512
maintate
monocor
zebeta

Long synonyms
1 [[alpha (2 isopropoxyethoxy) para tolyl]oxy] 3 isopropylamino 2 propanol fumarate
bis[1 [4 [(2 isopropoxyethoxy)methyl]phenoxy] 3 isopropylamino 2 propanol] fumarate
1 [4 [(2 isopropoxyethoxy)methyl]phenoxy] 3 isopropylamino 2 propanol fumarate

bisoprolol fumarate plus hydrochlorothiazide

WADA group
S8. MASKING AGENTS
P2. BETA-BLOCKERS
P3. DIURETICS

Trade names and research codes
maxsoten
ziac

Long synonyms
hydrochlorothiazide plus bisoprolol fumarate

bis(perfluorohexyl)ethylene

WADA group
M1. ENHANCEMENT OF OXYGEN TRANSFER

CAS Registry number
56523-43-4

Trade names and research codes
f 66e
f66e

Terms and Synonyms

bitolterol

WADA group
S6. BETA-2 AGONISTS

CAS Registry number
30392-40-6

Short synonyms
colterol 3,4 di para toluate
s 1540

Long synonyms
alpha (tert butylaminomethyl) 3,4 dihydroxybenzyl alcohol 3,4 di para toluate
4 [2 (1,1 dimethylethylamino) 1 hydroxyethyl] 1,2 phenylene bis(4 methylbenzoate)
4 [2 (1,1 dimethylethylamino) 1 hydroxymethyl] 1,2 phenylene bis(4 methylbenzoate)

bitolterol mesilate

WADA group
S6. BETA-2 AGONISTS

CAS Registry number
30392-41-7

Trade names and research codes
biterol
tornalate
win 32784

Short synonyms
bitolterol mesylate
bitolterol methanesulfonate
effectin

blood derivative

WADA group
S8. MASKING AGENTS
M1. ENHANCEMENT OF OXYGEN TRANSFER

blood extract

WADA group
S8. MASKING AGENTS
M1. ENHANCEMENT OF OXYGEN TRANSFER

Short synonyms
deproteinized blood extract

blood substitute

WADA group
S8. MASKING AGENTS
M1. ENHANCEMENT OF OXYGEN TRANSFER

MeSH descriptor
blood substitutes

Short synonyms
blood substitutes

bolandiol

WADA group
S4. ANABOLIC AGENTS

CAS Registry number
19793-20-5

Short synonyms
estr 4 ene 3beta,17beta diol
19 nor 4 androstenediol
19 norandrodiol
19 norandrostenediol
19 nordiol

Long synonyms
3beta,17beta dihydroxyestr 4 ene
19 nor 4 androstene 3beta,17beta diol
19 norandrost 4 ene 3beta,17beta diol

bolasterone

WADA group
S4. ANABOLIC AGENTS

CAS Registry number
1605-89-6

Trade names and research codes
myagen
nsc 66233
u 19763

Short synonyms
7alpha,17 dimethyltestosterone

Long synonyms
7alpha,17alpha dimethyltestosterone

boldenone

WADA group
S4. ANABOLIC AGENTS

CAS Registry number
846-48-0

Trade names and research codes
boldane
ciba 29038
ciba29038

Short synonyms
dehydrotestosterone
1 dehydrotestosterone
1,2 dehydrotestosterone

Long synonyms
androsta 1,4 dien 17 beta ol 3 one
androsta 1,4 dien 17beta ol 3 one
androsta 1,4 dien 3 one 17alpha ol
1,4 androstadien 17beta ol 3 one
17beta hydroxy 1,4 androstadien 3 one
17beta hydroxyandrost 1,4 dien 3 one
17beta hydroxyandrosta 1,4 dien 3 one
17 beta hydroxyandrosta 1,4 diene 3 one
3 oxo 17beta hydroxy 1,4 androstadiene

boldenone undecenoate

WADA group
S4. ANABOLIC AGENTS

CAS Registry number
13103-34-9

Trade names and research codes
ba 29038
ba29038
equipois
equipoise

hubernol
vebenol

Short synonyms
boldenone 10 undecenoate
boldenone undecylenate
parenabol

Long synonyms
17beta hydroxyandrosta 1,4 diene 3 one undecylenate
dehydrotestosterone undecylenate
1 dehydrotestosterone undecylenate

boldione

WADA group
S4. ANABOLIC AGENTS

CAS Registry number
897-06-3

Short synonyms
1,4 androstadien 3,17 dione
androsta 1,4 dien 3,17 dione
androstadiendione
1,4 androstadiene 3,17 dione
androsta 1,4 diene 3,17 dione
androstadienedione

Long Synonyms
delta 1,4 androstadiene 3,17 dione
delta1,4 androstadiene 3,17 dione

bopindolol

WADA group
P2. BETA-BLOCKERS

CAS Registry number
62658-63-3

Trade names and research codes
lt 31200
lt31200
sandonorm
wandonorm

Long synonyms
1 (tert butylamino) 3 [(2 methylindol 4 yl)oxy] 2 propanol benzoate

bornaprolol

WADA group
P2. BETA-BLOCKERS

CAS Registry number
69319-47-7

Trade names and research codes
fm 24
fm24

Long synonyms
1 (2 bicyclo[2.2.1]hept 2 ylphenoxy) 3 [(1 methylethyl)amino] 2 propanol
1 (2 bicyclo[2.2.1]hept 2 ylphenoxy) 3 isopropylamino 2 propanol
1 (2 exo bicyclo[2.2.1]hept 2 ylphenoxy) 3 [(1 methylethyl)amino] 2 propanol
1 isopropylamino 3 [2 (2 norbornyl)phenoxy] 2 propanol
1 (isopropylamino) 3 (o 2 exo norbornylphenoxy) 2 propanol

bovine insulin

WADA group
S5. PEPTIDE HORMONES

CAS Registry number
11070-73-8

Short synonyms
beef insulin
insulin,beef
insulin,bovine

brefonalol

WADA group
P2. BETA-BLOCKERS

CAS Registry number
104051-20-9

Trade names and research codes
bdf 8186
bdf8186

Short synonyms
brefanolol

Long synonyms
3,4 dihydro 6 [1 hydroxy 2 [(1,1 dimethyl 3 phenylpropyl)amino]ethyl] 2(1h) quinolinone
3,4 dihydro 6 [1 hydroxy 2 [(1,1 dimethyl 3 phenylpropyl)amino]ethyl]carbostyril

brimonidine

WADA group
S1. STIMULANTS

CAS Registry number
59803-98-4

Trade names and research codes
agn 190342
agn190342
alphagen
uk 14,304
uk14,304
uk 14304
uk14304
uk 14304 18
uk1430418
uk 14304-18
uk14304-18

Short synonyms
brimonidine tartrate

Long synonyms
5 bromo 6 (2 imidazolin 2 ylamino)quinoxaline
5 bromo n (4,5 dihydro 1h imidazol 2 yl)quinoxalinamine
5 bromo n (4,5 dihydro 2 imidazolyl)quinoxalinamine
2 (5 bromoquinoxalin 6 ylimino) 2 imidazoline
2 (8 bromoquinoxalin 7 ylimino) 2 imidazoline

briserin

WADA group
S8. MASKING AGENTS
P3. DIURETICS

CAS Registry number
55128-93-3

92355-74-3

Trade names and research codes
brinedine
brinerdin
brinerdine
briserim
briserin
briserine
cristepin
crystepin
kristepin

Long synonyms
clopamide plus dihydroergocristine plus reserpine

brocrinat

WADA group
S8. MASKING AGENTS
P3. DIURETICS

CAS Registry number
72481-99-3

Trade names and research codes
hp 3522

Short synonyms
halocrinic acid
hp 522

Long synonyms
[7 bromo 3 (2 fluorophenyl) 1,2 benzisoxazol 6 yloxy]acetic acid
[[7 bromo 3 (2 fluorophenyl) 1,2 benzisoxazol 6 yl]oxy]acetic acid

brolamfetamine

WADA group
S1. STIMULANTS

CAS Registry number
32156-26-6
51261-87-1

Long synonyms
2 amino 1 (2,5 dimethoxy 4 bromophenyl)propane
2 amino 1 (4 bromo 2,5 dimethoxyphenyl)propane
4 bromo 2,5 dimethoxy alpha methylphenethylamine
4 bromo 2,5 dimethoxyamphetamine
4 bromo 2,5 dimethoxyamphetamine hydrochloride
1 (4 bromo 2,5 dimethoxyphenyl) 2 aminopropane
4 bromo 2,5 dimethoxyphenylisopropylamine
4 bromo 2,5 dimethyloxyamphetamine
2,5 dimethoxy 4 bromoamphetamine
1 (2,5 dimethoxy 4 bromophenyl) 2 aminopropane

bromantan

WADA group
S1. STIMULANTS

Short synonyms
2 (4 bromoanilino)adamantane

Long synonyms
2 (4 bromophenylamino)adamantane

8 bromoacetamido 1 [2 hydroxy 3 (4 indolyloxy)propylamino] para menthane

WADA group
P2. BETA-BLOCKERS

CAS Registry number
106469-51-6

Long synonyms
1 (1 bromoacetamido para menth 8 ylamino) 3 (4 indolyloxy) 2 propanol
n8 bromoacetyl n1 [3 (4 indolyloxy) 2 hydroxypropyl] 1,8 diamino para menthane

bromoacetylalprenololmenthane

WADA group
P2. BETA-BLOCKERS

CAS Registry number
82870-40-4

4 [n (4 bromobenzyl) n (1,2,4 triazol 4 yl)amino]benzonitrile

WADA group
S7. AGENTS WITH ANTI-OESTROGENIC ACTIVITY

CAS Registry number
148869-05-0

Trade names and research codes
ym 511

Long synonyms
4 [n (4 bromobenzyl) n (4 cyanophenyl)amino] 4h 1,2,4 triazole

broxaterol

WADA group
S6. BETA-2 AGONISTS

CAS Registry number
76596-57-1

Trade names and research codes
summair

Short synonyms
broxaterol hydrochloride
z 1170

Long synonyms
1 (3 bromo 5 isoxazolyl) 2 (tert butylamino)ethanol
3 bromo alpha [(tert butylamino)methyl] 5 isoxazolemethanol

brucine

WADA group
S1. STIMULANTS

CAS Registry number
357-57-3

bucindolol

WADA group
P2. BETA-BLOCKERS

CAS Registry number
71119-11-4

Short synonyms
bucindolol hydrochloride
mj 13105
mj 13,105 1
mj 13105 1

Long synonyms
1 (2 cyanophenoxy) 3 [(2 indol 3 yl 1,1 dimethylethyl)amino] 2 propanol
2 [2 hydroxy 3 [(2 indol 3 yl 1,1 dimethylethyl)amino]propoxy]benzonitrile

bucumolol

WADA group
P2. BETA-BLOCKERS

CAS Registry number
36556-75-9
58409-59-9

Trade names and research codes
cs 359
cs359

Short synonyms
bucumarol
bukumolol

Long synonyms
coumarin,8 [3 (tert butylamino) 2 hydroxypropoxy] 5 methyl
8 [3 (tert butylamino) 2 hydroxypropoxy] 5 methylcoumarin

budesonide

WADA group
S9. GLUCOCORTICOSTEROIDS

MeSH descriptor
budesonide

CAS Registry number
51333-22-3

Trade names and research codes
budecol
budecort
budefat
budes
budeson
budiair
budon
entocort
entocort ec
olfex
olfex bucal
pulmaxan
pulmicort
pulmicort respules
pulmicort turbuhaler
respicort
rhinocort
rhinocort aqua
spirocort

Short synonyms
budenoside
preferid
s 1320

Long synonyms
16alpha,17beta butylidenedioxy 11beta,21 dihydroxypregna 1,4 diene 3,20 dione
11beta,16alpha,17,21 tetrahydroxypregn 1,4 diene 3,20 dione 16,17 butyraldehyde cyclic acetal
11beta,16alpha,17,21 tetrahydroxypregna 1,4 diene 3,20 dione 16,17 butyraldehyde cyclic acetal
11beta,16alpha,17,21 tetrahydroxypregna 1,4 diene 3,20 dione cyclic 16,17 acetal with butyraldehyde
pregna 1,4 diene 3,20 dione 16,17 butyraldehyde cyclic acetal,11beta,16alpha,17,21 tetrahydroxy

budesonide plus formoterol

WADA group
S6. BETA-2 AGONISTS
S9. GLUCOCORTICOSTEROIDS

Trade names and research codes
symbicort

Short synonyms
formoterol plus budesonide

bufetolol

WADA group
P2. BETA-BLOCKERS

CAS Registry number
53684-49-4

Short synonyms
adbiol

bufuralol

WADA group
P2. BETA-BLOCKERS

CAS Registry number
54340-62-4

Trade names and research codes
ro 3 4787

Short synonyms
angium
bufarolol

Long synonyms
2 tert butylamino 1 (7 ethylbenzofuran 2 ylethyl)ethanol
2 (2 tert butylamino 1 hydroxyethyl) 7 ethylbenzofuran

bumetanide

WADA group
S8. MASKING AGENTS
P3. DIURETICS

MeSH descriptor
bumetanide

CAS Registry number
28395-03-1

Trade names and research codes
bumex

burinex
fordiuran
ro 10 6338
ro 10-6338
ro10 6338
ro10-6338

Short synonyms
bumetamide
bumetidine
bymex
lixil
lunetoron

Long synonyms
3 butylamino 4 phenoxy 5 sulfamoylbenzoic acid

bunitrolol

WADA group
P2. BETA-BLOCKERS

CAS Registry number
23093-74-5
29876-08-2
34915-68-9

Trade names and research codes
ko 1366
stresson

Short synonyms
betrilol
bunitrolol hydrochloride
2 nitrilophenoxypropanolamine
tilcant

Long synonyms
2 nitrilo n t butyl phenoxypropanolamine
2 nitrilo n (tert butyl)phenoxypropanolamine
2 (3 tert butylamino 2 hydroxypropoxy)benzonitrile
1 tert butylamino 3 (2 cyanophenoxy) 2 propanol

bunolol

WADA group
P2. BETA-BLOCKERS

CAS Registry number
27591-01-1
31969-05-8

Trade names and research codes
w 6412 a
w 6412a

Short synonyms
bunolol hydrochloride
bunulol
bunulol hydrochloride
d bunolol
d bunolol hydrochloride
dextro bunolol

Long synonyms
5 (3 tert butylamino 2 hydroxypropoxy) 3,4 dihydro 1(2h) naphthalenone

buphenine

WADA group
S1. STIMULANTS

MeSH descriptor
nylidrin

CAS Registry number
447-41-6
849-55-8

Trade names and research codes
agyrase
arlibide
arlidin
belidrin
bufedon
buphedrin
certadyn
circovenil
dilatal
dilatol
dilatropin
dilatropon
dilydrin
ditalyl
flumil
mefeprol
nalide
nilvitam
nyderal
nylin
penitardon
perdilat
perdilatal
pervadil
pharmadil
rinarol
rudilin
rydrin
shatorn
skf 1700a
suprifen psb
tocodrin
vasiten

Short synonyms
bufenine
buphenin
buphenine hydrochloride
buphenin hydrochloride
nilidrine
nylhydrine
nylidrin
nylidrine
nylidrin hydrochloride
phenylsec.butylnorsuprifen

Long synonyms
para hydroxy n (3 phenylisobutyl)norephedrine
1 (para hydroxyphenyl) 2 (1 methyl 3 phenylpropylamino)propanol
1 (para hydroxyphenyl) 2 (1 methyl 3 phenylpropylamino) 1 propanol
1 (para hydroxyphenyl) 2 (1 methyl 3 phenylpropylamino)propanol hydrochloride

bupranolol

WADA group
P2. BETA-BLOCKERS

MeSH descriptor
bupranolol

CAS Registry number
14556-46-8
15148-80-8

Trade names and research codes
b 1312
b1312
betadrenol
kl255

ophtorenin

Short synonyms
bupranolol hydrochloride
kl 255
panimit

Long synonyms
1 (6' chloro 3' methylphenoxy) 3 tert butylaminopropan 2 ol hydrochloride
1 (6 chloro 3 methylphenoxy) 3 tert butylaminopropanol 2 hydrochloride
1 (6 chloro 3 methylphenoxy) tert (butylaminopropane 2 ol)
3 tert butylamino 1 (2 chloro 5 methylphenoxy) 2 propanol
1 tert butylamino 3 (2 chloro 5 methylphenoxy) 2 propanol hydrochloride
1 tert butylamino 3 (2 chloro 5 methylphenoxy)propan 2 ol
1 tert butylamino 3 (6 chloro 3 methylphenoxy) 2 propanol

buprenorphine

WADA group
S2. NARCOTICS

MeSH descriptor
buprenorphine

CAS Registry number
52485-79-7
53152-21-9

Trade names and research codes
buprenex
buprex
cl 112,302
cl 112302
cl112,302
cl112302
lepetan
nih 8805
nih8805
rx 6029 m
rx 6029m
rx6029m
subutex
temgesic
um 952
um952

Short synonyms
finibron

buserelin

WADA group
S5. PEPTIDE HORMONES

MeSH descriptor
buserelin

CAS Registry number
57982-77-1

Trade names and research codes
bigonist
receptal
superfact
suprefact

Short synonyms
busereline

Long synonyms
6 dextro serine tert butyl 10 desglycinamide luteinizing hormone releasing factor ethylamide
gnrh[1-9]ethylamide [6 (o tert butyl dextro serine)]
gonadorelin[1-9]ethylamide[6 (o tert butyl dextro serine)]
gonadorelin[6 dextro o tert butylserine 10 deglycine n ethylamide]
gonadorelin[6 dextro o tert butylserine 10 deglycine] n ethylamide
gonadorelin ethylamide[6 dextro tert butylserine 10 deglycine]
lhrh ethylamide[6 dextro o tert butylserine 10 deglycinamide]
luteinizing hormone releasing factor[6 [o (1,1 dimethylethyl) dextro serine] 9 (n ethylprolinamide) 10 deglycinamide]
5 oxoprolylhistidyltryptophylseryltyrosyl(o tert butyl dextro seryl)leucylarginyl n ethylprolinamide

buserelin acetate

WADA group
S5. PEPTIDE HORMONES

CAS Registry number
68630-75-1

Trade names and research codes
hoe 706
hoe 766
hoe 766 mp
suprecur
supremon

Short synonyms
buserelin monoacetate

butizide

WADA group
S8. MASKING AGENTS
P3. DIURETICS

CAS Registry number
2043-38-1

Trade names and research codes
saltucin

Short synonyms
buthiazide
eunephran
eunepran
isobutylhydrochlorothiazide
modenol
s 3500
sn 6187
thiabulazid
thiabutazide
thiobulazid
tiabutazide

Long synonyms
6 chloro 3,4 dihydro 3 isobutyl 2h 1,2,4 benzothiadiazine 7 sulfonamide 1,1 dioxide
6 chloro 3 isobutyl 3,4 dihydro (2h) 1,2,4 benzothiadiazine 7 sulfonamide 1,1 dioxide

butizide plus spironolactone

WADA group
S8. MASKING AGENTS
P3. DIURETICS

Trade names and research codes
aldactone saltucin
aldozone
aldozone forte
sali spiroctan

Short synonyms
butizide with spironolactone
spironolactone plus butizide
spironolactone with butizide

butofilolol

WADA group
P2. BETA-BLOCKERS

CAS Registry number
64552-17-6

Long synonyms
2' (3 tert butylamino 2 hydroxypropoxy) 5' fluorobutyrophenone
1 tert butylamino 3 (4 fluoro 2 propionylphenoxy) 2 propanol

butoxamine

WADA group
P2. BETA-BLOCKERS

MeSH descriptor
butoxamine

CAS Registry number
1937-89-9

Trade names and research codes
bw 64 9
bw 64-9
bw 649
bw64-9
bw649
nsc 106565
nsc106565

Short synonyms
butaxamine
butoxamide
butoxomine hydrochloride

Long synonyms
alpha (1 tert butylaminoethyl) 2,5 dimethoxybenzyl alcohol
2 tert butylamino 1 (2,5 dimethoxyphenyl) 1 propanol

n butyl 11 (16alpha chloro 3,17beta dihydroxyestra 1,3,5(10) trien 7alpha yl) n methylundecanamide

WADA group
S7. AGENTS WITH ANTI-OESTROGENIC ACTIVITY

CAS Registry number
131811-54-6

Trade names and research codes
em 139
em139

n butyl 11 (3,17beta dihydroxyestra 1,3,5(10) trien 7alpha yl) n methylundecanamide

WADA group
S7. AGENTS WITH ANTI-OESTROGENIC ACTIVITY

CAS Registry number
98007-99-9

Trade names and research codes
ici 164,384
ici 164384

Long synonyms
n butyl n methyl 11 (3,17beta dihydroxyestra 1,3,5(10) trien 7alpha yl)undecanamide

4 (3 tert butylamino 2 hydroxypropoxy) 2 benzimidazolone

WADA group
P2. BETA-BLOCKERS

CAS Registry number
81047-99-6

Trade names and research codes
cgp 12177
cgp12177
cgp 12177a
cgp12177a

Long synonyms
4 (3 tert butylamino 2 hydroxypropoxy) 2h benzimidazol 2 one
4 (3 tert butylamino 2 hydroxypropoxy)benzimidazol 2 one
4 (3 tert butylamino 2 hydroxypropoxy)benzimidazol 2 one hydrochloride

1 tert butylamino 3 (2 chlorophenoxy) 2 propanol

WADA group
P2. BETA-BLOCKERS

Trade names and research codes
kl 105

Long synonyms
2 (3 tert butylamino 2 hydroxypropoxy)chlorobenzene

1 tert butylamino 3 (2 methyl 4 indolyloxy) 2 propanol

WADA group
P2. BETA-BLOCKERS

CAS Registry number
23869-98-9
62658-85-9

Trade names and research codes
18-502

Long synonyms
4 (3 tert butylamino 2 hydroxypropoxy) 2 methylindole
1 tert butylamino 3 [(2 methylindol 4 yl)oxy] 2 propanol

1 tert butylamino 3 (3 methyl 2 nitrophenoxy) 2 propanol

WADA group
P2. BETA-BLOCKERS

CAS Registry number
72620-20-3

Trade names and research codes
zami 1305

Long synonyms
1 (2 nitro 3 methylphenoxy) 3 tert butylaminopropan 2 ol
3 tert butylamino 1 (3 methyl 2 nitrophenoxy) 2 propanol

9 (1 tert butylamino 3 hydroxy 2 propyloxyimino)fluorene

WADA group
P2. BETA-BLOCKERS

CAS Registry number
60979-28-4

Trade names and research codes
ips 339

Long synonyms
9 fluorenone oxime o (1 tert butylamino 3 hydroxy 2 propyl) ether
3 tert butylamino 2 (9 fluorenylideneaminoxy) 1 propanol
9 (1 tert butylamino 3 hydroxyprop 2 yloximido)fluorene

tert butylbicycloorthobenzoate

WADA group
S1. STIMULANTS

Long synonyms
tert butyl bicycloorthobenzoate

tert butylbicyclophosphorothioate

WADA group
S1. STIMULANTS

CAS Registry number
70636-86-1

Short synonyms
TBPS

Long synonyms
t butylbicyclophosphorothionate
tert butylbicyclophosphorothionate

cafedrine plus theodrenaline

WADA group
S1. STIMULANTS

CAS Registry number
69910-62-9
8004-31-7

Trade names and research codes
acrinor
akrinor
h 835
h835
praxinor

Short synonyms
cafedrine and theodrenaline
theodrenaline plus cafedrine

☝ caffeine

WADA group
S1. STIMULANTS

MeSH descriptor
caffeine

CAS Registry number
30388-07-9
58-08-2

Trade names and research codes
animine
no doz
nodoz

Short synonyms
anhydrous caffeine
cafeine
caffein
caffeine calcium complex
calcium caffeine
coffein
coffeine
guaranine
guarin
methyltheobromine
pac compound
thein
trimethylxanthine
1,3,7 trimethylxanthine
vivarin

Long synonyms
1,3,7 trimethyl 2,6 dioxopurine

☝ caffeine benzoate

WADA group
S1. STIMULANTS

CAS Registry number
5743-17-9
8000-95-1

Short synonyms
caffein benzoate
caffeine benzoate sodium
caffeine sodium benzoate
coffeine sodium benzoate
sodium caffeine benzoate

☝ caffeine citrate

WADA group
S1. STIMULANTS

CAS Registry number
69-22-7

Trade names and research codes
cafcit

Terms and Synonyms

calusterone

WADA group
S4. ANABOLIC AGENTS

CAS Registry number
17021-26-0

Short synonyms
methosarb
nsc 88536

Long synonyms
17beta hydroxy 7beta,17 dimethylandrost 4 en 3 one

cannabichromene

WADA group
S3. CANNABINOIDS

CAS Registry number
20675-51-8

cannabidiol

WADA group
S3. CANNABINOIDS

MeSH descriptor
cannabidiol

CAS Registry number
13956-29-1

Short synonyms
trans cannabidiol

cannabidiol derivative

WADA group
S3. CANNABINOIDS

cannabidiol dimethyl ether

WADA group
S3. CANNABINOIDS

CAS Registry number
1242-67-7

Short synonyms
dimethylcannabidiol

cannabidiol methyl ether

WADA group
S3. CANNABINOIDS

CAS Registry number
1972-05-0

Short synonyms
cannabidiol monomethyl ether
o methylcannabidiol

cannabielsoin

WADA group
S3. CANNABINOIDS

CAS Registry number
52025-76-0

cannabigerol

WADA group
S3. CANNABINOIDS

CAS Registry number
25654-31-3

cannabinoid

WADA group
S3. CANNABINOIDS

MeSH descriptor
cannabinoids

Short synonyms
cannabinoids

cannabinoid derivative

WADA group
S3. CANNABINOIDS

cannabinol

WADA group
S3. CANNABINOIDS

MeSH descriptor
cannabinol

CAS Registry number
521-35-7

Long synonyms
3 pentyl 6,6,9 trimethyl(6h)dibenzopyran 1 ol

cannabinol derivative

WADA group
S3. CANNABINOIDS

cannabis

WADA group
S3. CANNABINOIDS

MeSH descriptor
cannabis

CAS Registry number
8001-45-4
8063-14-7

Short synonyms
bhang
cannabis alkaloid
cannabis constituent
cannabis extract
cannabis herba
cannabis indica
cannabis indicae
cannabis leaf
cannabis sativa
cannabis sativa extract
cannabis sativa leaf

cannabis sativa var. indica
cannabis substitution
chara
charas
c.indica
ganja
ganjah
hashish
hemp
herba cannabis
indian bhang
indian ganja
indian hemp
marihuana
marijuana
mexican marihuana

cannabis derivative

WADA group
S3. CANNABINOIDS

CAS Registry number
38458-58-1

Short synonyms
cannabis component
cannabis sativa derivative
eucannabinolide
marihuana derivative

canrenoate potassium

WADA group
S8. MASKING AGENTS
P3. DIURETICS

MeSH descriptor
canrenoate potassium

CAS Registry number
6-4-2181

Trade names and research codes
8109 cb
8109cb
cb 8109
cb8109
kanrenol
mf 465 a
mf 465a
mf465a
saludactone
sc 14266
sc14266
soldactone

Short synonyms
aldadiene k
aldadiene kalium
aldadiene potassium
canrenol
potassium canrenoate
sincomen
soludactone

Long synonyms
beta (17alpha hydroxy 17beta oxo 3 androstadien 4,6 yl)propionate potassium

canrenoic acid

WADA group
S8. MASKING AGENTS
P3. DIURETICS

CAS Registry number
4138-96-9

Short synonyms
canrenoate
canrenoate sodium
caurenoate
caurenoic acid
venactone

Long synonyms
androsta 4,6 dien 17beta ol 3 on 17alpha ylpropionic acid

canrenone

WADA group
S8. MASKING AGENTS
P3. DIURETICS

MeSH descriptor
canrenone

CAS Registry number
976-71-6

Trade names and research codes
contaren
luvion
phanurane
rp 11614
rp11614
sc 9376
sc9376

Short synonyms
aldadiene
caurenone

Long synonyms
17alpha pregna 4,6 dien 17beta ol 3 one 21 carboxylic acid gamma lactone
17beta hydroxy 3 oxo 17alpha pregna 4,6 diene 21 carboxylic acid gamma lactone
17beta hydroxy 3 oxopregna 4,6 diene 21 carboxylic acid gamma lactone
17 hydroxy 3 oxo 17alpha pregna 4,6 diene 21 carboxylic acid 1,4 lactone
17 hydroxy 3 oxo 17alpha pregna 4,6 diene 21 carboxylic acid gamma lactone
17 hydroxy 3 oxo 17alpha pregna 4,6 diene 21 carboxylic acid lactone

canrenone derivative

WADA group
S8. MASKING AGENTS
P3. DIURETICS

captopril plus hydrochlorothiazide

WADA group
S8. MASKING AGENTS
P3. DIURETICS

Trade names and research codes
acediur

Terms and Synonyms

aceplus
capozide
captea
ecazide

Short synonyms
cozidocapt

Long synonyms
hydrochlorothiazide plus captopril

carazolol

WADA group
P2. BETA-BLOCKERS

CAS Registry number
57775-29-8

Trade names and research codes
bm 51052
bm51052
conducton

Short synonyms
suacron

Long synonyms
1 (carbazol 4 yloxy) 3 isopropylamino 2 propanol
4 (2 hydroxy 3 isopropylaminopropoxy)carbazole

n [1 carboxy 5 [4 (2 hydroxy 3 isopropylaminopropoxy)indole 2 carboxamido]pentyl]alanylproline

WADA group
P2. BETA-BLOCKERS

CAS Registry number
103221-88-1

Trade names and research codes
a575c
bw a575c
bwa575c
bw b385c
bwb385c

carboxyhemoglobin

WADA group
M1. ENHANCEMENT OF OXYGEN TRANSFER

MeSH descriptor
carboxyhemoglobin

CAS Registry number
9061-29-4

Short synonyms
carbon monoxide hemoglobin
carbon monoxyhemoglobin
carbonmonoxyhemoglobin
carbonyl hemoglobin
carbonylhemoglobin
carboxyhaemoglobin
carboxy hemoglobin
HbCO
hemoglobin carbon monoxide

carbuterol

WADA group
S6. BETA-2 AGONISTS

CAS Registry number
34866-46-1
34866-47-2

Trade names and research codes
pirem

Short synonyms
bronsecur
skf 40383

Long synonyms
1 [5 (2 tert butylamino 1 hydroxyethyl) 2 hydroxyphenyl]urea

carphedon

WADA group
S1. STIMULANTS

CAS Registry number
77472-70-9

Short synonyms
carfedon
carfedone
carphedone
karfedon
karphedon
4 phenylpiracetam
piracetam,4 phenyl

Long synonyms
2 oxo 4 phenyl 1 pyrrolidineacetamide

carteolol

WADA group
P2. BETA-BLOCKERS

MeSH descriptor
carteolol

CAS Registry number
51781-06-7
51781-21-6

Trade names and research codes
arteolol
arteoptic
arteoptik
carteol
cartrol
endak
endak mite
mikelan
ocupress
teoptic

Short synonyms
abbott 43326
carbonolol
carteolol hydrochloride
opc 1085

Long synonyms
5 [3 (1,1 dimethylethylamino) 2 hydroxypropoxy] 3,4 dihydro 2(1h)quinolinone
5 (3 tert butylamino 2 hydroxy)propoxy 3,4 dihydrocarbostyril

carvedilol

WADA group
P2. BETA-BLOCKERS

CAS Registry number
72956-09-3

Trade names and research codes
bm 14190
bm14190
coreg
dilatrend
dilbloc
dimitone
dq 2466
dq2466
eucardic
kredex
querto
skf 105517
skf105517

Long synonyms
1 (carbazol 4 yloxy) 3 [2 (2 methoxyphenoxy)ethylamino] 2 propanol
1 (4 carbazolyloxy) 3 [2 (2 methoxyphenoxy)ethylamino] 2 propanol

celestamine

WADA group
S9. GLUCOCORTICOSTEROIDS

CAS Registry number
62682-62-6

Trade names and research codes
celestamine

Long synonyms
betamethasone plus dexchlorpheniramine maleate
dexchlorpheniramine maleate plus betamethasone

celiprolol

WADA group
P2. BETA-BLOCKERS

MeSH descriptor
celiprolol

CAS Registry number
56980-93-9
57470-78-7

Trade names and research codes
abecor
celectol
dilanorm
rev 5320
rev 5320 a
rev 5320a
selecor
selectol
st 1396

Short synonyms
celiprolol hydrochloride

Long synonyms
3 [3 acetyl 4 [3 (tert butylamino) 2 hydroxypropoxy]phenyl] 1,1 diethylurea

centchroman

WADA group
S7. AGENTS WITH ANTI-OESTROGENIC ACTIVITY

MeSH descriptor
centchroman

CAS Registry number
31477-60-8

Trade names and research codes
centron
choice 7
saheh
saheli
shaeli

Short synonyms
levormeloxifene
ormeloxifene

Long synonyms
2,2 dimethyl 3 phenyl 4 [4 (2 pyrrolidinoethoxy)phenyl] 7 methoxychroman
7 methoxy 2,2 dimethyl 3 phenyl 4 [4 (2 pyrrolidin 1 ylethoxy)phenyl]chroman
1 [2 [4 (7 methoxy 2,2 dimethyl 3 phenylchroman 4 yl)phenoxy]ethyl]pyrrolidine
trans 2,2 dimethyl 3 phenyl 4 [4 (2 pyrrolidinoethoxy)phenyl] 7 methoxychroman
3,4 trans 2,2 dimethyl 3 phenyl 4 [4 (2 pyrrolidinoethoxy)phenyl] 7 methoxychroman

central stimulant agent

WADA group
S1. STIMULANTS

MeSH descriptor
central nervous system stimulants
stimulants (historical)

Short synonyms
analeptic
analeptic agent
analeptic combination
analeptic drug
analeptics
brain stimulant
central stimulant
central stimulating agent
CNS stimulant
psychoanaleptic agent
stimulant
stimulant agent
stimulant drug
stimulants (historical)
stimulating agent
stimulative agent

Long synonyms
central nervous stimulant agent
central nervous system stimulant
central nervous system stimulants

cetamolol

WADA group
P2. BETA-BLOCKERS

CAS Registry number
34919-98-7

Trade names and research codes
betacor

Short synonyms
ai 27,303
ai 27303
ici 72222

Long synonyms
2 [2 [3 [(1,1 dimethylethyl)amino] 2 hydroxypropoxy]phenoxy] n methylacetamide
2 [2 [3 (tert butylamino) 2 hydroxypropoxy]phenoxy] n methylacetamide

chloramphetamine

WADA group
S1. STIMULANTS

MeSH descriptor
p-chloroamphetamine

CAS Registry number
64-12-0

Short synonyms
chloroamphetamine
4 chloroamphetamine
levo para chloroamphetamine
para chloramphetamine
para chloroamphetamine
p Chloroamphetamine
p-chloroamphetamine

Long synonyms
2 amino 1 (4 chlorophenyl)propane

chlormerodrin

WADA group
S8. MASKING AGENTS
P3. DIURETICS

MeSH descriptor
chlormerodrin

CAS Registry number
62-37-3

Trade names and research codes
orimercur
merilid

Short synonyms
aramercur
asahydrin
chlomerodrin
chlormerodrine
chlormeroprin
chloromerodrin
chlorometrodrine
diurone
katonil
mercardox
mercloran
mercoral
merculest
mercuryluree
neohydrin
oramercur
oricur
percapyl
piurone
promeran

Long synonyms
1 [3 (chloromercuri) 2 methoxypropyl] urea
1 [3 (chloromercuri) 2 methoxypropyl]urea
(3 chloromercuri 2 methoxypropyl)urea

4 chloro 17beta hydroxy 17 methylandrosta 1,4 dien 3 one

WADA group
S4. ANABOLIC AGENTS

CAS Registry number
2446-23-3

Trade names and research codes
oral turinabol

Short synonyms
4 chlorometandienone
4 chloromethandienone
metandienone,4 chloro

Long synonyms
androsta 1,4 dien 17beta ol 3 one,4 chloro 17 methyl
4 chloro 17alpha methyl 1,4 androstadien 17beta ol 3 one
4 chloro 17alpha methyl 17beta hydroxy 1,4 androstadien 3 one
4 chloro 17alpha methyl 1,2 dehydrotestosterone
4 chloro 17beta hydroxy 17alpha methyl 1,4 androstadien 3 one
4 chloro 17beta hydroxy 17 methyl 1,4 androstadien 3 one
4 chloro 17beta hydroxy 3 oxo 17alpha methylandrosta 1,4 diene
4 chloro 17 methylandrosta 1,4 dien 17beta ol 3 one
clostebol,1,2 dehydro 17alpha methyl
1,2 dehydro 17alpha methylclostebol
dehydrochloromethyltestosterone

8 chloro 1 [alpha (2 dimethylaminoethyl)benzyl] 6 phenyl 4h 1,2,4 triazolo[4,3 a][1,4]benzodiazepine

WADA group
S8. MASKING AGENTS
P3. DIURETICS

8 chloro 3 (2 fluorophenyl) 5,6 dihydrofuro[3,2 f][1,2]benzisoxazole 6 carboxylate potassium

WADA group
S8. MASKING AGENTS
P3. DIURETICS

CAS Registry number
90247-09-9

Trade names and research codes
a 56234
a56234

Short synonyms
abbott 56234

Long synonyms
potassium 8 chloro 3 (2 fluorophenyl) 5,6 dihydrofuro[3,2 f][1,2]benzisoxazole 6 carboxylate

Terms and Synonyms

[[5 chloro 3 (2 methylphenyl) 4 oxo 4h benzopyran 7 yl]oxy]acetic acid

WADA group
S8. MASKING AGENTS
P3. DIURETICS

CAS Registry number
112953-47-6

Trade names and research codes
dr 3438
dr3438

8 chloro 3 methylnaringenin

WADA group
S7. AGENTS WITH ANTI-OESTROGENIC ACTIVITY

Trade names and research codes
be 14348d
be14348d
be 14348e
be14348e

Long synonyms
8 chloro 4',5,7 trihydroxy 3 methylflavanone

8 chloro 5 (4 chlorophenyl) 5h indeno[1,2 d]pyrimidine

WADA group
S7. AGENTS WITH ANTI-OESTROGENIC ACTIVITY

CAS Registry number
112959-07-6

Trade names and research codes
ly 113174

4 chloromethamphetamine

WADA group
S1. STIMULANTS

CAS Registry number
1199-85-5

Short synonyms
chlormethamphetamine
4 chlorodeoxyephedrine
4 chloro desoxyephedrine
4 chlorodesoxyephedrine
chloromethamphetamine
4 chloromethylamphetamine
para chloromethamphetamine
para chloro methylamphetamine
para chloromethylamphetamine
para chloro n methamphetamine

Long synonyms
dextro,levo para chloromethamphetamine
para chloro n,alpha dimethylphenethylamine
para chloro n methylamphetamine

3 chloro n (1,2,3,4 tetrahydro 7 hydroxy 2 naphthyl)phenylethanolamine

WADA group
S6. BETA-2 AGONISTS

CAS Registry number
120839-53-4

Trade names and research codes
sr 58572a

3 chloro n (7 ethoxycarbonylmethoxy 1,2,3,4 tetrahydro 2 naphthyl)phenylethanolamine

WADA group
S6. BETA-2 AGONISTS

CAS Registry number
120839-54-5

Trade names and research codes
sr 58539b

[[7 [[2 (3 chlorophenyl) 2 hydroxyethyl]amino] 5,6,7,8 tetrahydro 2 naphthyl]oxy]acetic acid ethyl ester

WADA group
S6. BETA-2 AGONISTS

CAS Registry number
121524-08-1
121524-09-2

Trade names and research codes
sr 58611
sr58611
sr 58611a
sr58611a

Long synonyms
2 (3 chlorophenyl) n (7 ethoxycarbonylmethoxy 1,2,3,4 tetrahydro 2 naphthyl) 2 hydroxyethylamine
ethyl [[7 [[2 (3 chlorophenyl) 2 hydroxyethyl]amino] 5,6,7,8 tetrahydronaphth 2 yl]oxy]acetate

5 [2 [[2 (3 chlorophenyl) 2 hydroxyethyl]amino]propyl] 1,3 benzodioxole 2,2 dicarboxylic acid

WADA group
S6. BETA-2 AGONISTS

CAS Registry number
138908-40-4

Trade names and research codes
bta 243
bta243
cl 314514
cl314514
cl 316243
cl316243

4 [2 [[2 (3 chlorophenyl) 2 hydroxyethyl]amino]propyl]phenoxy acetic acid

WADA group
S6. BETA-2 AGONISTS

CAS Registry number
114333-71-0

Trade names and research codes
brl 37344
brl37344

4 [2 [[2 (3 chlorophenyl) 2 hydroxyethyl]amino]propyl]phenoxy acetic acid methyl ester

WADA group
S6. BETA-2 AGONISTS

CAS Registry number
91097-81-3

Trade names and research codes
brl 35135
brl35135
brl 35135a
brl35135a

chloroprednisone

WADA group
S9. GLUCOCORTICOSTEROIDS

CAS Registry number
52080-57-6

Short synonyms
chlorprednisone

Long synonyms
6alpha chloro 17,21 dihydroxypregna 1,4 diene 3,11,20 trione
6alpha chloro 1,4 pregnadiene 17alpha,21 diol 3,11,20 trione

chlorothiazide

WADA group
S8. MASKING AGENTS
P3. DIURETICS

MeSH descriptor
chlorothiazide

CAS Registry number
58-94-6
7085-44-1

Trade names and research codes
chlotride
diachlor
diuril
saluric

Short synonyms
chlorosal
chlorothiazid
chlorothiazide sodium
chlorothiazide sodium salt
chlorothiazidum
chlorothiazine
chlorthiazide
diurilix
diuril lyovac
diuriwas wassermann milano
flumen
lyovac diuril
lyovac saluric
lyovac saluril
sodium chlorothiazide
warduzuide

Long synonyms
6 chloro 2h 1,2,4 benzothiadiazine 7 sulfamoyl 1,1 dioxide
6 chloro 2h 1,2,4 benzothiadiazine 7 sulfonamide 1,1 dioxide
6 chloro 7 sulfamoyl 2h 1,2,4 benzothiadiazin 2 yl sodium 1,1 dioxide
6 chloro 7 sulfamoyl 2h 1,2,4 benzothiadiazine 1,1 dioxide
6 chloro 7 sulfamyl 2h 1,2,4 benzothiazine 1,1 dioxide

chlorothiazide derivative

WADA group
S8. MASKING AGENTS
P3. DIURETICS

Short synonyms
chlorothiazide diuretic agent
hydroxychlorothiazide

chlorphentermine

WADA group
S1. STIMULANTS

MeSH descriptor
chlorphentermine

CAS Registry number
151-06-4
461-78-9

Short synonyms
avicol
avipron
chlorfentermine
chlorophentermine
chlorphentarmine hydrochloride
chlorphentermin
chlorphentermine hydrochloride
chlorphentermine sl
chlorphenterminumhydrochlorid
clorfentermina
desopimon
lucofen
lucofene
pre sate
presate
s 62
wx 2426
wx 2462

Long synonyms
alpha,alpha dimethyl para chlorophenethylamine
4 chloro alpha,alpha dimethylphenethylamine
chlorphentermine dihydrochloride
para chloro alpha,alpha dimethylphenethylamine
2 (para chlorobenzyl) 2 propylamine
1 (para chlorophenyl) 2 methyl 2 aminopropane
1 (para chlorophenyl) 2 methyl 2 propylamine

chlortalidone

WADA group
S8. MASKING AGENTS
P3. DIURETICS

MeSH descriptor
chlorthalidone

CAS Registry number
77-36-1

Trade names and research codes
g 33128
g33128
g 33 182
g 33182
g33 182
g33182
hygroton
hylidone
igroton
oxodolin
thalitone

Short synonyms
aquadon
chlorphthalidolone
chlorphthalidone
chlortalidon
chlorthalidine
chlorthalidon
chlorthalidone
chlorthialidone
clortalidone
edemdal
hidronal
higroton
higrotona
hydro-long tablinen
hygroton k
igrolina
isoren
natriuran
phthalamidine
phthalamodine
phthalamudine
renon
servidone
urofinil
zambesil

Long synonyms
2 chlor 5 (1 hydroxy 3 oxo 1 isoindolinyl) benzolsulfonamid
3 (4 chloro 3 sulfamoyl) 3 hydroxyphthalimidine
3 (4 chloro 3 sulfamoylphenyl) 3 hydroxyisoindolin 1 one
3 (4 chloro 3 sulfamoylphenyl) 3 hydroxyphthalimidine
3 (4' chloro 3' sulfamoyl phenyl) 3 hydroxyphthalimidine
3(4 chloro 3 sulfamoylphenyl) 3 hydroxyphthalimidine
3 (4 chloro 3 sulfanoylphenyl) 3 hydroxyisoindolin 1 one
2 chloro 5 (3 hydroxy 1 oxoisoindolin 3 yl)benzenesulfonamide
3 hydroxy 3 (3 sulfamoyl 4 chlorphenyl) isoindolin 1 on
3 hydroxy 3 (4 chloro 3 sulfamylphenyl)phthalimidine
1 keto 3 (3' sulfamyl 4' chlorophenyl) 3 hydroxyisoindoline
1 oxo 3 (3 sulfamyl 4 chlorophenyl) 3 hydroxyisoindoline
1 oxy 3 (3' sulfamyl 4' chlorophenyl) 3 hydroxyisoindole

chlortalidone plus metoprolol

WADA group
S8. MASKING AGENTS
P2. BETA-BLOCKERS
P3. DIURETICS

Trade names and research codes
igroton lopresor
logotron
logroton
lopresoretic
lopresor igroton
prelis comp

Short synonyms
metoprolol plus chlortalidone

chlortalidone plus reserpine

WADA group
S8. MASKING AGENTS
P3. DIURETICS

CAS Registry number
8058-25-1

Trade names and research codes
darebon
demi regroton
demi-regroton
demiregroton
hygroton reserpine
igroton reserpina
regroton
reserpine hygroton

Short synonyms
reserpine plus chlortalidone

chorionic gonadotropin

WADA group
S5. PEPTIDE HORMONES

MeSH descriptor
chorionic gonadotropin

CAS Registry number
9002-61-3

Trade names and research codes
chorigon
chorulon
endocorion
follutein
gonabion
gonadex
gonadotrophon
hcg endo
homosten
physex
praedyn
predalon
pregnesin
pregnyl
primogonyl
profasi
prymogonyl

Short synonyms
antuitrin s
apl
beta chorionic gonadotropin
choragon

choriogonadotrophin
choriogonadotropin
choriogonin
chorion gonadotrophic hormone
chorion gonadotrophin
chorion gonadotropin
chorionic gonadotrophin
chorionic gonadotropic hormone
chorionic gonadropin
choron
coriantin
gestasol dry
gonadotraphon l.h.
gonadotropin,human chorionic
gonadotropins, chorionic
h.c.g.
hCG
human choriogonadotropin
human chorion gonadotrophin
human chorion gonadotropin
human chorionic gonadotrophin
human chorionic gonadotropin
human gonadotrophin
human placental gonadotropin
libigen
pranturon
promogonyl
prophasi
puberogen

Long synonyms
chorionic gonadotrophic hormone
urinary chorionic gonadotrophin

chorionic gonadotropin alpha subunit

WADA group
S5. PEPTIDE HORMONES

Short synonyms
alpha hcg
hCG alpha subunit

Long synonyms
choriogonadotropin alpha subunit
human chorionic gonadotropin alpha subunit

chorionic gonadotropin beta subunit

WADA group
S5. PEPTIDE HORMONES

MeSH descriptor
chorionic gonadotropin, beta subunit, human

Short synonyms
beta hcg
beta subunit hcg
hCG beta subunit

Long synonyms
beta human chorionic gonadotrophin
beta human chorionic gonadotropin
choriogonadotropin beta subunit
chorionic gonadotropin, beta subunit, human
human chorionic gonadotropin beta subunit

ciclesonide

WADA group
S9. GLUCOCORTICOSTEROIDS

CAS Registry number
126544-47-6

Trade names and research codes
b 9207 015
b 9207015
b9207 015
b9207015
by 9010
by9010

Long synonyms
16alpha,17alpha cyclohexylmethylenedioxy 11beta,21 dihydroxypregna 1,4 dien 3 one 21 isobutyrate
16alpha,17alpha cyclohexylmethylenedioxy 11beta hydroxy 21 (isobutyryloxy)pregna 1,4 dien 3 one

cicloprolol

WADA group
S6. BETA-2 AGONISTS

CAS Registry number
63659-12-1

Trade names and research codes
sl 75177 10

Short synonyms
cycloprolol

Long synonyms
1 [4 [2 (cyclopropylmethoxy)ethoxy]phenoxy] 3 isopropylamino 2 propanol

cilazapril plus hydrochlorothiazide

WADA group
S8. MASKING AGENTS
P3. DIURETICS

Trade names and research codes
ro 23 9982

Long synonyms
hydrochlorothiazide plus cilazapril

cimaterol

WADA group
S6. BETA-2 AGONISTS

CAS Registry number
54239-37-1

Trade names and research codes
ab a 663
aba 663
aba663
ac 263780
ac263780
cl 263780
cl263780

Short synonyms
cimatrol

Long synonyms
1 (4 amino 3 cyanophenyl) 2 (isopropylamino)ethanol
2 amino 5 [1 hydroxy 2 [(1 methylethyl)amino]ethyl]benzonitrile
2 amino 5 [1 hydroxy 2 (isopropylamino)ethyl]benzonitrile
2 cyano 4 [1 hydroxy 2 (isopropylamino)ethyl]aniline
5 [1 hydroxy 2 (isopropylamino)ethyl]anthranilonitrile

ciprocinonide

WADA group
S9. GLUCOCORTICOSTEROIDS

CAS Registry number
58524-83-7

Trade names and research codes
rs 2386
rs2386

Long synonyms
fluocinolone acetonide 21 cyclopropanecarboxylate

citicoline

WADA group
S1. STIMULANTS

MeSH descriptor
cytidine diphosphate choline

CAS Registry number
56257-85-3
987-78-0

Trade names and research codes
brassel 1000
ceraxon
nicholin
rexort
sauran
sinkron
sintoclar
somazina

Short synonyms
CDP choline
cidifos
cidiphos
citicholine
citicolin
citicolina
cyticholine
cytidine diphosphate choline
cytidine 5 diphosphocholine
cytidine 5' diphosphocholine
cytidine diphosphocholine
cytocholine

Long synonyms
cytidine diphosphate choline ester
cytidine 5' diphosphorylcholine

clenbuterol

WADA group
S4. ANABOLIC AGENTS
S6. BETA-2 AGONISTS

MeSH descriptor
clenbuterol

CAS Registry number
21898-19-1
37148-27-9

Trade names and research codes
clenasma
clenbuterol pharmachim
clenbutol
contrasmina
contraspasmin
monores
nab 365
novegan
p 5369
prontovent
spiropent
ventipulmin
ventolase

Short synonyms
clenbuterol hydrochloride

Long synonyms
4 amino 3,5 dichloro alpha (tert butylaminomethyl)benzyl alcohol
1 (4 amino 3,5 dichlorophenyl) 2 tert butylaminoethanol
4 amino alpha (tert butylaminomethyl) 3,5 dichlorobenzyl alcohol

clioquinol plus dexamethasone

WADA group
S9. GLUCOCORTICOSTEROIDS

Trade names and research codes
millicortenol vioform
millicorten vioform
vioform millicorten
vioform millicortenol

Short synonyms
dexamethasone plus clioquinol

clioquinol plus flumetasone pivalate

WADA group
S9. GLUCOCORTICOSTEROIDS

Trade names and research codes
locacorten vioform
locorten vioform

Long synonyms
clioquinol plus flumethasone pivalate
flumetasone pivalate plus clioquinol
flumethasone pivalate plus clioquinol

clobenzorex

WADA group
S1. STIMULANTS

CAS Registry number
13364-32-4

Trade names and research codes
asenlix
dinintel
rexigen
sd 271 12

Short synonyms
amphetamine,n (2 chlorobenzyl)
clobenzorex hydrochloride
n (2 chlorobenzyl)amphetamine
sd 171 12

Long synonyms
n (2 chlorobenzyl) alpha methylphenethylamine

clobetasol

WADA group
S9. GLUCOCORTICOSTEROIDS

MeSH descriptor
clobetasol

CAS Registry number
25122-41-2

Long synonyms
21 chloro 9alpha fluoro 11beta,17alpha dihydroxy 16beta methylpregna 1,4 diene 3,20 dione

clobetasol butyrate

WADA group
S9. GLUCOCORTICOSTEROIDS

clobetasol propionate

WADA group
S9. GLUCOCORTICOSTEROIDS

CAS Registry number
25122-46-7

Trade names and research codes
cci 4725
cci4725
clobederm
clovate
dermoval
dermovate
gr 2 925
gr 2-925
gr 2925
gr2 925
gr2-925
gr2925
olux
temovate
tenovate

Short synonyms
clobesol
clobetasol 17 propionate

clobetasone

WADA group
S9. GLUCOCORTICOSTEROIDS

CAS Registry number
54063-32-0

clobetasone butyrate

WADA group
S9. GLUCOCORTICOSTEROIDS

CAS Registry number
25122-57-0

Trade names and research codes
cci 5537
cci5537
emovate
eumovate
gr 2 1214
gr 2-1214
gr 21214
gr2-1214

Short synonyms
clobetasone 17 butyrate
kindavate
sn 203

clocortolone

WADA group
S9. GLUCOCORTICOSTEROIDS

CAS Registry number
4828-27-7

Short synonyms
clocortolon

Long synonyms
9 chloro 6alpha fluoro 11beta,21 dihydroxy 16alpha methylpregna 1,4 diene 3,20 dione
9 chloro 6alpha fluoro 16alpha methylpregna 1,4 diene 11beta,21 diol 3,20 dione

clocortolone pivalate

WADA group
S9. GLUCOCORTICOSTEROIDS

CAS Registry number
34097-16-0

Trade names and research codes
cl 68
cl68
cl 68 creme
cl68 creme
cloderm
purantix
sh 863
sh863

Short synonyms
cilder
clocortolone 21 pivalate
clocortolone trimethylacetate

clomifene

WADA group
S7. AGENTS WITH ANTI-OESTROGENIC ACTIVITY

MeSH descriptor
clomiphene

CAS Registry number
911-45-5

Trade names and research codes
clomifen
kyliformin
nsc 35770
omnifen

Short synonyms
clomifene acid
clomifene isomer
clomiphen
clomiphene
trans cisclomiphene

Long synonyms
alpha chloro alpha' [para (2 diethylaminoethoxy)phenyl]stilbene
2 chloro 1,2 diphenyl 1 [para (2 diethylaminoethoxy)phenyl]ethylene
2 [para (beta chloro alpha phenylstyryl)phenoxy]triethylamine

clomifene citrate

WADA group
S7. AGENTS WITH ANTI-OESTROGENIC ACTIVITY

CAS Registry number
50-41-9

Trade names and research codes
clomid
clomivid
clostilbegyt
dyneric
fertyl
gravosan
ikaclomin
ikaklomin
omifin
pergotime
serophene

Short synonyms
clomifene citrate isomer
clomifene dihydrogen citrate
clomiphene citrate
clomiphene citrate isomer
mer 41
mrl 41

clopamide

WADA group
S8. MASKING AGENTS
P3. DIURETICS

MeSH descriptor
clopamide

CAS Registry number
636-54-4

Trade names and research codes
adurix
aquex
brinaldix
dt 327
dt327

Short synonyms
chlosudimeprimylum
clopamid
clopamidum
clopamine

Long synonyms
3 (aminosulfonyl) 4 chloro n (2,6 dimethyl 1 piperidinyl)benzamide
1 (4 chloro 3 sulfamoylbenzamido) 2,6 dimethylpiperidine
4 chloro n (2',6' dimethyl 1' piperidyl) 3 sulfamoylbenzamide
4 chloro n (2,6 dimethyl 1 piperidyl) 3 sulfamoylbenzamide
4 chloro n (cis 2,6 dimethylpiperid 1 yl) 3 sulfamoylbenzamide
n (2',6' dimethyl 1' piperidyl) 3 sulfamoyl 4 chlorobenzamide

cloprednol

WADA group
S9. GLUCOCORTICOSTEROIDS

CAS Registry number
5251-34-3

Trade names and research codes
syntestan

Short synonyms
rs 4691

Long synonyms
6 chloro 11alpha,17beta,21 trihydroxypregna 1,4,6 triene 3,10 dione
pregna 1,4,6 triene 11alpha,17beta,21 triol 3,10 dione,6 chloro

cloranolol

WADA group
P2. BETA-BLOCKERS

CAS Registry number
39563-28-5
54247-25-5

Trade names and research codes
gyki 41099
tobanum

Long synonyms
1 (2,5 dichlorophenoxy) 3 (tert butylamino) 2 propanol
3 tert butylamino 1 (2,5 dichlorophenoxy) 2 propanol
1 (tert butylamino) 3 (2,5 dichlorophenoxy) 2 propanol

clorprenaline

WADA group
S1. STIMULANTS
S6. BETA-2 AGONISTS

CAS Registry number
3811-25-4
6933-90-0
8061-63-0

Trade names and research codes
asthone
e 241
e241
l 20025
l20025
vortel

Short synonyms
chlorprenaline
clorprenaline hydrochloride
isoprofenamine
isoprophenamine

Long synonyms
1 (2 chlorophenyl) 2 isopropylaminoethanol
ortho chloro alpha (isopropylaminomethyl)benzyl alcohol

clortermine

WADA group
S1. STIMULANTS

CAS Registry number
10389-72-7
10389-73-8

Trade names and research codes
voranil

Short synonyms
chlortermine
clortermine hydrochloride
su 10568

Long synonyms
ortho chloro alpha,alpha dimethylphenethylamine

clostebol

WADA group
S4. ANABOLIC AGENTS

CAS Registry number
1093-58-9
51023-23-5

Short synonyms
chlorotestosterone
4 chlorotestosterone
chlortestosterone
4 chlortestosterone

Long synonyms
4 chloro 17beta hydroxy 4 androsten 3 one

clostebol acetate

WADA group
S4. ANABOLIC AGENTS

CAS Registry number
855-19-6

Trade names and research codes
megagrisevit

Short synonyms
chlorotestosterone acetate
4 chlorotestosterone acetate
chlortestosterone acetate
4 chlortestosterone acetate
macrobin
steranabol
turinabol

Long synonyms
4 chloro 17beta hydroxy 4 androstene 3 one acetate
4 chloro delta 4 androsten 17beta ol 3 one acetate

cocaine

WADA group
S1. STIMULANTS

MeSH descriptor
cocaine
crack cocaine

CAS Registry number
50-36-2
53-21-4
5937-29-1

Short synonyms
benzoylmethyl ecgonine
beta cocaine
cocain
cocaine hydrochloride
cocaine methiodide
cocain hydrochloride
codrenine
'crack'
crack cocaine
ecgonine methyl ester benzoate
erythroxylin
l cocaine
levo cocaine
locosthetic
neurocaine
sterilocaine

Long synonyms
2beta carbomethoxy 3beta benzoxytropane
l ecgonine 3 benzoate 2 methyl ester

combivent

WADA group
S6. BETA-2 AGONISTS

Trade names and research codes
combivent

Long synonyms
ipratropium bromide plus salbutamol sulfate
salbutamol sulfate plus ipratropium bromide

continuous erythropoiesis receptor activator

WADA group
M1. ENHANCEMENT OF OXYGEN TRANSFER

Short synonyms
CERA

convulsant agent

WADA group
S1. STIMULANTS

MeSH descriptor
convulsants

Short synonyms
convulsant
convulsant compound
convulsant drug
convulsants
convulsive agent

corticotropin

WADA group
S5. PEPTIDE HORMONES

MeSH descriptor
corticotropin

CAS Registry number
11136-52-0
9002-60-2
9061-27-2

Trade names and research codes
acortan
acthar
acton prolongatum
cortrophin
procortan forte
s cortophin
synacthen retard

Short synonyms
acethropan
acetophran
acetylated corticotropin
acortan prolongatum

acorto
ACTH
acth 40
acth 80
acth,acetylated
acth depot
acthon
acton
actonar
actrope
adactan
adrenal cortex trophic hormone
adrenal cortex tropic hormone
adrenocorticaltrophormon
adrenocorticotrope hormone
adrenocorticotrophic hormone
adrenocorticotrophin
adrenocorticotropic hormone
adrenocorticotropin
adrenocorticotropin hormone
adrenomone
adrenotropin
beta corticotropin
bird acth
bird corticotropin
cibacthen
corticotrophin
1,39 corticotrophin
corticotrophine
corticotrophin gelatin
corticotropic hormone
corticotropine
corticotropin hormone
cortigel
cortilin
cortiphyson
cortrophin gel acth
cortropin
cotrophin
depo acth
exactin
hp acthar gel
humacthid
humactid
porcine acth
porcine corticotropin
procortan
reacthin
solacthyl

Long synonyms
beta alanine 1 alpha 1 23nh2 acth

corticotropin[1-10]

WADA group
S5. PEPTIDE HORMONES

CAS Registry number
1-5-2791

Short synonyms
acth 1 10
acth[1-10]
adrenocorticotropin[1-10]
corticotropin 1 10
corticotropin [1-10]

corticotropin[11-24]

WADA group
S5. PEPTIDE HORMONES

CAS Registry number
4237-93-8

Short synonyms
acth [11-24]
acth(11 24)
acth[11 24]
acth[11-24]
adrenocorticotropin[11-24]
corticotropin [11-24]

corticotropin[1-17]

WADA group
S5. PEPTIDE HORMONES

CAS Registry number
7266-47-9

Short synonyms
ACTH[1-17]
acth 1-17
adrenocorticotropin 1-17
corticotropin 1 17

corticotropin[1-39]

WADA group
S5. PEPTIDE HORMONES

CAS Registry number
11137-42-1

Short synonyms
acth 1 39
acth 1-39
acth [1-39]
acth[1-39]
corticotropin (1-39)
corticotropin 1 39
corticotropin 1-39
corticotropin [1 39]
corticotropin [1-39]

corticotropin[18-39]

WADA group
S5. PEPTIDE HORMONES

CAS Registry number
66676-67-3

Short synonyms
acth 18 39
acth 18-39
acth [18-39]
acth[18-39]
c.l.i.p.
corticotropin [18 39]

Long synonyms
corticotropin like intermediate lobe peptide
corticotropin like intermediate lobe peptide[18-39]

corticotropin[4-10]

WADA group
S5. PEPTIDE HORMONES

CAS Registry number
8-1-4037

Short synonyms
ACTH 4-10
acth (4-10)
acth(4 10)

acth[4-10]
corticotropin (4-10)
corticotropin 4 10
corticotropin 4-10
corticotropin [4 10]

corticotropin[7-10]

WADA group
S5. PEPTIDE HORMONES

Short synonyms
acth [7-10]
acth[7-10]

corticotropin[7-16]

WADA group
S5. PEPTIDE HORMONES

Short synonyms
acth[7-16]

Long synonyms
phe arg trp gly lys pro val gly lys lys

corticotropin derivative

WADA group
S5. PEPTIDE HORMONES

Short synonyms
acth albumin polymer
ACTH analog
acth analogue
ACTH derivative
acth peptide
acth synthetic analog
acth synthetic analogue
adrenocorticotropin derivative
alpha 1-19 acth
alpha 1 23 nh2 acth
alpha 4 23 acth
alpha 4 23 adrenocorticotropin
alpha 4 23 corticotropin
alpha 5 23 acth
alpha 5 23 adrenocorticotropin
alpha 5 23 corticotropin
alpha 6 24 acth
alpha 6 24 adrenocorticotropin
alpha 6 24 corticotropin
alpha 7 23 acth
alpha 7 23 adrenocorticotropin
alpha 7 23 corticotropin
corticotrophin analog
corticotropin analog
corticotropin analogue
corticotropin peptide
corticotropin synthetic analog
decapeptide corticotropin 1-10
d phe 7 corticotropin 1-10
5 glutamine alpha 1-19 acth
7 leucyl alpha 1 24 acth
synacthen 1-39 peptide

Long synonyms
corticotropin (1-18) octadecapeptide amide
corticotropin synthetic analogue 1-39 peptide
glutamine beta (pyrazol 3 yl)alanine beta corticotropinamide
glutamine beta (pyrazolyl 3)alanine beta corticotropin amide
glutamine phenylalanine beta corticotropinamide
5 glutamyl acth (1-10) nonadecapeptide
7 leucyl alpha 1 24 adrenocorticotropin
7 leucyl alpha 1 24 corticotropin
n alpha 9 methyltryptophanyl alpha 1 24 acth
n alpha 9 methyltryptophanyl alpha 1 24 adrenocorticotropin
n alpha 9 methyltryptophanyl alpha 1 24 corticotropin

corticotropin releasing factor

WADA group
S5. PEPTIDE HORMONES

MeSH descriptor
corticotropin-releasing hormone

CAS Registry number
9015-71-8

Trade names and research codes
amunine
corticobiss

Short synonyms
ACTH releasing factor
acth releasing hormone
corticoliberin
corticorelin
corticotropin release factor
CRF
c rf
crf 41
release factor,corticotropin

Long synonyms
corticotrophin releasing factor
corticotrophin releasing hormone
corticotropin releasing hormone
corticotropin-releasing hormone

corticotropin releasing factor[9-41]

WADA group
S5. PEPTIDE HORMONES

Short synonyms
crf 9-41

Long synonyms
corticotropin releasing factor (9-41)
corticotropin releasing factor 9-41

corticotropin releasing factor derivative

WADA group
S5. PEPTIDE HORMONES

Short synonyms
crf analog
crf derivative

Long synonyms
corticotrophin releasing factor analog
corticotropin releasing factor analog
corticotropin releasing hormone derivative

cortisone

WADA group
S9. GLUCOCORTICOSTEROIDS

MeSH descriptor
cortisone

Terms and Synonyms

CAS Registry number
53-06-5

Trade names and research codes
adrenalex
corlin
cortadren
cortagen
cortandren
cortane
cortisate
cortison
cortistal
cortivite
cortogen
cortone
incorlin
incortin
nsc 9703
ricortex
scheroson
scherosone

Short synonyms
compound e (kendall)
cortisal
cortisone sodium
17 hydroxy 11 dehydrocortisone
kendall compound e
reichstein substance fa
wintersteiner compound f

Long synonyms
17alpha,21 dihydroxy 4 pregnene 3,11,20 trione
11 dehydro 17 hydroxy corticosterone
11 dehydro 17 hydroxycorticosterone
delta4 pregnene 17alpha,21 diol 3,11,20 trione
pregn 4 en 17 alpha, 21 diol 3,11,20 trione
pregn 4 ene 17alpha,21 diol 3,11,20 trione
4 pregnene 17alpha,21 diol 3,11,20 trione

cortisone acetate

WADA group
S9. GLUCOCORTICOSTEROIDS

CAS Registry number
50-04-4

Trade names and research codes
adreson
atriona
cortal
cortelan
cortistab
cortisyl
cortone acetate

Short synonyms
cortisone 21 acetate
cortisone 2' acetate
cortogen acetate

Long synonyms
4 pregnen 3,11,20 trione 17alpha,21 diol 21 acetate

cortisone derivative

WADA group
S9. GLUCOCORTICOSTEROIDS

Short synonyms
cortisone derivatives
17 hydroxycortisone

cortisporin

WADA group
S9. GLUCOCORTICOSTEROIDS

CAS Registry number
8024-64-4

Trade names and research codes
cortisporin
otosporin

Short synonyms
cortisporin otic

cortivazol

WADA group
S9. GLUCOCORTICOSTEROIDS

CAS Registry number
1110-40-3

Trade names and research codes
altim
diaster
nsc 80998
nsc80998

Short synonyms
cortivazol acetate

cromoglycate disodium plus reproterol

WADA group
S6. BETA-2 AGONISTS

Trade names and research codes
aarane
allergospasmin

Long synonyms
reproterol plus cromoglycate disodium

cropropamide

WADA group
S1. STIMULANTS

CAS registry number
633-47-6

Long synonyms
alpha (n' crotonyl n' propyl)amino n,n dimethylbutyramide
2 (crotonoylpropylamino) n,n dimethylbutyramide
2 crotonoylpropylamino n,n dimethylbutyramide
n [1 (dimethylaminocarbonyl)propyl] n propyl 2 butenamide
n (1 dimethylcarbamoylpropyl) n propylcrotonamide

crotamiton plus hydrocortisone

WADA group
S9. GLUCOCORTICOSTEROIDS

Trade names and research codes
eurax hc
eurax hydrocortisone

Short synonyms
hydrocortisone plus crotamiton

crotetamide

WADA group
S1. STIMULANTS

CAS Registry number
6168-76-9

Short synonyms
crotethamide
crothetamide

Long synonyms
alpha (n' crotonyl n' ethyl)amino n,n dimethylbutyramide
2 (crotonoylethylamino) n,n dimethylbutyramide
2 crotonoylethylamino n,n dimethylbutyramide
n [1 (dimethylaminocarbonyl)propyl] n ethyl 2 butenamide
n (1 dimethylcarbamoylpropyl) n ethylcrotonamide

cyanoiodopindolol

WADA group
P2. BETA-BLOCKERS

MeSH descriptor
iodocyanopindolol

CAS Registry number
83498-72-0

Short synonyms
iodocyanopindolol

1 (2 cyanophenoxy) 3 [2 (3 phenylureido)ethylamino] 2 propanol

WADA group
P2. BETA-BLOCKERS

CAS Registry number
53671-71-9

Trade names and research codes
ici 89,406
ici 89406

Long synonyms
1 (2 cyanophenoxy) 3 [2 (3 phenylureido)ethylamino]propan 2 ol
1 (2 cyanophenoxy) 3 [[2 (phenylureido)ethyl]amino]propan 2 ol
[2 hydroxy 3 [(3 phenylureido)ethylamino] 1 propoxy] 2 benzenecarbonitrile

cyanopindolol

WADA group
P2. BETA-BLOCKERS

CAS Registry number
69906-85-0

cyclofenil

WADA group
S7. AGENTS WITH ANTI-OESTROGENIC ACTIVITY

MeSH descriptor
cyclofenil

CAS Registry number
2624-43-3

Trade names and research codes
f 6066
f6066
fertodur
h 3452
h3452
neoclym
ondogyne
sexovid

Short synonyms
cyclofenyl
cyclophenil
cyclophenyl

Long synonyms
4 [[4 (acetyloxy)phenyl]cyclohexylidenemethyl]phenyl acetate
bis (4 acetoxyphenyl)cyclohexylidenemethane
bis(4 acetoxyphenyl)cyclohexylidene methane
bis(4 acetoxyphenyl)cyclohexylidenemethane
bis(para acetoxyphenyl)cyclohexilidene methane
bis(para acetoxyphenyl) cyclohexylidenemethane
bis(para acetoxyphenyl)cyclohexylidene methane
bis(para acetoxyphenyl)cyclohexylidenemethane
cyclohexylidenebis(4 acetoxyphenyl)methane

cyclohexyl[4 [2 [2 hydroxy 3 (4 hydroxyphenoxy)propylamino]ethyl] phenoxymethyl]phosphinic acid

WADA group
S6. BETA-2 AGONISTS

Trade names and research codes
sb 226552

Long synonyms
[4 [2 [2 hydroxy 3 (4 hydroxyphenoxy)propylamino]ethyl]phenoxymethy l]cyclohexylphosphinic acid

4 cyclohexylamino 1 (1 naphthyloxy) 2 butanol

WADA group
P2. BETA-BLOCKERS

CAS Registry number
57281-35-3

Trade names and research codes
ch 103
ch103
chinoin 103
chinoin103
te 176
te176

Long synonyms
1 cyclohexylamino 4 (1 naphthyloxy) 3 butanol

5 (2 cyclohexylideneethyl) 5 ethylbarbituric acid

WADA group
S1. STIMULANTS

Terms and Synonyms

☝ *probably not prohibited*

CAS Registry number
22173-64-4

Long synonyms
5 (2 cyclohexylideneethyl) 5 ethylbarbiturate
5 (2 cyclohexylideneethyl) 5 ethyl barbituric acid
5 ethyl 5 (2 cyclohexylideneethyl)barbituric acid

cyclopentamine

WADA group
S1. STIMULANTS

CAS registry number
102-45-4
1-6-3459
538-02-3

Trade names and research codes
cyclonarol
cyklosan

Short synonyms
clopane
clopane hydrochloride
cyclopentadrin
cyclopentamine hydrochloride

Long synonyms
1 cyclopentyl 2 methylaminopropane
1 cyclopentyl n methylisopropylamine
n,alpha dimethylcyclopentaneethylamine

cyclopenthiazide

WADA group
S8. MASKING AGENTS
P3. DIURETICS

MeSH descriptor
cyclopenthiazide

CAS Registry number
742-20-1

Trade names and research codes
navidex k
navidrex
navidrex k
navidrex serpasil k
navidrix
su 8341

Short synonyms
cyclomethiazide
cyclopenthiazine
cyclopentiazide
cyclophenthiazide
tsiklometiazid

Long synonyms
6 chloro 3 cyclopentylmethyl 3,4 dihydro 7 sulfamoyl 2h 1,2,4 benzothiadiazine 1,1 dioxide

cyclopenthiazide plus guanethidine

WADA group
S8. MASKING AGENTS
P3. DIURETICS

Trade names and research codes
ismelin navidrex
navidrex ismelin

Long synonyms
guanethidine plus cyclopenthiazide

cyclopenthiazide plus oxprenolol

WADA group
S8. MASKING AGENTS
P2. BETA-BLOCKERS
P3. DIURETICS

CAS Registry number
71265-68-4

Trade names and research codes
trasidex
trasidrex

Short synonyms
co prenozide
co-prenozide
coprenozide

Long synonyms
oxprenolol plus cyclopenthiazide

n [2 [3 [4 [2 (2 cyclopropylmethoxyethoxy)ethyl]phenoxy] 2 hydroxypropylamino]ethyl] 4 hydroxy 1 piperidinecarboxamide

WADA group
P2. BETA-BLOCKERS

CAS Registry number
108495-27-8

Trade names and research codes
h 216 44

6 [4 [3 [[3 [4 [2 (cyclopropylmethoxy)ethyl]phenoxy] 2 hydroxypropyl]amino]propionamido] phenyl] 4,5 dihydro 5 methyl 3(2h) pyridazinone

WADA group
P2. BETA-BLOCKERS

CAS Registry number
111794-31-1

Trade names and research codes
skf 95018

cycloteriam

WADA group
S8. MASKING AGENTS
P3. DIURETICS

Trade names and research codes
cycloteriam

Short synonyms
cyclothiazide plus triamterene
triamterene plus cyclothiazide

cyclothiazide

WADA group
S8. MASKING AGENTS
P3. DIURETICS

CAS Registry number
2259-96-3

Trade names and research codes
anhydron
fluidil
l 35483
l35483
mdi 193
mdi193

Short synonyms
doburil

Long synonyms
6 chloro 3,4 dihydro 3 (5 norbornen 2 yl) 2h 1,2,4 benzothiadiazine 7 sulfonamide 1,1 dioxide

daktacort

WADA group
S9. GLUCOCORTICOSTEROIDS

Trade names and research codes
daktacort

Short synonyms
hydrocortisone plus miconazole
miconazole plus hydrocortisone

danazol

WADA group
S4. ANABOLIC AGENTS

MeSH descriptor
danazol

CAS Registry number
17230-88-5

Trade names and research codes
chronogyn
cyclomen
danatrol
danocrine
danokrin
danol
mastodanatrol
win 17757
win17757
winobanin

Short synonyms
isoxozol

Long synonyms
17alpha pregna 2,4 dien 20 yno[2,3 d]isoxazol 17 ol

deacetyllevonantradol

WADA group
S3. CANNABINOIDS

CAS Registry number
80286-75-5

Short synonyms
desacetyllevonantradol
levonantradol,deacetyl

deacetylmetipranolol

WADA group
P2. BETA-BLOCKERS

CAS Registry number
57193-14-3

Trade names and research codes
vufb 6502

Short synonyms
desacetylmetipranolol
metipranolol,deacetyl

Long synonyms
1 (4 hydroxy 2,3,5 trimethylphenoxy) 3 isopropylamino 2 propanol

deanol

WADA group
S1. STIMULANTS

MeSH descriptor
deanol

CAS Registry number
108-01-0
2498-25-1

Trade names and research codes
recrein

Short synonyms
beta (dimethylamino)ethanol
beta dimethylaminoethanol
deanol teststreifen g
demanol
dimethylaminoethanol
2 (dimethylamino)ethanol
2 dimethyl amino ethanol
2 dimethylaminoethanol
2(dimethylamino)ethanol
dimethylethanolamine
2 hydroxyethyldimethylamine
n,n dimethylethanolamine

Long synonyms
beta dimethylaminoethyl alcohol
2 dimethylaminoethanol hydrochloride
n,n dimethyl 2 hydroxyethylamine

deflazacort

WADA group
S9. GLUCOCORTICOSTEROIDS

CAS Registry number
14484-47-0

Trade names and research codes
dl 458
dl458
dl 458 it
dl 458it
dl458it
dl 5458
dl5458
flantadin
rosilar

Short synonyms
azacort

probably not prohibited

calcort
deflan
defluorofluazacort
9 defluorofluazacort
fluazacort,defluoro

Long synonyms
21 acetoxy 11beta hydroxy 2' methyl 5'beta h pregna 1,4 dieno[17,16 d]oxazole 3,20 dione

deglycochorionic gonadotropin

WADA group
S5. PEPTIDE HORMONES

Long synonyms
deglycosylated chorionic gonadotrophin
deglycosylated chorionic gonadotropin

denopamine

WADA group
S6. BETA-2 AGONISTS

CAS Registry number
71771-90-9

Trade names and research codes
kalgut
kargut
ta 064

Long synonyms
alpha (3,4 dimethoxyphenethylaminomethyl) 4 hydroxybenzyl alcohol
alpha [[(3,4 dimethoxyphenethyl)amino]methyl] 4 hydroxybenzyl alcohol
1 (4 hydroxyphenyl) 2 (3',4' dimethoxyphenethylamino)ethanol
1 (4 hydroxyphenyl) 2 [(3,4 dimethoxyphenethyl)amino]ethanol
1 (para hydroxyphenyl) 2 [(3,4 dimethoxyphenethyl)amino]ethanol

deoxycorticosterone

WADA group
S5. PEPTIDE HORMONES

MeSH descriptor
desoxycorticosterone

Trade names and research codes
cecostrate
cortarmour
cortifat
decortacete
decorton
dohycamon
krinocort
nsc 11319

Short synonyms
cortexon
cortexone
deoxycortan
deoxycorten
11 deoxycorticosterone
deoxycortone
desoxycortane
desoxycorticosteron
desoxycorticosterone
11 desoxycorticosterone
desoxycortone
doc
21 hydroxyprogesterone
kendall deoxy compound b
pregn 4 en 21 ol 3,20 dione
4 pregnen 21 ol 3,20 dione
reichstein substance q

Long synonyms
21 hydroxypregn 4 en 3,20 dione
21 hydroxy 4 pregnene 3,20 dione
21 hydroxypregn 4 ene 3,20 dione

deoxycorticosterone acetate

WADA group
S5. PEPTIDE HORMONES

CAS Registry number
56-47-3

Trade names and research codes
arcort
cortate
cortenil
cortesan
cortigen
cortinaq
cortiron
cortivis
cortixyl
decosterone
descorterone
descotone
dorcostrin
doxo
doxycamon
ocriten
percorten
percorten acetate
primicort
primocorten
sincortex
steraq

Short synonyms
dca
deoxycortone acetate
desoxicorticosterone acetate
desoxycorticosterone acetate
desoxycortone acetate
doca
doca acetate
surenosterone
syncort
syncorta
syncortyl
unidocan

Long synonyms
11 deoxycorticosterone 21 acetate
11 deoxycorticosterone acetate
deoxycorticosterone acetate sodium chloride

deoxycorticosterone phenpropionate plus nandrolone phenpropionate

WADA group
S4. ANABOLIC AGENTS
S5. PEPTIDE HORMONES

Trade names and research codes
docabolin
energital

Terms and Synonyms

Long synonyms
nandrolone phenpropionate plus deoxycorticosterone phenpropionate
nandrolone phenpropionate with deoxycortone phenpropionate

deoxycorticosterone pivalate

WADA group
S5. PEPTIDE HORMONES

CAS Registry number
808-48-0

Trade names and research codes
percorten m
percorten pivalate

Short synonyms
deoxycortone pivalate
desoxycortone pivalate
desoxycortone trimethylacetate

Long synonyms
deoxycorticosterone 21 pivalate
11 deoxycorticosterone pivalate
deoxycorticosterone trimethylacetate
desoxycorticosterone trimethylacetate

deoxyhemoglobin

WADA group
M1. ENHANCEMENT OF OXYGEN TRANSFER

Short synonyms
deoxyhaemoglobin

deslorelin

WADA group
S5. PEPTIDE HORMONES

CAS Registry number
70235-53-9

Trade names and research codes
somagard

Short synonyms
lhrh t

Long synonyms
gonadorelin[1-9] ethylamide[6 dextro tryptophan 9 dextro proline]
gonadorelin[6 dextro tryptophan 9 dextro proline 10 deglycine n ethylamide]

desonide

WADA group
S9. GLUCOCORTICOSTEROIDS

MeSH descriptor
desonide

CAS Registry number
638-94-8

Trade names and research codes
'apolar'
d 2083
d2083
desowen
locapred
prenacid
sterax
topifug
tridesilon
tridesonit

Short synonyms
prednacinolone

Long synonyms
16alpha hydroxyprednisolone 16,17 acetonide
16alpha hydroxyprednisolone acetonide
16 hydroxyprednisolone 16,17 acetonide
16 hydroxyprednisolone acetonide

desoximetasone

WADA group
S9. GLUCOCORTICOSTEROIDS

MeSH descriptor
desoximetasone

CAS Registry number
382-67-2

Trade names and research codes
a 41 304
a 41304
a41304
esperson
flubason
hoe 304
hoe304
ibaril
r 2113
r2113
stiedex
topicort
topicorte
topisolone

Short synonyms
17 deoxydexamethasone
deoxymethasone
17 deoxymethasone
deoxymethazone
desoximethasone
desoxydexamethasone
17 desoxydexamethasone
desoxymetasone
desoxymethasone
r 17 desoxy dexamethasone

Long synonyms
9 fluoro 11beta,21 dihydroxy 16alpha methylpregna 1,4 diene 3,20 dione
pregna 1,4 diene 11beta,21 diol 3,20 dione,9 fluoro 1alpha methyl

dexamethasone

WADA group
S9. GLUCOCORTICOSTEROIDS

MeSH descriptor
dexamethasone

CAS Registry number
50-02-2

Trade names and research codes
azium
cebedex
colofoam
dalalone
decadion

decadran
decadron
decadronal
decadrone
decadron la
decaesadril
decaspray
decilone
dectancyl
dexacort
dexacortin
dexahelvacort
dexalocal
dexamecortin
fluormone
fortecortin
hexadrol
isopto dex
isoptodex
lokalison f
maxidex
mephamesone
millicorten
millicortenol
opticortinol
oradexan
oradexon
visumethazone

Short synonyms
aeroseb dex
aflucoson
aflucosone
anaflogistico
anaflogistico novobios
arcodexan
arcodexane
calonat
cortidrona
cortidrone
cortisumman
dacortina fuerte
dacortine fuerte
decacortin
decadeltosona
decadeltosone
decamethasone
decasone
decasterolone
decofluor
dekacort
delladec
deltafluoren
deltafluorene
dergramin
deronil
desacort
desacortone
desadrene
desalark
desameton
desametone
dexachel
dexacortal
dexacorten
dexa cortisyl
dexacortisyl
dexa dabrosan
dexadabroson
dexadecadrol
dexadrol
dexagen
dexa korti
dexakorti
dexameson
dexamesone
dexametason
dexametasone
dexameth
dexamethason
dexamethasone alcohol
dexamethazon
dexamethazone
dexamethonium
dexan
dexane
dexapot
dexa scherosan
dexascheroson
dexa scherozon
dexascherozon
dexa scherozone
dexascherozone
dexason
dexasone
dexinoral
dexionil
dexone
dextelan
dezone
doxamethasone
esacortene
exadion
exadione
ex s1
firmalone
fluormethylprednisolon
fluormethyl prednisolone
fluormethylprednisolone
fluorocort
fluorodelta
fluoromethylprednisolone
gammacorten
gammacortene
grosodexon
grosodexone
hexadecadiol
hexadecadrol
hexadiol
isnacort
isopto maxidex
isoptomaxidex
luxazone
marvidione
mediamethasone
megacortin
mephameson
metasolon
metasolone
methazone ion
methazon ion
methazonion
methazonione
metisone lafi
mk 125
nisomethasona
novocort
nsc 34521
opticorten
oradexone
orgadrone
policort
predni f tablinen
prednisolone f
prodexona
prodexone
sanamethasone
spoloven
triamcimetil

Long synonyms
9alpha fluoro 11beta,17alpha,21 trihydroxy 16alpha methyl 1,4 pregnadiene 3,20 dione

Terms and Synonyms

9alpha fluoro 11beta,17alpha,21 trihydroxy 16alpha methylpregna 1,4 diene 3,20 dione
9 alpha fluoro 16 alpha methyl delta corticosterone
9alpha fluoro 16alpha methyl delta corticosterone
16alpha methyl 9alpha fluoroprednisolone

dexamethasone 17,21 dipropionate

WADA group
S9. GLUCOCORTICOSTEROIDS

CAS Registry number
55541-30-5

Short synonyms
ths 101

dexamethasone 17 valerate

WADA group
S9. GLUCOCORTICOSTEROIDS

CAS Registry number
33755-46-3

Short synonyms
anaflogistico 17 valerate
calonat 17 valerate
corson 17 valerate
decacortin 17 valerate
decadron 17 valerate
decasone 17 valerate
dectanyl 17 valerate
dekacort 17 valerate
delta fluorene 17 valerate
dergramin 17 valerate
derolin 17 valerate
deseronil 17 valerate
dexacortal 17 valerate
dexameson 17 valerate
dexameth 17 valerate
dexamethasone valerate
dexascherosan 17 valerate
dexason 17 valerate
dexinoral 17 valerate
dextelan 17 valerate
fluormone 17 valerate
fortecortin 17 valerate
gammacorten 17 valerate
hexadecadrol 17 valerate
hexadrol 17 valerate
luxazone 17 valerate
millicorten 17 valerate
oradexon 17 valerate
policort 17 valerate
spoloven 17 valerate

Long synonyms
9alpha fluoro 16alpha methylprednisolone 17 valerate
16alpha methyl 9alpha fluoro 1,4 pregnadiene 11beta,17alpha 21 triol 3,20 dione 17 valerate
16alpha methyl 9alpha fluoro delta hydrocortisone 17 valerate
16alpha methyl 9alpha fluoro prednisolone 17 valerate
1 dehydro 16alpha methyl 9alpha fluorohydrocortisone 17 valerate
9 fluoro 11beta 17,21 trihydroxy 16alpha methyl pregna 1,4 diene 3,20 dione 17 valerate

dexamethasone 21 mesilate

WADA group
S9. GLUCOCORTICOSTEROIDS

CAS Registry number
2265-22-7

Short synonyms
dexamethasone 21 mesylate

Long synonyms
dexamethasone 21 methanesulfonate
21 methanesulfonyldexamethasone

dexamethasone acetate

WADA group
S9. GLUCOCORTICOSTEROIDS

CAS Registry number
1177-87-3

Trade names and research codes
supertendin

Short synonyms
dexamethasone 21 acetate

Long synonyms
9 fluoro 11beta 17,21 trihydroxy 16alpha methylpregna 1,4 diene 3.20 dione 21 acetate

dexamethasone derivative

WADA group
S9. GLUCOCORTICOSTEROIDS

Short synonyms
dexamethasone ester

dexamethasone isonicotinate

WADA group
S9. GLUCOCORTICOSTEROIDS

MeSH descriptor
dexamethasone isonicotinate

CAS Registry number
2265-64-7

Trade names and research codes
auxiloson
auxison
dosauxison
he 111
voren

Short synonyms
dexamethason 21 isonicotinate
dexamethasone 21 isonicotinate
dexamethasone 2 isonicotinate
21 dexamethasone isonicotinate
dexamethasone isonioatinate

Long synonyms
dexamethasone 21 (4 pyridine carboxylate)
dexamethasone 21 (4 pyridinecarboxylate)
dexamethasone 21 isonicotinoate
dexamethasone 21 pyridine 4 carboxylate

dexamethasone plus tobramycin

WADA group
S9. GLUCOCORTICOSTEROIDS

Trade names and research codes
tobradex

Short synonyms
tobramycin plus dexamethasone

dexamethasone sodium phosphate

WADA group
S9. GLUCOCORTICOSTEROIDS

CAS Registry number
2392-39-4
312-93-6

Trade names and research codes
dexadreson
dexair
dexavet
hexadrol phosphate
soldesam
soludecadron
spersadex
totocortin

Short synonyms
dexamethasone 21 phosphate
dexamethasone phosphate
dexamethasone phosphate sodium
dexamethazone phosphate
maxidex ointment
neodecadron ophthalmic
soludecadrol
solu decadron
turbinaire
wymesone
wymesone sodium

Long synonyms
dexamethasone 21 disodiumphosphate
dexamethasone 21 mono sodium phosphate
dexamethasone 21 phosphate disodium
dexamethasone 21 phosphate sodium
dexamethasone disodium phosphate
dexamethasonium sodium phosphate

dexamphetamine

WADA group
S1. STIMULANTS

MeSH descriptor
dextroamphetamine

CAS Registry number
1462-73-3
51-63-8
51-64-9

Trade names and research codes
biphetamine
dexadrine
dexedrine
dexedrine spansules
dextrostat
doxedrine

Short synonyms
afatin
afettine
albemap
amfetasul
amitrene
amphedrine
amphex
amsustain
ardex
betafedrina
betaphedrine d
carboxyphen
d 1 phenyl 2 aminoproprane
dadex
d alpha methylphenethylamin
d amfetasul
d amphetamine
d amphetamine sulfate
d amphetamine sulphate
daprisal
d ate
d beta phenylisopropylamine
dephadren
dexaline
dexalme
dexalone
dexamed
dexamfetamine
dexamphetamine sulfate
dexamphetamin sulphate
dexamphethamine
dexamphoid
dexamyl
dexaspan b
dexeamphetanine
dexedrine sulfate
dexoval
dextro amphetamine
dextroamphetamine
dextro amphetamine sulfate
dextroamphetamine sulfate
diocarb
diocurb
domafate
domefate
dynaphenyl
evrodex
hetamine
nsc 73713
obesedrin
obesonil
phetadex
simpamina d
sympamin

Long synonyms
d 1 phenyl 2 aminopropane hydrochloride
d 1 phenyl 2 aminopropane sulfate
d alpha methylphenethylamine sulfate
d alpha methylphenethylamin hydrochloride
d alpha methylphenethylamin sulfate
d beta phenylisopropylamine sulfate
dextroamphetamine hydrochloride

dexanabinol

WADA group
S3. CANNABINOIDS

CAS Registry number
112924-45-5

Trade names and research codes
hu 210
hu 211

Long synonyms
3 (1,1 dimethylheptyl) 11 hydroxy delta8 tetrahydrocannabinol
7 hydroxy delta6 tetrahydrocannabinol dimethylheptyl homolog

Terms and Synonyms

dexatopic

WADA group
S4. ANABOLIC AGENTS
S9. GLUCOCORTICOSTEROIDS

Trade names and research codes
dexatopic

Long synonyms
chlorhexidine plus dexamethasone plus nandrolone decanoate
dexamethasone plus nandrolone decanoate plus chlorhexidine

dexfenfluramine

WADA group
S1. STIMULANTS

MeSH descriptor
dexfenfluramine

CAS Registry number
3239-44-9
3239-45-0

Trade names and research codes
adifax
glypolix
isomeride
redux
s 5614

Short synonyms
dexfenfluramine hydrochloride
dextro fenfluramine
d fenfluramine
fenfluramine,dextro

dexmethylphenidate

WADA group
S1. STIMULANTS

CAS Registry number
19262-68-1

Trade names and research codes
focalin

Short synonyms
d threo methylphenidate

Long synonyms
dexmethylphenidate hydrochloride
d threo methylphenidate hydrochloride

dexnorfenfluramine

WADA group
S1. STIMULANTS

CAS Registry number
19036-73-8

Short synonyms
nordexfenfluramine

dexoxadrol

WADA group
S1. STIMULANTS

CAS Registry number
4741-41-7

Trade names and research codes
cl 911 c
cl 911c
cl911c

Short synonyms
d dioxadrol
dexoxadrol hydrochloride
nsc 526062
relane

Long synonyms
d 2,2 diphenyl 4 piperid 2 yl 1,3 dioxolane

dextran

WADA group
S8. MASKING AGENTS

MeSH descriptor
dextrans

CAS Registry number
87915-38-6
9014-78-2

Trade names and research codes
dextraven 150
dialens
gentran
longasteril
macrodex
onkovertin
plasmaclair
promit
rheomacrodex

Short synonyms
alpha 1,6 glucan
dextran 45
dextrane
dextran k 300000
dextran k 40000
dextran k 500000
dextran k 70000
dextrans
dextraven
expandex
hemodex
high molecular weight dextran
intradex
lmw dextran
low molecular dextran
low molecular weight dextran
macrodex 500
macrose
neoplasmafusin
neoschiwadex
oncovertin
onkotin
pharmodex
plavolex
polyglucin
polyglucine
polyglucinum
polyglusol
polyglusole
promiten
pvtd
sinkol

Long synonyms
cyanogen bromide activated dextran
sodium meta periodate activated dextran

Terms and Synonyms

dextran 40

WADA group
S8. MASKING AGENTS

CAS Registry number
86220-87-3

Trade names and research codes
dextran ebewe
infucoll m 40
infukoll m 40
plasmacair
plasmodex
schiwadex 40

Short synonyms
deltaplasmat 40
dextran 40,000
dextran 40000
gentran 40
hemodex 40
lmd
lmwd
longasteril 40
lvd

dextran 60

WADA group
S8. MASKING AGENTS

Trade names and research codes
schiwadex 60

dextran 70

WADA group
S8. MASKING AGENTS

Trade names and research codes
deltaplasmat 70
gentran 70
hemodex 70
hyskon

dextromethorphan plus morphine

WADA group
S2. NARCOTICS

Trade names and research codes
morphidex

Short synonyms
morphine plus dextromethorphan

Long synonyms
dextromethorphan hydrobromide plus morphine sulfate
morphine sulfate plus dextromethorphan hydrobromide

dextromoramide

WADA group
S2. NARCOTICS

MeSH descriptor
dextromoramide

CAS Registry number
2922-44-3
357-56-2

Trade names and research codes
dimorlin
jetrium
palfium
palphium
r 875
sk and f 5137
skf 5137

Short synonyms
dextro moramide
dextromoramide bitartras
dextromoramide bitartrate
dextromoramide tartrate
dextromoramine
d moramide
d moramide bitartrate
moramide
pyrrolamidole
pyrroloamidol
r 875

Long synonyms
1 (3 methyl 4 morpholino 2,2 diphenylbutyryl)pyrrolidine
4 [2 methyl 4 oxo 3,3 diphenyl 4 (1 pyrrolidinyl)butyl]morpholine

dextronantradol

WADA group
S3. CANNABINOIDS

CAS Registry number
74430-97-0

Trade names and research codes
cp 53870 1
cp 538701
cp53870 1
cp538701

Short synonyms
nantradol,dextro

diacetolol

WADA group
P2. BETA-BLOCKERS

CAS Registry number
28197-69-5
69796-04-9

Trade names and research codes
eu 4891
eu4891
m and b 16 942
m and b 16942
m and b 16942 a
m and b 16942a

Short synonyms
diacetolol hydrochloride

Long synonyms
3' acetyl 4' [2 hydroxy 3 (isopropylamino)propoxy]acetanilide
n [3 acetyl 4 [2 hydroxy 3 [(1 methylethyl)amino]propoxy]phenyl]acetamide

Terms and Synonyms

3,5 diamino 6 chloro n [1 [n [2 [2 hydroxy 3 (1 naphthoxy)propylamino]ethyl]carbamoyl] 1 methylethyl]pyrazine 2 carboxamide

WADA group
S8. MASKING AGENTS
P2. BETA-BLOCKERS
P3. DIURETICS

CAS Registry number
83812-65-1

Trade names and research codes
ici 147,798
ici 147798

diamorphine

WADA group
S2. NARCOTICS

MeSH descriptor
heroin

CAS Registry number
1502-95-0
561-27-3

Short synonyms
acetomorphine
diacephine
diacetyl morphine
diacetylmorphine
3,6 diacetylmorphine
diacetylmorphine hydrochloride
diamorphine hydrochloride
diaphorin
heroin
heroine
heroine hydrochloride
heroin hydrochloride
morphacetin
morphine 3,6 diacetate

diaspirin crosslinked hemoglobin

WADA group
M1. ENHANCEMENT OF OXYGEN TRANSFER

Trade names and research codes
hemassist

Long synonyms
diaspirin cross linked hemoglobin

dichlorisoprenaline

WADA group
S6. BETA-2 AGONISTS

CAS Registry number
51-29-6
59-61-0

Trade names and research codes
l 20522

Short synonyms
dci
dichlorisopropylnoradrenalin
dichlorisoproterenol
dichloroisoprenalin
dichloro isoprenaline
dichloroisoprenaline
dichloro isoproterenol
dichloroisoproterenol

Long synonyms
beta hydroxy n isopropyl 3,4 dichlorophenethylamine
3,4 bis(desoxy) 3,4 dichloroisoprenaline
dichlorisoprenaline hydrochloride
dichlorisoprenaline phosphoric acid
3,4 dichloro alpha (isopropylaminomethyl)benzyl alcohol
dichloroisoprenaline hydrochloride
dichloroisoproterenol hydrochloride
1 (3,4 dichlorophenyl) 2 isopropylaminoethanol
phosphoric acid dichlorisoprenaline

6,7 dichloro 2,3 dihydro 5 (n,n dimethylsulfamoyl)coumarilic acid

WADA group
S8. MASKING AGENTS
P3. DIURETICS

CAS Registry number
103968-87-2

Trade names and research codes
s 8666

Long synonyms
6,7 dichloro 2,3 dihydro 5 (n,n dimethylsulfamoyl) 2 benzofurancarboxylic acid
6,7 dichloro 2,3 dihydro 5 (n,n dimethylsulfamoyl)benzofuran 2 carboxylic acid
6,7 dichloro 5 dimethylsulfamoyl 2,3 dihydrobenzofuran 2 carboxylic acid
6,7 dichloro 5 (n,n dimethylsulfamoyl) 2,3 dihydrobenzofuran 2 carboxylic acid
5 (n,n dimethylsulfamoyl) 6,7 dichloro 2,3 dihydrobenzofuran 2 carboxylic acid

1,1 dichloro 2,3 diphenylcyclopropane

WADA group
S7. AGENTS WITH ANTI-OESTROGENIC ACTIVITY

CAS Registry number
33044-82-5
36611-98-0
59130-21-1

Short synonyms
analog ii
tamoxifen analog ii

2,6 dichloro 4 dimethylaminoamphetamine

WADA group
S1. STIMULANTS

CAS Registry number
67759-58-4

Trade names and research codes
fla 365
fla365

Long synonyms
amphetamine,2,6 dichloro 4 dimethylamino

2,6 dichloro 4 dimethylamino alpha methylphenethylamine
(2,6 dichloro 4 dimethylaminophenyl)isopropylamine

1 (2,4 dichlorophenoxy) 3 [2 (3,4 dimethoxyphenyl)ethylamino] 2 propanol

WADA group
P2. BETA-BLOCKERS

CAS Registry number
104970-08-3

Trade names and research codes
b 24 76
b 2476
b2476

diclofenamide

WADA group
S8. MASKING AGENTS
P3. DIURETICS

MeSH descriptor
dichlorphenamide

CAS Registry number
120-97-8

Trade names and research codes
daranide
fenamide
oralcon
oratrol

Short synonyms
dichlorofenamide
dichlorophenamide
dichlorphenamide

Long synonyms
4,5 dichloro 1,3 benzenedisulfonamide
1,2 dichloro 3,5 disulfamoylbenzene

1 (4,4' dicyanobenzhydryl)imidazole

WADA group
S7. AGENTS WITH ANTI-OESTROGENIC ACTIVITY

CAS Registry number
112808-99-8

Trade names and research codes
cgs 18320b
cgs18320b

Long synonyms
1 [bis(4 cyanophenyl)methyl]imidazole

4 (2 diethylaminoethoxy) alpha' ethyl alpha (4 hydroxyphenyl) 4' methoxystilbene

WADA group
S7. AGENTS WITH ANTI-OESTROGENIC ACTIVITY

CAS Registry number
71868-47-8

Trade names and research codes
h 1285

Long synonyms
4 [2 (n,n diethylamino)ethoxy] 4' methoxy alpha (4 hydroxyphenyl) alpha' ethylstilbene
4 [2 (n,n diethylamino)ethoxy] 4' methoxy alpha (para hydroxyphenyl) alpha' ethylstilbene

diflorasone

WADA group
S9. GLUCOCORTICOSTEROIDS

CAS Registry number
2557-49-5

Short synonyms
6alpha fluorobetamethasone

Long synonyms
6alpha,9 difluoro 11beta,17,21 trihydroxy 16beta methylpregna 1,4 diene 3,20 dione
6alpha,9 difluoro 16beta methylprednisolone

diflorasone diacetate

WADA group
S9. GLUCOCORTICOSTEROIDS

CAS Registry number
33564-31-7

Trade names and research codes
diacort
diflal
florone
maxiflor
psorcon
u 34865
u34865

Short synonyms
diflorasone 17,21 diacetate

diflucortolone

WADA group
S9. GLUCOCORTICOSTEROIDS

MeSH descriptor
diflucortolone

CAS Registry number
9-6-2607

Short synonyms
difluocortolone

Long synonyms
6alpha,9 difluoro 11beta,21 dihydroxy 16alpha methylpregna 1,4 diene 3,20 dione

diflucortolone valerate

WADA group
S9. GLUCOCORTICOSTEROIDS

CAS Registry number
59198-70-8

Trade names and research codes
nerisona
nerisona forte
nerisone

ro 10 7614
shl 183a
temetex
travocort

Short synonyms
difluocortolone 21 valerate
diflucortolone valerianate
difluocortolone valerate
difluorocortolone valerate
difluorocortolone valerianate
neriforte
temetex c

6alpha,9alpha difluoro 11beta,17alpha dihydroxy 16beta methyl 17beta methylthiocarbonylandrosta 1,4 dien 3 one 17 acetate

WADA group
S9. GLUCOCORTICOSTEROIDS

CAS Registry number
125709-03-7

Trade names and research codes
rs 21314

6alpha,9alpha difluoro 11beta,17alpha dihydroxy 16beta methyl 17beta methylthiocarbonylandrosta 1,4 dien 3 one 17 propionate

WADA group
S9. GLUCOCORTICOSTEROIDS

CAS Registry number
79578-12-4

Trade names and research codes
rs 85095

difluprednate

WADA group
S9. GLUCOCORTICOSTEROIDS

CAS Registry number
23674-86-4

Trade names and research codes
cm 9155
cm9155
epitopic
myser
w 6309
w6309
warner 6309

Long synonyms
6alpha,9alpha difluoroprednisolone 21 acetate 17 butyrate
6alpha,9 difluoro 11beta,17,21 trihydroxypregna 1,4 diene 3,20 dione 21 acetate 17 butyrate
6alpha,9 difluoroprednisolone 21 acetate 17 butyrate

dihydralazine plus hydrochlorothiazide plus reserpine

WADA group
S8. MASKING AGENTS
P3. DIURETICS

Trade names and research codes
adelfan esidrex
adelphane esidrex
adelphan esidrex
adepresol
elfanex

Long synonyms
hydrochlorothiazide plus dihydralazine plus reserpine
reserpine plus dihydralazine plus hydrochlorothiazide

dihydralazine plus oxprenolol

WADA group
P2. BETA-BLOCKERS

Trade names and research codes
trasipresol
trasipressol

Short synonyms
oxprenolol plus dihydralazine

2,3 dihydro 5 methyl 3 (morpholinomethyl) 6 (1 naphthoyl)pyrrolo[1,2,3 de][1,4]benzoxazine

WADA group
S3. CANNABINOIDS

CAS Registry number
134959-51-6

Trade names and research codes
win 55212
win 55212 2
win 55212 3

2,4 dihydro 6,8 dinitro 1,2,4 triazolo[3,4 c][1,4]benzoxazin 1 one

WADA group
S8. MASKING AGENTS
P3. DIURETICS

CAS Registry number
96753-85-4

Trade names and research codes
idph 8032

dihydroalprenolol

WADA group
P2. BETA-BLOCKERS

MeSH descriptor
dihydroalprenolol

CAS Registry number
60106-89-0

Short synonyms
alprenolol,dihydro

Long synonyms
3 isopropylamino 1 (2 propylphenoxy)propan 2 ol

6,7 dihydrocanrenone

WADA group
S8. MASKING AGENTS
P3. DIURETICS

CAS Registry number
976-70-5

Trade names and research codes
ru 22092
sc 5233

Short synonyms
canrenone,6,7 dihydro

Long synonyms
3 (17beta hydroxy 3 oxoandrost 4 en 17 yl)propionic acid gamma lactone
17 testosteronepropionic acid gamma lactone

20 dihydroprednisolonic acid methyl ester

WADA group
S9. GLUCOCORTICOSTEROIDS

CAS Registry number
57073-10-6

Long synonyms
20alpha dihydroprednisolonecarboxylic acid methyl ester
20beta dihydroprednisolonecarboxylic acid methyl ester
20 dihydroprednisolonecarboxylic acid methyl ester
methyl 20alpha dihydroprednisolonate
methyl 20beta dihydroprednisolonate
methyl 20 dihydroprednisolonate

11beta,17beta dihydroxy 17 (1 propynyl)androsta 1,4,6 trien 3 one

WADA group
S9. GLUCOCORTICOSTEROIDS

CAS Registry number
74915-58-5

Trade names and research codes
ru 26988

Long synonyms
11beta,17beta dihydroxy 17 (1 propynyl) 1,4,6 androstatrien 3 one
11beta,17beta dihydroxy 17alpha (1 propynyl)androsta 1,4,6 trien 3 one
11beta,17beta dihydroxy 21 methyl 17alpha pregna 1,4,6 trien 20 yn 3 one

11beta,17beta dihydroxy 6 methyl 17alpha (1 propynyl)androsta 1,4,6 trien 3 one

WADA group
S9. GLUCOCORTICOSTEROIDS

CAS Registry number
74915-64-3

Trade names and research codes
ru 28362

1 (3,4 dihydroxyphenoxy) 3 (3,4 dimethoxyphenethylamino) 2 propanol

WADA group
S6. BETA-2 AGONISTS

CAS Registry number
74513-77-2

Trade names and research codes
ro 363

Long synonyms
3 (3,4 dihydroxyphenoxy) 1 (3,4 dimethoxyphenethylamino) 2 propanol
1 (3,4 dihydroxyphenoxy) 2 hydroxy 3 (3,4 dimethoxyphenethylamino)propane
1 (3,4 dimethoxyphenethylamino) 3 (3,4 dihydroxyphenoxy) 2 propanol
n [2 hydroxy 3 (3,4 dihydroxyphenoxy)prop 1 yl] 3,4 dimethoxyphenethylamine

3 (3,4 dihydroxyphenyl) 2 [3 (4 fluorophenyl)propylamino] 3 hydroxypropionic acid pyrrolidine amide

WADA group
S6. BETA-2 AGONISTS

CAS Registry number
142784-65-4

Trade names and research codes
sm 11044

6 [2 (3,4 dihydroxyphenyl) 2 hydroxyethylamino] n [4 (trifluoromethyl)phenyl]heptanamide

WADA group
S6. BETA-2 AGONISTS

CAS Registry number
83086-14-0

Trade names and research codes
ro 17 2218
ro 17 8648
ro 17 9651

dilevalol

WADA group
P2. BETA-BLOCKERS

CAS Registry number
75659-07-3

Trade names and research codes
dilevalon
levadil
unicard

Short synonyms
ah 19501
(R,R) labetalol
sch 19927

dimefline

WADA group
S1. STIMULANTS

CAS Registry number
1165-48-6
7-4-2740

Trade names and research codes
dw 62
dw62
nsc 114650
nsc114650
rec 7 0267
rec 7-0267
rec 70267
rec7 0267
rec7-0267
rec70267

Short synonyms
dimefline chloride
dimefline hydrochloride
remeflin

Long synonyms
8 dimethylaminomethyl 7 methoxy 3 methylflavone

dimetamfetamine

WADA group
S1. STIMULANTS

CAS Registry number
4075-96-1

Trade names and research codes
metromin

Short synonyms
dimethylamphetamine
n,n dimethylamphetamine

Long synonyms
n,n,alpha trimethylphenethylamine

2,5 dimethoxy 4 methylamphetamine

WADA group
S1. STIMULANTS

MeSH descriptor
2,5-dimethoxy-4-methylamphetamine

CAS Registry number
15588-95-1
26011-50-7

Short synonyms
dimethoxy 4 methylamphetamine
DOM
stp

Long synonyms
2 amino 1 (2,5 dimethoxy 4 methylphenyl)propane
amphetamine,2,5 dimethoxy 4 methyl
2,5 dimethoxy 4,alpha dimethylphenethylamine
2,5 dimethoxy 4 methyl amphetamine
2,5-dimethoxy-4-methylamphetamine
1 (2,5 dimethoxy 4 methylphenyl) 2 aminopropane
1 (2,5 dimethoxy 4 methylphenyl) 2 propanamine
2,5 dimethoxy 4 methylphenylisopropylamine
1 (4 methyl 2,5 dimethoxyphenyl) 2 aminopropane
4 methyl 2,5 dimethoxyphenylisopropylamine

n (3,5 dimethoxyphenethyl) 5 methoxy 2 (phenylethynyl)amphetamine

WADA group
S1. STIMULANTS

CAS Registry number
119615-65-5

Trade names and research codes
mcn 6186

Long synonyms
n (3,5 dimethoxyphenethyl) 5 methoxy alpha methyl 2 (phenylethynyl)phenethylamine

11 [4 (2 dimethylaminoethoxy)phenyl]estradiol

WADA group
S7. AGENTS WITH ANTI-OESTROGENIC ACTIVITY

CAS Registry number
120382-04-9

Trade names and research codes
ru 39411

Long synonyms
estradiol,11 [4 (2 dimethylaminoethoxy)phenyl]

5 (1,3 dimethylbutyl) 5 ethylbarbituric acid

WADA group
S1. STIMULANTS

CAS Registry number
9-6-2964

Short synonyms
diberal

Long synonyms
barbituric acid,5 ethyl 5 (1',3' dimethylbutyl)
5 (1,3 dimethylbutyl) 5 ethylbarbiturate
5 (1',3' dimethylbutyl) 5 ethylbarbituric acid
5 ethyl 5 (1',3' dimethylbutyl)barbituric acid
5 ethyl 5 (1,3 dimethylbutyl)barbituric acid
5 ethyl 5 (4' methylpent 2 yl)barbituric acid

4 (1,1 dimethylheptyl) 1',2',3',4',5',6' hexahydro 2,3' dihydroxy 6' (3 hydroxypropyl)biphenyl

WADA group
S3. CANNABINOIDS

CAS Registry number
83003-12-7

Trade names and research codes
cp 55940
cp55940
cp 56667

cp56667

Long synonyms
4 (1,1 dimethylheptyl) 2,3' dihydroxy 6' (3 hydroxypropyl) 1',2',3',4',5',6' hexahydrobiphenyl
3 [2 hydroxy 4 (1,1 dimethylheptyl)phenyl] 4 (3 hydroxypropyl)cyclohexanol

5 (1,1 dimethylheptyl) 2 (3 hydroxy 7 hydroxymethyldecahydro 1 naphthyl)phenol

WADA group
S3. CANNABINOIDS

CAS Registry number
79678-32-3

Trade names and research codes
cp 55243
cp55243
cp 55244
cp55244
cp 97587
cp97587

Long synonyms
3 (1,1 dimethylheptyl) 6 (3 hydroxy 7 hydroxymethyldecahydronaphthalen 1 yl)phenol

dimethylstilbestrol

WADA group
S7. AGENTS WITH ANTI-OESTROGENIC ACTIVITY

CAS Registry number
552-80-7

dimetofrine

WADA group
S1. STIMULANTS

CAS Registry number
22950-29-4

Short synonyms
dimethofrine
dimethophrine
dimetophrine

☝ diphenylpyraline plus phenylpropanolamine

WADA group
S1. STIMULANTS

Trade names and research codes
eskornade

Long synonyms
phenylpropanolamine plus diphenylpyraline

dipivefrine

WADA group
S1. STIMULANTS

CAS Registry number
52365-63-6
52698-24-9

Trade names and research codes
diopine
epifrin
glaucothil
k 30081
pivalephrine
propine

Short synonyms
adrenalin dipivalate
adrenaline dipivalate
dipivaloyl epinephrine
dipivalyladrenalin
dipivalylepinephrine
dipivefrin
dpe
epinephrine dipivalate

Long synonyms
4 [1 hydroxy 2 (methylamino)ethyl] 1,2 phenylene bis(2,2 dimethylpropanoate)

ditec

WADA group
S6. BETA-2 AGONISTS

Trade names and research codes
ditec

Long synonyms
cromoglycate disodium plus fenoterol

diucomb

WADA group
S8. MASKING AGENTS
P3. DIURETICS

Trade names and research codes
diucomb

Short synonyms
bemetizide plus triamterene
triamterene plus bemetizide

diuretic agent

WADA group
S8. MASKING AGENTS
P3. DIURETICS

MeSH descriptor
diuretics, sulfamyl
diuretics

Short synonyms
diuretic
diuretic drug
diuretics
diuretics, mercurial
diuretics, sulfamyl
diureticum
mercurial diuretic
mercury diuretic
mercury diuretic agent
organomercurial diuretic
saluretic agent

dobutamine

WADA group
S1. STIMULANTS

MeSH descriptor
dobutamine

CAS Registry number
34368-04-2
52663-81-7

Trade names and research codes
compound 81929
dobuject
dobutrex
inotres
inotrex

Short synonyms
dobutamide
dobutamine hydrochloride

Long synonyms
2,3 dihydroxy n [3 (4 hydroxyphenyl) 1 methylpropyl]phenethylamine
4 [2 [3 (4 hydroxyphenyl) 1 methylpropylamino]ethyl]pyrocatechol
n [2 (3,4 dihydroxyphenyl)ethyl] 4 (4 hydroxyphenyl) 2 butylamine

domoprednate

WADA group
S9. GLUCOCORTICOSTEROIDS

CAS Registry number
66877-67-6

Trade names and research codes
ro 12 7024
stermonid

Long synonyms
11beta,17alpha dihydroxy d homopregna 1,4 diene 3,20 dione 17alpha butyrate

☝ dopamine

WADA group
S1. STIMULANTS

MeSH descriptor
dopamine

CAS Registry number

Trade names and research codes
asl 279
asl279
catabon
dopastat
dopmin
giludop
inotropin
inovan
intropin
revivan
tensamin

Short synonyms
4 (2 aminoethyl)pyrocatechol
3,4 dihydroxyphenethylamine
dihydroxyphenylethylamine
3,4 dihydroxyphenylethylamine
dopamin
dopamine hydrochloride
3 hydroxytyramine
hydroxytyramine
l dopamine
levo dopamine

Long synonyms
alpha (3,4 dihydroxyphenyl) beta aminoethane
4 (2 aminoethyl)pyrocatechol hydrochloride
2 (3,4 dihydroxyphenyl)ethylamine

dopexamine

WADA group
S1. STIMULANTS
S6. BETA-2 AGONISTS

CAS Registry number
86197-47-9
86484-91-5

Trade names and research codes
dopacard
fpl 60278
fpl60278
fpl 60278 ar
fpl 60278ar
fpl60278ar

Short synonyms
dopachard
dopexamine dihydrochloride
dopexamine hydrochloride

Long synonyms
4 [2 [6 (phenethylamino)hexylamino]ethyl]pyrocatechol

doxaminol

WADA group
S6. BETA-2 AGONISTS

CAS Registry number
55286-56-1

Trade names and research codes
bm 10188
bm10188

Long synonyms
1 [2 (6,11 dihydrodibenz[b,e]oxepin 11 yl) n methylethylamino] 3 phenoxy 2 propanol
6,11 dihydro n (2 hydroxy 3 phenoxypropyl) n methyldibenz[b,e]oxepin 11 ethylamine

doxapram

WADA group
S1. STIMULANTS

MeSH descriptor
doxapram

CAS Registry number
113-07-5
309-29-5
7081-53-0

Trade names and research codes
ahr 619
ahr619
dopram
dopram v
doxapril

Terms and Synonyms

stimulexin

Short synonyms
doxapram chlorhydrate
doxapram hydrochloride
doxapram hydrochloride hydrate
doxopram

Long synonyms
3,3 diphenyl 1 ethyl 4 (2 morpholinoethyl) 2 pyrrolidinone
3,3 diphenyl 1 ethyl 4 (beta morpholinoethyl) 2 pyrrolidinone
1 ethyl 4 (2 morpholinoethyl) 3,3 diphenyl 2 pyrrolidinone
1 ethyl 4 (2 morpholinoethyl) 3,3 diphenyl 2 pyrrolidinone hydrochloride hydrate

drocinonide

WADA group
S9. GLUCOCORTICOSTEROIDS

CAS Registry number
36637-22-6

Trade names and research codes
sq 17409

Long synonyms
drocinonide phosphate potassium

droloxifene

WADA group
S7. AGENTS WITH ANTI-OESTROGENIC ACTIVITY

CAS Registry number
82413-20-5

Trade names and research codes
fk 435
fk435
k 060
k060
k 21060e
k21060e

Short synonyms
3 hydroxytamoxifen
tamoxifen,3 hydroxy

Long synonyms
alpha [4 [2 (dimethylamino)ethoxy]phenyl] alpha' ethyl 3 stilbenol
1 [4 (2 dimethylaminoethoxy)phenyl] 1 (3 hydroxyphenyl) 2 phenylbut 1 ene
3 [1 [4 (2 dimethylaminoethoxy)phenyl] 2 phenyl 1 butenyl]phenol

dronabinol

WADA group
S3. CANNABINOIDS

CAS Registry number
7663-50-5

Trade names and research codes
ea 1477
ea1477
marinol

Short synonyms
delta 1,2 tetrahydrocannabinol
delta 1 tetrahydrocannabinol
delta1 tetrahydrocannabinol
delta1 thc
delta 9 tetrahydrocannabinol
delta9 tetrahydro cannabinol
delta9 tetrahydrocannabinol
qcd 84924
tetrahydrocannabinol 1 ene
tetrahydrocannabinol delta1
tetrahydrocannabinol delta9
u1 tetrahydrocannabinol
u9 tetrahydrocannabinol

Long synonyms
delta 1 3,4 trans tetrahydrocannabinol
delta1 3,4 trans tetrahydrocannabinol
delta1 cis tetrahydrocannabinol
delta 1 trans tetrahydrocannabinol
delta1 trans tetrahydrocannabinol
delta 9 trans tetrahydrocannabinol
delta9 trans tetrahydrocannabinol
l delta 9 trans tetrahydrocannabinol
levo delta 1 tetrahydrocannabinol
levo delta 9 tetrahydrocannabinol
trans delta 9 tetrahydrocannabinol
1 trans delta 9 tetrahydrocannabinol

☝ drospirenone

WADA group
S8. MASKING AGENTS
P3. DIURETICS

CAS Registry number
67392-87-4

Trade names and research codes
sh 470
sh470
zk 30595
zk30595

Short synonyms
1,2 dihydrospirorenone
spirorenone,1,2 dihydro

☝ drospirenone plus estradiol

WADA group
S8. MASKING AGENTS
P3. DIURETICS

Trade names and research codes
angeliq

Short synonyms
estradiol plus drospirenone

☝ drospirenone plus ethinylestradiol

WADA group
S8. MASKING AGENTS
P3. DIURETICS

CAS Registry number
164017-31-6

Trade names and research codes
petibelle
yasmin

Short synonyms
ethinylestradiol plus drospirenone

☝ *probably not prohibited*

drostanolone

WADA group
S4. ANABOLIC AGENTS

CAS Registry number
3232-69-7
58-19-5

Short synonyms
dromostanolone
dromstanolone
2 methyldihydrotestosterone

Long synonyms
2 alpha methyldihydrotestosterone
2alpha methyldihydrotestosterone

drostanolone propionate

WADA group
S4. ANABOLIC AGENTS

CAS Registry number
521-12-0

Trade names and research codes
drolban
masterid
masteril
masteron
masterone
nsc 12198
permastril
permastryl

Short synonyms
dromostanolone propionate
l 32379
metholone

Long synonyms
2alpha methylandrostan 17beta ol 3 one propionate
2alpha methyl dihydrotestosterone propionate
2alpha methyldihydrotestosterone propionate

dutimelan

WADA group
S9. GLUCOCORTICOSTEROIDS

CAS Registry number
56939-84-5

Trade names and research codes
dutimelan
dutimelan 8 15
dutimelan 815

ebiratide

WADA group
S5. PEPTIDE HORMONES

CAS Registry number
105250-86-0

Trade names and research codes
hoe 427

Long synonyms
acth[4-9][4 (methionine sulfone) 8 dextro lysine 9 phenylalanine (8 aminooctyl)amide]
corticotropin[4-9][4 (methionine sulfone) 8 dextro lysine 9 phenylalanine (8 aminooctyl)amide]

ebiratide acetate

WADA group
S5. PEPTIDE HORMONES

CAS Registry number
115994-46-2

efaproxiral

WADA group
M1. ENHANCEMENT OF OXYGEN TRANSFER

CAS Registry number
131179-95-8

Trade names and research codes
rsr 13
rsr13

Short synonyms
efaproxiral sodium

Long synonyms
2 [4 [[(3,5 dimethylanilino)carbonyl]methyl]phenoxy] 2 methylpropionic acid
2 [4 [2 [(3,5 dimethylphenyl)amino] 2 oxoethyl]phenoxy] 2 methylpropanoic acid

enalapril plus hydrochlorothiazide

WADA group
S8. MASKING AGENTS
P3. DIURETICS

Trade names and research codes
co renitec
co retinec
renacor
renidur
vaseretic
vasoretic

Long synonyms
hydrochlorothiazide plus enalapril

enclomifene

WADA group
S7. AGENTS WITH ANTI-OESTROGENIC ACTIVITY

CAS Registry number
15690-57-0

Short synonyms
en clomiphene
enclomiphene
isomer b
rmi 16,289
rmi 16289
trans clomifene
transclomifene
trans clomiphene
transclomiphene

Long synonyms
2 [4 (2 chloro trans 1,2 diphenylvinyl)phenoxy]triethylamine
(e) 2 [4 (2 chloro 1,2 diphenylvinyl)phenoxy]triethylamine

enclomifene citrate

WADA group
S7. AGENTS WITH ANTI-OESTROGENIC ACTIVITY

CAS Registry number
7599-79-3

Trade names and research codes
mdl 16289f

Short synonyms
enclomiphene citrate
trans clomifene citrate
trans clomiphene citrate

epanolol

WADA group
S6. BETA-2 AGONISTS
P2. BETA-BLOCKERS

CAS Registry number
86880-51-5

Trade names and research codes
ici 141292
visacor

Long synonyms
n [2 [3 (2 cyanophenoxy) 2 hydroxypropylamino]ethyl] 4 hydroxyphenylacetamide
n [2 [3 (ortho cyanophenoxy) 2 hydroxypropylamino]ethyl] 4 hydroxyphenylacetamide

ephedrine

WADA group
S1. STIMULANTS

MeSH descriptor
ephedrine

CAS Registry number
50-98-6

Trade names and research codes
biophedrin
eciphin
efedra orion
ephadrosan
ephalone
ephedral
ephedra orion
ephedrosan
ephedrosst
i sedrin
kratedyn
mandrin
primatene
sanedrin
sanedrine
zephrol

Short synonyms
dl ephedrine
efedrin
efedrine
efidrin
eggophedrin
ephedrin
ephedrine hydrochloride
fedrin
l ephedrine
levo ephedrine
neo fedrin

Long synonyms
l erythro 2 methylamino 1 phenylpropan 1 ol
l 2 methylamino 1 phenyl 1 propanol
2 methylamino 1 phenyl 1 propanol
1 phenyl 1 hydroxy 2 methylaminopropane
1 phenyl 2 methylaminopropanol

epiandrosterone

WADA group
S4. ANABOLIC AGENTS

CAS Registry number
481-29-8

Short synonyms
androstan 3beta ol 17 one
5 androstan 3beta ol 17 one
3beta hydroxyandrostan 17 one
isoandrosterone

Long synonyms
5alpha androstan 3beta ol 17 one
3beta hydroxy 5alpha androstan 17 one

epihydrocortisone

WADA group
S9. GLUCOCORTICOSTEROIDS

CAS Registry number
566-35-8

Short synonyms
11alpha cortisol
11alpha hydrocortisone
11alpha hydroxycortexolone
11alpha hydroxycortodoxone
epicortisol
11 epicortisol
11 epihydrocortisone
hydrocortisone,11 epi

Long synonyms
11alpha,17,21 trihydroxyprogesterone
11alpha,17alpha,21 trihydroxypregn 4 ene 3,20 dione
11alpha,17alpha,21 trihydroxyprogesterone

☝ epimestrol

WADA group
S7. AGENTS WITH ANTI-OESTROGENIC ACTIVITY

MeSH descriptor
epimestrol

CAS Registry number
7004-98-0

Trade names and research codes
nsc 55975
nsc55975
org 817
org817
stimovul

Short synonyms
3 methoxy 17 epiestriol

Terms and Synonyms

Long synonyms
3 methoxyestra 1,3,5(10) triene 16alpha,17alpha diol

epinine

WADA group
S6. BETA-2 AGONISTS
S8. MASKING AGENTS
P3. DIURETICS

MeSH descriptor
deoxyepinephrine

CAS Registry number
501-15-5
62-32-8

Trade names and research codes
skf 1085 a

Short synonyms
alpha desoxyadrenalin
deoxyadrenalin
deoxyadrenaline
deoxyepinephrine
desoxyepinephrine
epinine hydrochloride
n methyldopamine

Long synonyms
3,4 dihydroxy n methylphenethylamine
4 (2 methylaminoethyl)pyrocatechol
4 [(2 methylamino)ethyl]pyrocatechol
n [2 (3,4 dihydroxyphenyl)ethyl]methylamine
n methyl 2 (3,4 dihydroxyphenyl)ethylamine
n methyl 2 (3,4 dihydroxyphenyl)ethylamine hydrochloride

epitestosterone

WADA group
S8. MASKING AGENTS

MeSH descriptor
epitestosterone

CAS Registry number
481-30-1

Short synonyms
alpha testosterone
17alpha testosterone
4 androsten 17alpha ol 3 one
androst 4 en 17alpha ol 3 one
17 epitestosterone

Long synonyms
17alpha hydroxy 4 androsten 3 one
17alpha hydroxyandrost 4 en 3 one

epitizide

WADA group
S8. MASKING AGENTS
P3. DIURETICS

CAS Registry number
1764-85-8

Short synonyms
epithiazide
nsc 108164
p 2105
thiaver

Long synonyms
6 chloro 3,4 dihydro 7 sulfamoyl 3 (2,2,2 trifluoroethylthiomethyl) 2h 1,2,4 benzothiadiazine 1,1 dioxide

eplerenone

WADA group
S8. MASKING AGENTS
P3. DIURETICS

CAS Registry number
107724-20-9

Trade names and research codes
cgp 30 083
cgp 30083
cgp30083
inspra
sc 66110
sc66110

Short synonyms
9alpha,11alpha epoxymexrenone
9,11alpha epoxymexrenone
mexrenone,9,11alpha epoxy

Long synonyms
9alpha,11alpha epoxy 17beta hydroxy 3 oxo 17alpha pregn 4 ene 7alpha,21 dicarboxylic acid gamma lactone 7 methyl ester

erythrocruorin

WADA group
M1. ENHANCEMENT OF OXYGEN TRANSFER

MeSH descriptor
erythrocruorins

Short synonyms
erythrocruorins

erythropoietin

WADA group
S5. PEPTIDE HORMONES
M1. ENHANCEMENT OF OXYGEN TRANSFER

MeSH descriptor
erythropoietin

CAS Registry number
11096-26-7

Short synonyms
erthropoietin
erythropoietic factor
hematopoietin
hemopoietin
kidney erythropoietic factor
renal erythropoietic factor

Long synonyms
erythropoiesis stimulating factor
erythropoietic stimulation factor

esmolol

WADA group
P2. BETA-BLOCKERS

CAS Registry number
81147-92-4

probably not prohibited

81161-17-3

Trade names and research codes
asl 8052
asl8052
asl 8052 001
asl 8052-001
asl8052-001
asl8052001
brevibloc

Short synonyms
esmolol hydrochloride

Long synonyms
4 (2 hydroxy 3 isopropylaminopropoxy)hydrocinnamic acid methyl ester
3 [4 (2 hydroxy 3 isopropylaminopropoxy)phenyl]propionic acid methyl ester
3 [4 [2 hydroxy 3 (isopropylamino)propoxy]phenyl]propionic acid methyl ester
para (2 hydroxy 3 isopropylaminopropoxy)hydrocinnamic acid methyl ester

estr 4 ene 3,17 dione

WADA group
S4. ANABOLIC AGENTS

CAS Registry number
734-32-7

Short synonyms
estra 4 ene 3,17 dione
4 estrene 3,17 dione
19 nor 4 androstenedione
19 norandrost 4 enedione
19 norandrostenedione
norandrostenedione

Long synonyms
19 nor 4 androstene 3,17 dione

estratest

WADA group
S4. ANABOLIC AGENTS

Trade names and research codes
estratest

Long synonyms
esterified estrogen plus methyltestosterone
methyltestosterone plus esterified estrogen

etacrynic acid

WADA group
S8. MASKING AGENTS
P3. DIURETICS

MeSH descriptor
ethacrynic acid

CAS Registry number
58-54-8

Trade names and research codes
edecril
edecrin
endecril
hydromedin
mk 595
nsc 85791
reomax
uregit
uregyt

Short synonyms
etacrinic acid
etacrynate
ethacrinic acid
ethacrynate
ethacrynic acid
ethacryonic acid
ethocrynic acid
ethycrynic acid

Long synonyms
2,3 dichloro 4 (2 ethylacryloyl)phenoxyacetic acid
2,3 dichloro 4 (2 methylenebutyryl)phenoxyacetic acid
[2,3 dichloro 4 (2 methylenebutyryl)phenoxy]acetic acid

etafedrine

WADA group
S1. STIMULANTS
S6. BETA-2 AGONISTS

CAS Registry number
48141-64-6
530-35-8
5591-29-7
7681-79-0

Trade names and research codes
menethyl
menetyl
nethamine
novedrin

Short synonyms
etafedrine hydrochloride
ethylephedrine
ethylephrine
etilphrine
levo n ethylephedrine
n ethylephedrine
1 n ethylephedrine

Long synonyms
1 2 (ethylmethylamino) 1 phenylpropan 1 ol
levo alpha [1 (ethylmethylamino)ethyl]benzyl alcohol
2 methylethylamino 1 phenyl 1 propanol

etamivan

WADA group
S1. STIMULANTS

CAS Registry number
304-84-7

Trade names and research codes
analepticon
cardiovanil
clairvan
corivanil
divanal
emiran
emivan
nsc 406087
nsc406087
romecor
sevanil
simaron

Terms and Synonyms

vandid

Short synonyms
etamivam
etamivanum
ethamivan
n,n diethylvanillamide
vanillic acid diethylamide

etanterol

WADA group
S6. BETA-2 AGONISTS

CAS Registry number
93047-39-3

ethamoxytriphetol

WADA group
S7. AGENTS WITH ANTI-OESTROGENIC ACTIVITY

MeSH descriptor
ethamoxytriphetol

CAS Registry number
67-98-1

Trade names and research codes
mer 25

Short synonyms
ethamoxy triphetol
ethanoxytriphetol

Long synonyms
4 (2 diethylaminoethoxy) alpha hydroxy 4 methoxy alpha phenylbibenzyl
4 (2 diethylaminoethoxy) alpha hydroxy 4' methoxy alpha phenylbibenzyl
4 (2 diethylaminoethoxy) alpha hydroxy 4'methoxy alpha phenylbibenzyl
1 [4 (2 diethylaminoethoxy)phenyl] 1 phenyl 2 (4 methoxyphenyl)ethanol
1 [4 (2 diethylaminoethoxy)phenyl] 2 (4 methoxyphenyl) 1 phenylethanol
1 (para 2 diethylaminoethoxyphenyl) 1 phenyl 2 para methoxyphenylethanol
1 [para (2 diethylaminoethoxy)phenyl] 2 (para methoxyphenyl) 1 phenylethanol

ethiazide

WADA group
S8. MASKING AGENTS
P3. DIURETICS

CAS Registry number
1824-58-4

Trade names and research codes
hypertane

Long synonyms
6 chloro 3,4 dihydro 3 ethyl 7 sulfamoyl 1,2,4 benzothiadiazine 1,1 dioxide
6 chloro 3 ethyl 3,4 dihydro 2h 1,2,4 benzothiadiazine 7 sulfonamide 1,1 dioxide

ethimizole

WADA group
S1. STIMULANTS

MeSH descriptor
etimizol

CAS Registry number
64-99-3

Short synonyms
aethimizol
aethimizole
ethimizol
ethymisol
ethymizol
etimizol
etimizole

Long synonyms
1 ethyl 4,5 bis(methylcarbamoyl)imidazole
1 ethyl 4,5 imidazoledicarboxylic acid bis(methylamide)
1 ethylimidazole 4,5 dicarboxylic acid bis(methylamide)

ethinylestradiol plus methyltestosterone

WADA group
S4. ANABOLIC AGENTS

Trade names and research codes
mixogen

Long synonyms
methyltestosterone plus ethinylestradiol

2beta ethoxy 3alpha hydroxy 11alpha isopentylamino 5alpha androstane 17beta carboxylic acid methyl ester

WADA group
S4. ANABOLIC AGENTS

CAS Registry number
82663-16-9

Trade names and research codes
cci 22277
cci22277

Long synonyms
2beta ethoxy 3alpha hydroxy 11alpha (3 methylbutylamino) 5alpha androstane 17beta carboxylic acid methyl ester
methyl 2beta ethoxy 3alpha hydroxy 11alpha (3 methylbutylamino) 5alpha androstane 17beta carboxylate

ethoxzolamide

WADA group
S8. MASKING AGENTS
P3. DIURETICS

MeSH descriptor
ethoxzolamide

CAS Registry number
452-35-7

Trade names and research codes
cardrase

cardrax
cardraze

Short synonyms
ethoxazolamide
ethoxyzolamide
etoxzolamide

Long synonyms
6 ethoxy 2 benzothiazolesulfonamide
6 ethoxybenzothiazole 2 sulfonamide

13beta ethyl 17beta hydroxygon 4 en 3 one

WADA group
S4. ANABOLIC AGENTS

Short synonyms
18 methylnandrolone

Long synonyms
17beta hydroxy 18a homoestr 4 en 3 one
18a homo 17beta hydroxyestr 4 en 3 one

n ethyl 3,4 methylenedioxyamphetamine

WADA group
S1. STIMULANTS

CAS Registry number
14089-52-2

Short synonyms
MDEA

Long synonyms
amphetamine,3,4 methylenedioxy n ethyl
amphetamine,n ethyl 3,4 methylenedioxy
3,4 methylenedioxyamphetamine,n ethyl
3,4 methylenedioxy n ethylamphetamine
n ethyl alpha methyl 3,4 methylenedioxyphenethylamine

5 ethyl 5 (3 methyl 2 butenyl)barbituric acid

WADA group
S1. STIMULANTS

Long synonyms
barbituric acid,5 ethyl 5 (3' methylbut 2' enyl)
5 ethyl 5 (3' methylbut 2' enyl)barbituric acid

4 ethyl 6,7 dimethoxy beta carboline 3 carboxylic acid methyl ester

WADA group
S1. STIMULANTS

CAS Registry number
82499-00-1

Trade names and research codes
zk 90798

Short synonyms
DMCM

Long synonyms
3 carbomethoxy 4 ethyl 6,7 dimethoxy beta carboline
3 carbomethoxy 6,7 dimethoxy 4 ethyl beta carboline
6,7 dimethoxy 4 ethyl 3 carbomethoxy beta carboline
6,7 dimethoxy 4 ethyl beta carboline 3 carboxylic acid methyl ester
methyl 4 ethyl 6,7 dimethoxy beta carboline 3 carboxylate
methyl 6,7 dimethoxy 4 ethyl beta carboline 3 carboxylate

n ethylamphetamine

WADA group
S1. STIMULANTS

CAS Registry number
457-87-4

Short synonyms
adiparthrol
apetinil
ethyl amphetamine
ethylamphetamine
etilamphetamine
n ethyl amphetamine
1 phenyl 2 ethylaminopropane

Long synonyms
n ethyl alpha methylphenethylamine

ethylestrenol

WADA group
S4. ANABOLIC AGENTS

MeSH descriptor
ethylestrenol

CAS Registry number
965-90-2

Trade names and research codes
artoron
duraboral
maxibolin
orabolin
orgabolin

Short synonyms
ethylestranol
ethylestrenal
ethyl estrenol
ethylestrenole
ethylnandrol
ethyloestrenol

1 (2 ethylphenoxy) 3 (1,2,3,4 tetrahydro 1 naphthylamino) 2 propanol oxalate

WADA group
P2. BETA-BLOCKERS

CAS Registry number
174689-39-5

Trade names and research codes
sr 59230
sr 59230a
sr 59483a

Long synonyms
3 (2 ethylphenoxy) 1 (1,2,3,4 tetrahydronaphth 1 ylamino) 2 propanol oxalate

etilefrine

WADA group
S1. STIMULANTS
S6. BETA-2 AGONISTS

MeSH descriptor
etilefrine

CAS Registry number
10128-36-6
534-87-2
709-55-7
943-17-9

Trade names and research codes
bioflutin
circupon
confidol
effontil
effortil
efortil
ethyl adrianol
ethyladrianol
etipuren
fetanol
fetanyl
m 1 36
phetanol
phetanyl
thomasin
thomasin retard

Short synonyms
ethyladrianol hydrochloride
ethyl norphenylephrine
ethylnorphenyl ephrine
ethylnorphenylephrine
ethylphenylephrine
etilefrine acetate
etilefrine butyrate
etilefrine hydrochloride
etilefrine propionate
etilefrine sulfate

Long synonyms
alpha ethylaminomethyl 3 hydroxybenzyl alcohol
2 ethylamino 1 hydroxy 1 (3 hydroxyphenyl)ethane
ethylphenylephrine hydrochloride
1 (3 hydroxyphenyl) 2 ethylaminoethanol hydrochloride

etilefrine pivalate

WADA group
S1. STIMULANTS
S6. BETA-2 AGONISTS

CAS Registry number
85750-39-6

Trade names and research codes
k 30 052
k 30052

Long synonyms
etilefrine pivalate hydrochloride

etiocholanone

WADA group
S4. ANABOLIC AGENTS

CAS Registry number
1912-61-4

Short synonyms
5beta androstan 17 one
5beta androstanone
ethiocholanone

etozolin

WADA group
S8. MASKING AGENTS
P3. DIURETICS

CAS Registry number
73-09-6

Trade names and research codes
elkapin
go 687
go687
goe 687
goe687
w 2900
w2900

Short synonyms
etazolin
etozoline
ozolinone ethyl ester

Long synonyms
2 carbethoxymethylene 3 methyl 5 piperid 1 yl 4 thiazolidinone
2 carbethoxymethylene 3 methyl 5 piperidino 4 thiazolidone
ethyl 3 methyl 4 oxo 5 piperid 1 ylthiazolidinylidene 2 acetate
ethyl 3 methyl 4 oxo 5 piperidino 2 thiazolidinylideneacetate

exaprolol

WADA group
P2. BETA-BLOCKERS

CAS Registry number
55837-19-9
59333-90-3

Trade names and research codes
mg 8823

Long synonyms
3 (2 cyclohexylphenoxy) 1 (isopropylamino)propan 2 ol
1 (2 cyclohexylphenoxy) 3 (isopropylamino) 2 propanol
1 (2 cyclohexylphenoxy) 3 (isopropylamino)propan 2 ol

exemestane

WADA group
S7. AGENTS WITH ANTI-OESTROGENIC ACTIVITY

CAS Registry number
107868-30-4

Trade names and research codes
aromasin
fce 24304
fce24304
nikidess
pnu 155971
pnu155971

Long synonyms
6 methyleneandrosta 1,4 diene 3,17 dione

fadrozole

WADA group
S7. AGENTS WITH ANTI-OESTROGENIC ACTIVITY

MeSH descriptor
fadrozole

CAS Registry number
102676-31-3

Trade names and research codes
afema
arensin
cgs 16949
cgs16949
cgs 16949 a
cgs 16949a
cgs16949a

Short synonyms
fadrozole hydrochloride

Long synonyms
5 (4 cyanophenyl) 3,6,7,8 tetrahydro 5h imidazo[1,5 a]pyridine
4 (3,6,7,8 tetrahydro 5h imidazo[1,5 a]pyridin 5 yl)benzonitrile

falintolol

WADA group
P2. BETA-BLOCKERS

CAS Registry number
90581-63-8

Long synonyms
o [3 (tert butylamino) 2 hydroxypropyl]cyclopropyl methyl ketone oxime

falintolol oxalate

WADA group
P2. BETA-BLOCKERS

CAS Registry number
96479-88-8
96479-90-2
96479-92-4
96479-94-6

felodipine plus metoprolol

WADA group
P2. BETA-BLOCKERS

Trade names and research codes
logimax
mobloc

Short synonyms
metoprolol plus felodipine

fencamfamin

WADA group
S1. STIMULANTS

CAS Registry number
1209-98-9
2240-14-4

Trade names and research codes
euvitol
glucoenergan
h 610
n 610
reactivan

Short synonyms
fenacamfamine
fencamfamine
fencamfamine hydrochloride
fencamfamin hydrochloride

Long synonyms
2 ethylamino 3 phenylbicyclo[2.2.1]heptane
2 ethylamino 3 phenylnorbornane
2 ethylamino 3 phenylnorcamphane
n ethyl 3 phenylbicyclo[2.2.1]heptan 2 amine
n ethyl 3 phenylbicyclo[2.2.1]hept 2 ylamine
n ethyl 3 phenyl 2 norbornanamine
n ethyl 3 phenyl 2 norcamphanamine
2 phenyl 3 ethylaminobicyclo[2.2.1]heptane
2 phenyl 3 ethylaminonorbornane

fenetylline

WADA group
S1. STIMULANTS

CAS Registry number
1892-80-4
1-8-3736

Trade names and research codes
biocapton
captagon
r 720 11

Short synonyms
amfetyline
amphetyline
fenethylline
fenethylline hydrochloride
fenetyllin
phenetylline
theophyllineethylamphetamine

Long synonyms
7 [2 [(alpha methylphenethyl)amino]ethyl]theophylline
7 [beta (alpha methyl beta phenylethylamino)ethyl]theophylline
7 (3 phenyl 2 propylaminoethyl)theophylline
7 (phenylisopropylaminoethyl)theophylline

fenfluramine

WADA group
S1. STIMULANTS

MeSH descriptor
fenfluramine

CAS Registry number
404-82-0
458-24-2

Trade names and research codes
ahr 965
ahr965
dimafen
fenured
kataline

minifage
moderex
pesos
ponderal
ponderax
ponderex
pondimin
ponflural
ponflural retard
val 1177
val1177

Short synonyms
dextro levo fenfluramine
dl fenfluramine
fenfluramide
fenfluramin
fenfluramine hydrochloride
l fenylfluramine
phenfluoramine

Long synonyms
2 ethylamino 1 (3 trifluoromethylphenyl)propane
n ethyl alpha methyl 3 (trifluoromethyl)phenethylamine
n ethyl alpha methyl 3 trifluoromethylphenylethylamine
n ethyl meta trifluoromethylamphetamine
phenylethylamine,n ethyl alpha methyl 3 trifluoromethyl

fenoldopam

WADA group
S1. STIMULANTS

MeSH descriptor
fenoldopam

CAS registry number
67227-56-9

Trade names and research codes
skf 82526
skf r 82526

Long synonyms
6 chloro 7,8 dihydroxy 1 (4 hydroxyphenyl) 2,3,4,5 tetrahydro 1h 3 benzazepine
6 chloro 7,8 dihydroxy 1 (para hydroxyphenyl) 2,3,4,5 tetrahydro 1h 3 benzazepine
6 chloro 2,3,4,5 tetrahydro 7,8 dihydroxy 1 (4 hydroxyphenyl) 1h 3 benzazepine
6 chloro 2,3,4,5 tetrahydro 1 (4 hydroxyphenyl) 1h 3 benzazepine 7,8 diol
6 chloro 2,3,4,5 tetrahydro 1 (para hydroxyphenyl) 1h 3 benzazepine 7,8 diol

fenoldopam 7,8 bis(n ethylcarbamate)

WADA group
S1. STIMULANTS

CAS Registry number
125375-99-7

Trade names and research codes
skf r 106114

fenoldopam mesilate

WADA group
S1. STIMULANTS

CAS Registry number
67227-57-0

Trade names and research codes
corlopam
skf 82526 j

Short synonyms
fenoldopam mesylate

Long synonyms
6 chloro 2,3,4,5 tetrahydro 1 (4 hydroxyphenyl) 1h 3 benzazepine 7,8 diol methanesulfonate

fenoterol

WADA group
S6. BETA-2 AGONISTS

MeSH descriptor
fenoterol

CAS Registry number
13392-18-2
3-12-1944

Trade names and research codes
berotec
dosberotec
dosberotec inhaletten
partusisten
partusisten perlongets
th 1165
th 1165 a
th 1165a

Short synonyms
diphenorciprenaline
fenoterol hydrobromide
hydroxyphenylorciprenaline
phenoterol

Long synonyms
beta',3',4,5' tetrahydroxy alpha methyldiphenethylamine
beta,3,4',5 tetrahydroxy alpha' methyldiphenethylamine
3,5 dihydroxy alpha (4 hydroxy alpha methylphenethylaminomethyl)benzyl alcohol
3,5 dihydroxy alpha [(4 hydroxy alpha methylphenethyl)aminomethyl]benzyl alcohol
3,5 dihydroxy alpha [((para hydroxy alpha methylphenethyl)amino)methyl]benzylalcohol
1 (3,5 dihydroxyphenyl) 2 (4 hydroxy alpha methylphenethylamino)ethanol
5 [1 hydroxy 2 [[2 (4 hydroxyphenyl) 1 methylethyl]amino]ethyl] 1,3 benzenediol

fenoterol plus ipratropium bromide

WADA group
S6. BETA-2 AGONISTS

Trade names and research codes
berodual
bronchodual
duovent
iprafen

Long synonyms
ipratropium bromide plus fenoterol

Terms and Synonyms

fenproporex

WADA group
S1. STIMULANTS

CAS Registry number
15686-61-0

Trade names and research codes
antiobes retard

Short synonyms
desobesi
dicel
n (2 cyanoethyl)amphetamine
phenproporex

fenquizone

WADA group
S8. MASKING AGENTS
P3. DIURETICS

CAS Registry number
20287-37-0

Trade names and research codes
idrolone
mg 13054

Long synonyms
7 chloro 1,2,3,4 tetrahydro 2 phenyl 6 sulfonamido 4 quinazolinone
7 chloro 1,2,3,4 tetrahydro 4 oxo 2 phenyl 6 quinazolinesulfonamide

finrozole

WADA group
S7. AGENTS WITH ANTI-OESTROGENIC ACTIVITY

CAS Registry number
160146-16-7
160146-17-8

Trade names and research codes
mpv 2213ad
mpv2213ad

Long synonyms
4 [3 (4 fluorophenyl) 2 hydroxy 1 (1,2,4 triazol 1 yl)propyl]benzonitrile

flerobuterol

WADA group
S6. BETA-2 AGONISTS

CAS Registry number
101687-91-6
101687-92-7
101687-94-9
82101-10-8

Long synonyms
alpha (tert butylaminomethyl) 2 fluorobenzyl alcohol
2 tert butylamino 1 (2 fluorophenyl)ethanol

flestolol

WADA group
P2. BETA-BLOCKERS

CAS Registry number
87721-62-8
88844-73-9

Trade names and research codes
acc 9089
acc9089

Short synonyms
flestolol sulfate

Long synonyms
3 [[2 [(aminocarbonyl)amino] 1,1 dimethylethyl]amino] 2 hydroxypropyl 2 fluorobenzoate
3 [[1,1 dimethyl 2 [(aminocarbonyl)amino]ethyl]amino] 2 hydroxypropyl 2 fluorobenzoate
3 [(1,1 dimethyl 2 ureidoethyl)amino] 2 hydroxypropyl 2 fluorobenzoate
1 (1,1 dimethyl 2 ureidoethylamino) 3 (2 fluorobenzoyloxy) 2 propanol
n (1,1 dimethyl 2 ureidoethyl) 2 hydroxy 3 (2 fluorobenzoyloxy)propylamine
n (1,1 dimethyl 2 ureidoethyl) 2 hydroxy 3 (ortho fluorobenzoyloxy)propylamine

fluclorolone

WADA group
S9. GLUCOCORTICOSTEROIDS

CAS Registry number
3693-38-7

fluclorolone acetonide

WADA group
S9. GLUCOCORTICOSTEROIDS

CAS Registry number
3693-39-8

Trade names and research codes
rs 2252
topilar

Short synonyms
flucloronide

fludrocortisone

WADA group
S9. GLUCOCORTICOSTEROIDS

MeSH descriptor
fludrocortisone

CAS Registry number
127-31-1

Trade names and research codes
alflorone
astonin h
f cortef
florinef
fludrone
fludronef
flurinef

Short synonyms
9alpha fludrocortisone
9alpha fluorocortisal
9 alpha fluorocortisol
9alpha fluorocortisol
alpha fluorohydrocortisone
9alpha fluorohydro cortisone
9alpha fluorohydrocortisone
fludrocortisol
fludrocortone
fludrohydrocortisone
fluohydrisone
fluohydrocortisone
fluorhydrocortisonum
fluorocortisone
fluorohydrocortisone
flurohydrocortisone

fludrocortisone acetate

WADA group
S9. GLUCOCORTICOSTEROIDS

CAS Registry number
514-36-3

Trade names and research codes
alfafluorone
alfanonidrone
cortineff
f cortef acetate
florinef acetate
scherofluran
scherofluron

Short synonyms
9alpha fluorocortisol acetate
fludrocortisate
fludrocortisone 21 acetate
fluohydrisone acetate
fluohydrocortisone acetate
fluorhydrocortisone actetate
fluorohydrocortisone acetate

Long synonyms
9alpha fluorohydrocortisone acetate

fludroxycortide

WADA group
S9. GLUCOCORTICOSTEROIDS

MeSH descriptor
flurandrenolone

CAS Registry number
1524-88-5

Trade names and research codes
cordran
cordran n
drenison
drocort
haelan
l 33379
sermaka

Short synonyms
fluandrenalone
fluandrenolide
fluandrenolone
fluandrenolone acetonide
fludroxycordide
fludroxy cortide
fluorandrenolone
flurandrenolide
flurandrenolon
flurandrenolone
flurandrenolone acetonide

Long synonyms
fluorodihydroxycorticosterone acetonide

flumetasone

WADA group
S9. GLUCOCORTICOSTEROIDS

MeSH descriptor
flumethasone

CAS Registry number
2135-17-3

Trade names and research codes
cortexilar
flumilar
nsc 54702
nsc54702
rs 2177
rs2177

Short synonyms
6alpha fluorodexamethasone
dexamethasone,6alpha fluoro
flumethason
flumethasone

Long synonyms
6alpha,9alpha difluoro 11beta,17,21 trihydroxy 16alpha methylpregna 1,4 diene 3,20 dione
6alpha,9alpha difluoro 11beta,17alpha,21 trihydroxy 16alpha methylpregna 1,4 diene 3,20 dione
6alpha,9alpha difluoro 16alpha methylprednisolone
prednisolone,6alpha,9alpha difluoro 16alpha methyl

flumetasone acetate

WADA group
S9. GLUCOCORTICOSTEROIDS

Trade names and research codes
flucort
flucort cream
methagon

Short synonyms
flumethasone 21 acetate
flumethasone acetate

Long synonyms
6alpha fluorodexamethasone acetate

flumetasone pivalate

WADA group
S9. GLUCOCORTICOSTEROIDS

CAS Registry number
2002-29-1

Trade names and research codes
cerson
cersone
locacorten
locacorten tar
locorten
lorinden
nsc 107680
nsc107680

Short synonyms
flumetasone 21 pivalate
flumetasone trimethylacetate
flumetazone pivalate
flumethasone pivalate
flumethazone pivalate

flumetasone pivalate plus salicylic acid

WADA group
S9. GLUCOCORTICOSTEROIDS

CAS Registry number
57973-63-4

Trade names and research codes
locasalen
locosalen
losalen
salena

Long synonyms
flumetasone pivalate salicylic acid
flumethasone pivalate salicylic acid
salicylic acid plus flumetasone pivalate

flumetasone pivalate plus triclosan

WADA group
S9. GLUCOCORTICOSTEROIDS

Trade names and research codes
logamel

Long synonyms
flumethasone pivalate plus triclosan
triclosan plus flumetasone pivalate
triclosan plus flumethasone pivalate

flumoxonide

WADA group
S9. GLUCOCORTICOSTEROIDS

CAS Registry number
60135-22-0

Trade names and research codes
rs 40584
rs40584

Long synonyms
6alpha,9 difluoro 11beta hydroxy 21,21 dimethoxy 16alpha,17 [(1 methylethylidene)bis(oxy)]pregna 1,4 diene 3,20 dione

flunisolide

WADA group
S9. GLUCOCORTICOSTEROIDS

CAS Registry number
3-3-3385

Trade names and research codes
aerobid
bronalide
bronilide
cyntaris
inhacort
locasyn
lokilan
lunis
nasalide
nasarel
rhinalar
rs 3999
rs3999
synaclyn
syntaris
val 679
val679

Short synonyms
6beta flunisolide
flunisolide hemihydrate

Long synonyms
6alpha fluoro 11beta,16alpha,17,21 tetrahydroxypregna 1,4 diene 3,20 dione acetonide

flunisolide acetate

WADA group
S9. GLUCOCORTICOSTEROIDS

CAS Registry number
4533-89-5

Trade names and research codes
rs 1320
rs1320

fluocinolone

WADA group
S9. GLUCOCORTICOSTEROIDS

CAS Registry number
807-38-5

Short synonyms
flucinolone
fluocinolon

Long synonyms
6alpha,9alpha difluoro 11beta,16alpha,17,21 tetrahydroxypregna 1,4 diene 3,20 dione
6alpha,9alpha difluoro 11beta,16alpha,17alpha,21 tetrahydroxypregna 1,4 diene 3,20 dione
6alpha,9alpha difluoro 16alpha hydroxyprednisolone

fluocinolone acetonide

WADA group
S9. GLUCOCORTICOSTEROIDS

MeSH descriptor
fluocinolone acetonide

CAS Registry number
67-73-2

Trade names and research codes
fluolar
fluonid
fluonide
fluotrex
jellin
localyn
localyn glicole
nasal synalar
neosynalar
psoranide
retisert
rs 1401 at
rs1401 at
synalar

Terms and Synonyms

synalar forte
synalar gamma
synalar nasal
synandone
synemol
synotic
trisyn

Short synonyms
flucinolone acetonide
fluocinolon acetonid
fluocinolone 16,17 acetonide
nasal fluocinolone acetonide

fluocinonide

WADA group
S9. GLUCOCORTICOSTEROIDS

MeSH descriptor
fluocinonide

CAS Registry number
356-12-7

Trade names and research codes
flucinar
lidex
lidex e
lydex
lydex e
metosyn
nsc 101791
nsc101791
ruful
topsym
topsyn
topsyne

Short synonyms
fluocinolide
fluocinolone acetonide acetate

Long synonyms
fluocinole acetonide 21 acetate
fluocinolone acetonide 21 acetate

fluocortin

WADA group
S9. GLUCOCORTICOSTEROIDS

CAS Registry number
33124-50-4

Trade names and research codes
rhinolar

Long synonyms
6alpha fluoro 11beta hydroxy 16alpha methyl 3,20 dioxopregna 1,4 dien 21 oic acid
progesterone,1 dehydro 21 carboxy 6alpha fluoro 11beta hydroxy 16alpha methyl

fluocortin butyl

WADA group
S9. GLUCOCORTICOSTEROIDS

CAS Registry number
41767-29-7

Trade names and research codes
sh k 203
sh k203
vaspit

Short synonyms
flucortin butyl
fluocortin butyl ester
fluorocortin butyl ester

Long synonyms
6alpha fluoro 11beta hydroxy 16alpha methyl 3,20 dioxopregna 1,4 dien 21 oic acid butyl ester
butyl 6alpha fluoro 11beta hydroxy 16alpha methyl 3,20 dioxopregna 1,4 dien 21 oate
3,20 dioxo 6alpha fluoro 11beta hydroxy 16alpha methylpregna 1,4 dien 21 oic acid butyl ester

fluocortolone

WADA group
S9. GLUCOCORTICOSTEROIDS

MeSH descriptor
fluocortolone

CAS Registry number
152-97-6

Trade names and research codes
syracort
topodil
ultracur

Short synonyms
flucortolon
flucortolone
fluocortolone monohydrate
fluorocortolone

Long synonyms
6alpha fluoro 11beta,21 dihydroxy 16alpha methylpregna 1,4 diene 3,20 dione
6alpha fluoro 16alpha methyl 1 dehydrocorticosterone
6alpha fluoro 16alpha methyl delta1,4 pregnadiene 11beta,21 diol 3,20 dione

fluocortolone caproate

WADA group
S9. GLUCOCORTICOSTEROIDS

CAS Registry number
303-40-2

Trade names and research codes
ultralan

Short synonyms
flucortolon caproate
flucortolon capronate
flucortolone caproate
flucortolone capronate
flucortolone hexanoate
fluocortolon caproate
fluocortolone 21 caproate
fluocortolone 21 hexanoate
fluocortolone capronate
fluocortolone hexanoate
fluorcortolone 21 capronate
fluor cortolone caproate
fluorocortolone caproate

fluocortolone pivalate

WADA group
S9. GLUCOCORTICOSTEROIDS

CAS Registry number
29205-06-9

probably not prohibited

Short synonyms
flucortolone trimethyl acetate
flucortolonetrimethyl acetate
fluocortolone trimethylacetate

Long synonyms
fluocortolone trimethyl acetate
fluorocortolone trimethyl acetate

fluorometholone

WADA group
S9. GLUCOCORTICOSTEROIDS

MeSH descriptor
fluorometholone

CAS Registry number
426-13-1

Trade names and research codes
cortilet
delmeson
delmesone
efflumidex
fluaton
flucon
flumetholon
fluorlon
fluorlon lavsan
fml forte
fml liquifilm
isopto flucon
loticort
methasite
oxylone

Short synonyms
fluometholone
fluormetholon
fluoromethalone

Long synonyms
9alpha fluoro 11beta,17alpha dihydroxy 6alpha methylpregna 1,4 diene 3,20 dione
21 desoxy 6alpha methyl 9alpha fluoroprednisolone
21 desoxy 9alpha fluoro 6alpha methylprednisolone

2 [2 (4 fluorophenoxy)ethyl]phenol

WADA group
S8. MASKING AGENTS
P3. DIURETICS

CAS Registry number
132194-67-3

Trade names and research codes
cre 10904
cre10904

[2 [2 (4 fluorophenoxy)ethyl]phenyl] sulfate

WADA group
S8. MASKING AGENTS
P3. DIURETICS

Trade names and research codes
cre 11296
cre11296

fluosol

WADA group
M1. ENHANCEMENT OF OXYGEN TRANSFER

CAS Registry number
83271-20-9

Trade names and research codes
fluosol

fluosol da

WADA group
M1. ENHANCEMENT OF OXYGEN TRANSFER

CAS Registry number
75216-20-5

Trade names and research codes
fluosol da
fluosol da 20
perfucol

Long synonyms
perfluorodecalin plus perfluorotripropylamine

fluoxymesterone

WADA group
S4. ANABOLIC AGENTS

MeSH descriptor
fluoxymesterone

CAS Registry number
76-43-7

Trade names and research codes
androfluorene
androfluorone
android f
fluosterone
fluotestin
halotensin
halotestin
nsc 12165
nsc12165
oratestin
ora testryl
testoral
ultandren

Short synonyms
fluoroxymesterone
fluoximesterone
fluoxymesteron
fluoxymestrone

Long synonyms
9alpha fluoro 11beta,17beta dihydroxy 17 methylandrost 4 en 3 one
9alpha fluoro 11beta hydroxy 17alpha methyltestosterone
11beta,17beta dihydroxy 9alpha fluoro 17alpha methyl 4 androsten 3 one

fluprednidene

WADA group
S9. GLUCOCORTICOSTEROIDS

CAS Registry number
2193-87-5

Short synonyms
fluoprednilidene
fluorprednylidene
fluprednilidene
fluprednylidene

Long synonyms
9 fluoro 11beta,17,21 trihydroxy 16 methylenepregna 1,4 diene 3,20 dione

fluprednidene acetate

WADA group
S9. GLUCOCORTICOSTEROIDS

CAS Registry number
1255-35-2

Trade names and research codes
corticoderm
decoderm
stc 1106
stc1106
vobaderm

Short synonyms
decoderm trivalent
decoderm trivalent cream
emcortina
etacortin
fluoprednilidene 21 acetate
fluoprednylidene 21 acetate
fluoprednylidene acetate
fluoroprednilidene
fluoroprednylidene 21 acetate
fluprednidene 21 acetate
fluprednilene 21 acetate
flupredniliden acetate
fluprednilidene 21 acetate
fluprednilidene acetate
fluprednylen 21 acetate
fluprednyliden 21 acetate
fluprednylidene 21 acetate
fluprednylidene acetate
fluprednylidene acetate cream
r fluprednylidene acetate
sali decoderm

fluprednisolone

WADA group
S9. GLUCOCORTICOSTEROIDS

MeSH descriptor
fluprednisolone

CAS Registry number
53-34-9

Trade names and research codes
alphadrol
b 673
b673
lukrutor
nsc 47439
nsc47439

Short synonyms
6 alpha fluoroprednisolone
6alpha fluoroprednisolone

flurothyl

WADA group
S1. STIMULANTS

MeSH descriptor
flurothyl

CAS Registry number
333-36-8

Trade names and research codes
indoklon
indokolon

Short synonyms
bis(trifluoroethyl) ether
fluorothyl
flurothil
flurotyl
hexafluorodiethyl ether
hexafluorodiethylether
hfe

Long synonyms
bis (2,2,2 trifluoroethyl)ether
bis(2,2,2 trifluoroethyl) ether

flusoxolol

WADA group
P2. BETA-BLOCKERS

CAS Registry number
84057-96-5

Trade names and research codes
ro 31 1118
ro 31-1118
ro31 1118
ro31-1118
ro 31 1411
ro 31-1411
ro31 1411
ro31-1411

Long synonyms
1 [4 [2 (4 fluorophenethyloxy)ethoxy]phenoxy] 3 isopropylamino 2 propanol

fluticasone

WADA group
S9. GLUCOCORTICOSTEROIDS

CAS Registry number
90566-53-3

fluticasone propionate

WADA group
S9. GLUCOCORTICOSTEROIDS

CAS Registry number
80474-14-2

Trade names and research codes
atemur
axotide
cci 18781
cci18781
cutivate
flixonase
flixotide

flonase
flovent
flunase
fluspiral
flutide
flutide nasal
flutinase
flutivate
fluxonal
gr 18781
gr18781

fluticasone propionate plus salmeterol

WADA group
S6. BETA-2 AGONISTS
S9. GLUCOCORTICOSTEROIDS

Trade names and research codes
advair
seretide
viani

Long synonyms
salmeterol plus fluticasone propionate

folligen

WADA group
S5. PEPTIDE HORMONES

CAS Registry number
103631-79-4

Long synonyms
gonadorelin[1-9] ethylamide[6 dextro phenylalanine 8 glutamine]

follitropin

WADA group
S5. PEPTIDE HORMONES

MeSH descriptor
follicle stimulating hormone

CAS Registry number
9002-68-0

Trade names and research codes
fertiline
fertinom p
folltropin
fsh nosticon
ovagen
super ov

Short synonyms
follicle stimulating hormone
follicotropin
folliculostimulating hormone
follitrophin
follitropine
FSH
human follitropin
human fsh
ovine fsh
rat follitropin
rat fsh

Long synonyms
follicle stimulating hormone, human
human follicle stimulating hormone
ovine follicle stimulating hormone

follitropin beta subunit

WADA group
S5. PEPTIDE HORMONES

MeSH descriptor
follicle stimulating hormone, beta subunit

Short synonyms
follitropin beta fragment
FSH beta fragment
FSH beta subunit

Long synonyms
follicle stimulating hormone beta fragment
follicle stimulating hormone beta subunit
follicle stimulating hormone, beta subunit

follitropin derivative

WADA group
S5. PEPTIDE HORMONES

Short synonyms
fsh derivative

follitropin receptor binding inhibitor

WADA group
S5. PEPTIDE HORMONES

Short synonyms
fsh receptor binding inhibitor

Long synonyms
follicle stimulating hormone receptor binding inhibitor

follitropin releasing factor

WADA group
S5. PEPTIDE HORMONES

CAS Registry number
9034-38-2

Short synonyms
follitropin release factor
fsh releasing factor
fsh releasing hormone
fsh rf
fsh rh

Long synonyms
factor,follicle stimulating hormone releasing
follicle stimulating hormone release factor
follicle stimulating hormone releasing factor
follicle stimulating hormone rf
releasing factor,follicle stimulating hormone

fominoben

WADA group
S1. STIMULANTS

CAS Registry number
18053-31-1
24600-36-0

Trade names and research codes
pb 89
pb89
terion

Long synonyms
3' chloro 2' (methylmorpholinocarbonylmethylaminomethyl)benzanilide

formebolone

WADA group
S4. ANABOLIC AGENTS

CAS Registry number
7-11-2454

Trade names and research codes
esiclene

Short synonyms
formyldienolone

Long synonyms
2 formyl 11alpha,17beta dihydroxy 17 methyl 1,4 androstadien 3 one

formestane

WADA group
S7. AGENTS WITH ANTI-OESTROGENIC ACTIVITY

CAS Registry number
566-48-3

Trade names and research codes
cgp 32349
cgp32349
lentaron

Short synonyms
androst 4 en 4 ol 3,17 dione
androstenedione,4 hydroxy
4 hydroxyandrostene 3,17 dione
4 hydroxyandrostenedione

Long synonyms
4 hydroxy 4 androstene 3,17 dione
4 hydroxyandrost 4 ene 3,17 dione

formetorex

WADA group
S1. STIMULANTS

CAS Registry number
15302-18-8

Short synonyms
amphetamine,n formyl
formetamide
n formylamphetamine

Long synonyms
n formyl alpha methylphenethylamine

formocortal

WADA group
S9. GLUCOCORTICOSTEROIDS

CAS Registry number
2825-60-7

Trade names and research codes
deflamene
fluderma

Short synonyms
fluorofarmilone
formocortral
formoftil

formoterol

WADA group
S6. BETA-2 AGONISTS

CAS Registry number
73573-87-2

Trade names and research codes
oxis

Short synonyms
eformoterol

Long synonyms
2' hydroxy 5' [1 hydroxy 2 [(4 methoxy alpha methylphenethyl)amino]ethyl]formanilide

formoterol fumarate

WADA group
S6. BETA-2 AGONISTS

CAS Registry number
43229-80-7

Trade names and research codes
atock
bd 40a
bd40a
cgp 25827a
cgp25827a
cgp 25827 a-e
cgp 25827a-e
cgp25827a-e
foradil
fordilen
ym 08316
ym08316

Short synonyms
eformoterol fumarate
formoterol hemifumarate

Long synonyms
3 formamido 4 hydroxy alpha [[(4 methoxy alpha methylphenethyl)amino]methyl]benzenemethanol fumarate
3 formamido 4 hydroxy alpha [[(para methoxy alpha methylphenethyl)amino]methyl]benzylalcohol fumarate
3 formylamino 4 hydroxy alpha [[(para methoxy alpha methylphenethyl)amino]methyl]benzylalcohol hemifumarate
n [2 hydroxy 5 [1 hydroxy 2 [(4 methoxy alpha methylphenethyl)amino]ethyl]phenyl]methanamide fumarate

fresh frozen plasma

WADA group
S8. MASKING AGENTS
M1. ENHANCEMENT OF OXYGEN TRANSFER

Short synonyms
plasma,fresh frozen

frumil

WADA group
S8. MASKING AGENTS
P3. DIURETICS

CAS Registry number
92522-90-2

Trade names and research codes
frumil
frusamil

Short synonyms
amiloride plus furosemide
co amilofruse
furosemide plus amiloride

fulvestrant

WADA group
S7. AGENTS WITH ANTI-OESTROGENIC ACTIVITY

CAS Registry number
129453-61-8

Trade names and research codes
faslodex
ici 182780
ici182780
zd 182780
zd182780
zd 9238
zd9238
zm 182780
zm182780

Long synonyms
7alpha [9 (4,4,5,5,5 pentafluoropentylsulfinyl)nonyl]estra 1,3,5(10) triene 3,17beta diol

furazabol

WADA group
S4. ANABOLIC AGENTS

CAS Registry number
1239-29-8

Trade names and research codes
miotolon

Short synonyms
androfurazanol

Long synonyms
17beta hydroxy 17alpha methyl 5alpha androstano[2,3 c]furazan

furfenorex

WADA group
S1. STIMULANTS

CAS Registry number
3776-93-0

Trade names and research codes
frugalan

Short synonyms
furfurylmethylamphetamine
methamphetamine,n furfuryl
n furfurylmethamphetamine
n furfuryl n methylamphetamine

Long synonyms
n methyl n (1 phenyl 2 propyl)furfurylamine
n methyl n (alpha methylphenethyl)furfurylamine

furfurylamphetamine

WADA group
S1. STIMULANTS

Short synonyms
amphetamine,furfuryl

Long synonyms
2 furfurylamino 1 phenylpropane

furosemide

WADA group
S8. MASKING AGENTS
P3. DIURETICS

MeSH descriptor
furosemide

CAS Registry number
54-31-9

Trade names and research codes
diamazon
'discoid'
diural
diuresal
diurix
durafurid
fruzex
fumarenid
fumide
furanthril
furantril
furesis
furix
furobasan
furomide
furo puren
furopuren
furorese
furosemix
fusid
hydro rapid
impugan
lasilix
lasix
laxis
lb 502
lb502
luramide
oedemase
oedemex
sigasalur

Short synonyms
aluzine
diumide
eutensin
eutensine
flurosemide
frusemide
furasemide
furosamide
furose
furosemid
furosimide
fursemide

Terms and Synonyms

lasiletten
lasix retard
mirfat
salinex
seguril
vesix

Long synonyms
4 chloro n 2 furfuryl 5 sulfamoylanthranilic acid
4 chloro n (2 furylmethyl) 5 sulfamoylanthranilic acid
4 chloro n furfuryl 5 sulfamoylanthranilic acid

furosemide plus triamterene

WADA group
S8. MASKING AGENTS
P3. DIURETICS

Trade names and research codes
diutrix
dysemide
frusene
hydrotrix
salidur

Short synonyms
furosemide with triamterene
triamterene plus furosemide
triamterene with furosemide

gelatinol

WADA group
S8. MASKING AGENTS

CAS Registry number
39340-56-2

Trade names and research codes
gelatinol

gelatin succinate

WADA group
S8. MASKING AGENTS

CAS Registry number
39340-57-3

Trade names and research codes
gelofusine

Short synonyms
gelatin succinic anhydride
succinylated gelatin

gepefrine

WADA group
S1. STIMULANTS
S6. BETA-2 AGONISTS

CAS Registry number
18840-47-6

Short synonyms
alpha methyl meta tyramine
alpha methyl m tyramine
3 (2 aminopropyl)phenol
amphetamine,meta hydroxy
d,l alpha methyl meta tyramine
gepefrin
m (2 aminopropyl)phenol
meta (2 aminopropyl)phenol
meta hydroxyamphetamine

Long synonyms
2 amino 1 (3 hydroxyphenyl)propane
dextro levo alpha methyl meta tyramine
1 (3 hydroxyphenyl) 2 aminopropane

gepefrine tartrate

WADA group
S1. STIMULANTS
S6. BETA-2 AGONISTS

Trade names and research codes
pressionorm
wintonin

gestrinone

WADA group
S4. ANABOLIC AGENTS

MeSH descriptor
gestrinone

CAS Registry number
16320-04-0

Trade names and research codes
a 46 745
a 46745
a46745
dimetriose
dimetrose
nemestran
r 2323
r2323
ru 2323
ru2323
tridomose

Long synonyms
17alpha ethinyl 13beta ethyl 17 hydroxygona 4,9,11 trien 3 one
17alpha pregna 4,9,11 trien 17 ol 20 yn 3 one, 13 ethyl 18,19 nor
13beta ethyl 17alpha ethynyl 17 hydroxygona 4,9,11 trien 3 one
13 ethyl 17alpha ethynyl 17beta hydroxygona 4,9,11 trien 3 one
13 ethyl 17alpha ethynyl 17 hydroxygona 4,9,11 trien 3 one
13 ethyl 17 hydroxy 18,19 dinor 17alpha pregna 4,9,11 trien 20 yn 3 one

giractide

WADA group
S5. PEPTIDE HORMONES

CAS Registry number
24870-04-0

glucocorticoid

WADA group
S9. GLUCOCORTICOSTEROIDS

MeSH descriptor
glucocorticoids, synthetic
glucocorticoids, topical
glucocorticoids

Short synonyms
glucocorticoid drug
glucocorticoid hormone
glucocorticoids
glucocorticoids, synthetic
glucocorticoid steroid
glucocorticoidsteroid
glucocorticoids, topical
glucocorticosteroid
glucocortoid
glycocorticoid
glycocorticosteroid

glycosylated hemoglobin

WADA group
M1. ENHANCEMENT OF OXYGEN TRANSFER

MeSH descriptor
hemoglobin a, glycosylated

CAS Registry number
9062-63-9

Short synonyms
glycated hemoglobin
glycohemoglobin
glycosyl hemoglobin
glycosylhemoglobin
glycosylized hemoglobin
hb a 1
hb a1
hemoglobin A1
hemoglobin a 1
hemoglobin a, glycosylated
hemoglobin ai
hemoglobin alpha 1
hemoglobin glycoside
hemoglobin glycosylation

gonadorelin

WADA group
S5. PEPTIDE HORMONES

MeSH descriptor
gonadorelin

CAS Registry number
33515-09-2
9034-40-6

Trade names and research codes
ay 24,031
ay 24031
ay24,031
ay24031
cryptocur
factrel
fertagyl
fertiral
hoe 471
hoe471
ici 88262
ici88262
kryptocur
luforan
lutal
pulstim
relisorm

Short synonyms
gn rh
gnrh
gnrh serono
gonadoliberin
gonadotrophin releasing factor
gonadotropin release factor
gonadotropin releasing factor
gonadotropin releasing hormone
hoechst 471
lh releasing hormone
lhrf
LHRH
lrh
luliberin
luliberine
lutamin

Long synonyms
gonadotrophin releasing hormone
6 leucine 10 deglycine gonadotropin releasing factor ethylamide
[6 leucine 10 deglycine]gonadotropin releasing factor ethylamide
lrh luteinizing hormone releasing factor
luteinizing hormone release factor
luteinizing hormone releasing factor
luteinizing hormone releasing hormone

gonadorelin[1-9][6 dextro alanine]

WADA group
S5. PEPTIDE HORMONES

Long synonyms
gonadorelin[6 dextro alanine 10 deglycinamide]
luteinizing hormone releasing hormone[6 dextro alanine 10 deglycinamide]

gonadorelin[1-9] ethylamide[6 dextro alanine]

WADA group
S5. PEPTIDE HORMONES

CAS Registry number
52435-06-0

Trade names and research codes
surfagon
wy 18481

Long synonyms
[10 deglycine 6 dextro alanine]gonadorelin ethylamide
10 desglycyl 6 dextro alanyl gonadorelin ethylamide
6 dextro alanine 10 deglycine gonadorelin ethylamide
6 dextro alanine gonadotropin releasing hormone[1-9] ethylamide
gonadorelin[1-9]ethylamide[6 dextro alanine 9 proline]
gonadorelin[6 dextro alanine 10 deglycine n ethylamide]
gonadorelin ethylamide[10 deglycine 6 dextro alanine]
gonadorelin ethylamide[6 dextro alanine 10 deglycinamide]
gonadorelin ethylamide[6 dextro alanine 10 deglycine]
gonadorelin n ethylamide[6 dextro alanine 10 deglycine]
gonadotropin releasing hormone[6 dextro alanine 10 deglycine n ethylamide]
gonadotropin releasing hormone n ethylamide[6 dextro alanine 10 deglycine]
lhrh[6 dextro alanine 10 deglycine n ethylamide]
lhrh ethylamide[6 dextro alanine 10 deglycinamide]

gonadorelin[1-9] ethylamide[6 dextro tryptophan]

WADA group
S5. PEPTIDE HORMONES

CAS Registry number
57773-65-6

Trade names and research codes
tryptal
tryptex

Short synonyms
d trp 6 pro 9 net lhrh

Long synonyms
6 dextro tryptophan 9 proline aminoethyl gonadorelin
gonadorelin[1-9][6 dextro tryptophan] ethylamide
gonadorelin[6 dextro tryptophan 9 proline n ethylamide]
gonadorelin ethylamide[6 dextro tryptophan 10 deglycine]
gonadorelin ethylamide[6 dextro tryptophan 9 proline]
lhrh[6 dextro tryptophan 10 deglycinamide] ethylamide

gonadorelin[6 dextro [3 (2 naphthyl)alanine] 10 azaglycine]

WADA group
S5. PEPTIDE HORMONES

CAS Registry number
121897-30-1

Trade names and research codes
rs 49947

gonadorelin[6 dextro lysine] 2 pyrrolinodoxorubicin

WADA group
S5. PEPTIDE HORMONES

CAS Registry number
179910-83-9

Trade names and research codes
an 207
an-207
an207

Long synonyms
LHRH[6 dextro lysine] 2 pyrrolinodoxorubicin
2 pyrrolinodoxorubicin LHRH[6 dextro lysine]

gonadorelin[6 dextro lysine] doxorubicin

WADA group
S5. PEPTIDE HORMONES

CAS Registry number
139570-93-7

Trade names and research codes
an 152
an-152
an152

Long synonyms
doxorubicin LHRH[6 dextro lysine]
LHRH[6 dextro lysine] doxorubicin

gonadorelin[6 medphalan]

WADA group
S5. PEPTIDE HORMONES

Trade names and research codes
sb 05

Long synonyms
gonadorelin[6 dextro melphalan]

gonadorelin acetate

WADA group
S5. PEPTIDE HORMONES

CAS Registry number
52699-48-6

Trade names and research codes
abbott 41070
cryptolin
cystorelin
lutrelef
lutrepulse
ovarelin

Short synonyms
gonadorelin diacetate

gonadorelin agonist

WADA group
S5. PEPTIDE HORMONES

Short synonyms
gnrh agonist
LHRH agonist

Long synonyms
gonadotropin releasing hormone agonist
luteinizing hormone releasing hormone agonist

gonadorelin associated peptide

WADA group
S5. PEPTIDE HORMONES

CAS Registry number
124375-77-5

Short synonyms
gonadorelin associated protein

Long synonyms
gonadotropin releasing hormone associated peptide
gonadotropin releasing hormone associated protein

gonadorelin associated peptide derivative

WADA group
S5. PEPTIDE HORMONES

Long synonyms
gonadorelin associated protein derivative
gonadotropin releasing hormone associated peptide derivative
gonadotropin releasing hormone associated protein derivative

gonadorelin derivative

WADA group
S5. PEPTIDE HORMONES

Short synonyms
gnrh derivative
gonadoliberin analog
gonadoliberin derivative
gonadorelin analog
lh releasing hormone analog
lhrh a
lhrh analog
LHRH derivative
luliberin analog
luliberin derivative

Long synonyms
gonadotropin releasing factor derivative
gonadotropin releasing hormone derivative
luteinizing hormone releasing factor derivative
luteinizing hormone releasing hormone analog
luteinizing hormone releasing hormone derivative
luteinizing releasing hormone analog

gonadotropin

WADA group
S5. PEPTIDE HORMONES

MeSH descriptor
gonadotropins, pituitary
gonadotropins

CAS Registry number
63231-54-9

Trade names and research codes
ambinon
anthrogon
folistiman
gonan

Short synonyms
carp pituitary gonadotropin
gonadotrophic hormone
gonadotrophin
gonadotropic hormone
gonadotropine
gonadotropin,pituitary
gonadotropins
gonadotropins, pituitary
gonad stimulating hormone
gonad stimulatory hormone
human gonadotropin
hypophyseal gonadotropin
hypophysis gonadotropin
pituitary gonadotrophin
pituitary gonadotropin
pregonadotropin

gonadotropin derivative

WADA group
S5. PEPTIDE HORMONES

Short synonyms
gonadotrophin derivative

goserelin

WADA group
S5. PEPTIDE HORMONES

MeSH descriptor
goserelin

CAS Registry number
65807-02-5

Trade names and research codes
ici 118 630
ici 118630
ici118630
ici 118630 depot
zoladex
zoladex depot

Short synonyms
buserelin carbazamide
goserelin acetate

Long synonyms
gonadorelin[1-9][6 (o tert butyl dextro serine)]carbazamide
gonadorelin[1-9] carbazamide[6 (o tert butyl dextro serine)]
gonadorelin[6 dextro o tert butylserine 10 glycine azide]
lhrh[6 dextro o tert butylserine 10 glycine azide]
pyroglutamylhistidyltryptophylseryltyrosyl(o tert butyl dextro seryl)leucylarginylprolylcarbazamide

growth hormone

WADA group
S5. PEPTIDE HORMONES

MeSH descriptor
growth hormone

CAS Registry number
36992-73-1
37267-05-3
66419-50-9
9002-72-6

Trade names and research codes
grorm
nanormon

Short synonyms
antuitrin t
bovine growth hormone
gerohormetten
GH
growth hormone fraction
growth hormone,hypophysis
growth hormone treatment
hormone,growth
hypophysis growth hormone
immunoreactive growth hormone
leutrophin
ovine growth hormone
phyol
phyon
pituitary growth hormone
rat growth hormone
sf
somacton
somantin
somatotrofin
somatotrope hormone
somatotrophic hormone
somatotrophin
somatotropic hormone
somatotropin
somatropic hormone
st
sth

Terms and Synonyms

growth hormone derivative

WADA group
S5. PEPTIDE HORMONES

Short synonyms
growth hormone analog
somatotropin analog
somatotropin derivative

growth hormone releasing factor

WADA group
S5. PEPTIDE HORMONES

MeSH descriptor
somatotropin-releasing hormone

CAS Registry number
83930-13-6
9034-39-3

Trade names and research codes
somatobiss

Short synonyms
gh releasing factor
GHRF
gh rf
GHRH
GRF
growth hormone release factor
somatocrinin
somatocrinin 44
somatoliberin
somatorelin
somatotropin releasing factor
somatotropin-releasing hormone

Long synonyms
growth hormone releasing factor[1-44]
growth hormone releasing hormone
human pancreatic growth hormone releasing factor
pancreatic growth hormone releasing factor

growth hormone releasing factor[1-29]

WADA group
S5. PEPTIDE HORMONES

CAS Registry number
90830-28-7

Short synonyms
ghrf 1-29

Long synonyms
growth hormone releasing factor 1-29
somatotropin releasing hormone[1-29]

growth hormone releasing factor derivative

WADA group
S5. PEPTIDE HORMONES

Short synonyms
ghrf derivative
somatocrinin derivative

guanethidine plus hydrochlorothiazide

WADA group
S8. MASKING AGENTS
P3. DIURETICS

CAS Registry number
8015-24-5

Trade names and research codes
esidrex ismelin
esimil
ismelin esidrex

Long synonyms
hydrochlorothiazide plus guanethidine

halcinonide

WADA group
S9. GLUCOCORTICOSTEROIDS

MeSH descriptor
halcinonide

CAS Registry number
3093-35-4

Trade names and research codes
halciderm
halcimat
halcort
halog

Short synonyms
alcinonide
alcinonidel

Long synonyms
21 chloro 9alpha fluoro 11beta hydroxy 16alpha,17alpha isopropylidenedioxypregn 4 ene 3,20 dione
pregn 4 en 11beta ol 3,20 dione,21 chloro 9alpha fluoro 16alpha,17alpha isopropylidenedioxy

halometasone

WADA group
S9. GLUCOCORTICOSTEROIDS

CAS Registry number
50629-82-8

Trade names and research codes
sicorten

Short synonyms
alometasone

Long synonyms
2 chloro 6alpha,9 difluoro 11beta,17,21 trihydroxy 16alpha methylpregna 1,4 diene 3,20 dione
pregna 1,4 diene 11beta,17,21 triol 3,20 dione,2 chloro 6alpha,9 difluoro 16alpha methyl

halopredone

WADA group
S9. GLUCOCORTICOSTEROIDS

CAS Registry number
57781-15-4

Long synonyms
2 bromo 6beta,9 difluoro 11beta,17,21 trihydroxypregna 1,4 diene 3,20 dione
2 bromo 6beta,9 difluoroprednisolone

halopredone acetate

WADA group
S9. GLUCOCORTICOSTEROIDS

CAS Registry number
57781-14-3

Trade names and research codes
haloart
ths 201
topicon

Short synonyms
halopredone 17,21 diacetate

Long synonyms
17alpha,21 diacetoxy 2 bromo 6beta,9alpha difluoro 11beta hydroxy 1,4 pregnadiene 3,20 dione
2bromo 6beta,9 difluoro 11beta,17,21 trihydroxypregna 1,4 diene 3,20 dione 17,21 diacetate

hemodialysis fluid

WADA group
S8. MASKING AGENTS

MeSH descriptor
hemodialysis solutions

Short synonyms
hemodialysis solutions

hemoglobin

WADA group
M1. ENHANCEMENT OF OXYGEN TRANSFER

MeSH descriptor
hemoglobins

CAS Registry number
9008-02-0

Trade names and research codes
hemolink

Short synonyms
ferrohemoglobin
free hemoglobin
haemoglobin
Hb
hemoglobine
hemoglobins
hemoglobulin
unstable hemoglobin

hemoglobin A

WADA group
M1. ENHANCEMENT OF OXYGEN TRANSFER

MeSH descriptor
hemoglobin A

CAS Registry number
9034-51-9

Short synonyms
adult Hb
haemoglobin a
Hb A
hemoglobin alpha

hemoglobin A1c

WADA group
M1. ENHANCEMENT OF OXYGEN TRANSFER

CAS Registry number
62572-11-6

Short synonyms
glycated hemoglobin A1c
glycosylated hemoglobin A1c
Hb A1c
hb a(1c)
hba 1c
hba1c
hemoglobin a 1c
hemoglobin a(1c)
hemoglobin aic

hemoglobin A2

WADA group
M1. ENHANCEMENT OF OXYGEN TRANSFER

MeSH descriptor
hemoglobin A2

CAS Registry number
37203-64-8
37203-65-9
53262-80-9
9034-53-1
99493-07-9

Short synonyms
a2 hemoglobin
Hb A2
hb a 2
hemoglobin a 2
hemoglobin a2 babinga
hemoglobin a 2 indonesia
hemoglobin a 2 melbourne
hemoglobin a2 nyu
hemoglobin a2 sphakia
hemoglobin alpha 2

hemoglobin alpha chain

WADA group
M1. ENHANCEMENT OF OXYGEN TRANSFER

Short synonyms
alpha chain,hemoglobin
globin alpha chain
haemoglobin alpha chain
hb alpha chain

hemoglobin beta chain

WADA group
M1. ENHANCEMENT OF OXYGEN TRANSFER

Short synonyms
beta chain,hemoglobin
globin beta chain
haemoglobin beta chain

hb beta chain

hemoglobin C

WADA group
M1. ENHANCEMENT OF OXYGEN TRANSFER

MeSH descriptor
hemoglobin C

CAS Registry number
9008-00-8

Short synonyms
haemoglobin c
Hb C
hemoglobin gamma

hemoglobin chain

WADA group
M1. ENHANCEMENT OF OXYGEN TRANSFER

Short synonyms
haemoglobin chain
hemoglobin subunit

hemoglobin delta chain

WADA group
M1. ENHANCEMENT OF OXYGEN TRANSFER

Short synonyms
globin delta chain

hemoglobin derivative

WADA group
M1. ENHANCEMENT OF OXYGEN TRANSFER

hemoglobin E

WADA group
M1. ENHANCEMENT OF OXYGEN TRANSFER

MeSH descriptor
hemoglobin E

CAS Registry number
9034-61-1

Short synonyms
haemoglobin e
Hb E
hemoglobin e variant

hemoglobin F

WADA group
M1. ENHANCEMENT OF OXYGEN TRANSFER

MeSH descriptor
fetal hemoglobin

CAS Registry number
9034-63-3

Short synonyms
embryo hemoglobin
embryonic hemoglobin
fetal hb
fetal hemoglobin
fetus hemoglobin
foetal haemoglobin
foetal hemoglobin
haemoglobin f
HbF
hb f
hemoglobin f dammam
hemoglobin,fetal
neonatal hemoglobin f

hemoglobin gamma chain

WADA group
M1. ENHANCEMENT OF OXYGEN TRANSFER

Short synonyms
gamma chain,hemoglobin
globin gamma chain
haemoglobin gamma chain
hb gamma chain

hemoglobin H

WADA group
M1. ENHANCEMENT OF OXYGEN TRANSFER

MeSH descriptor
hemoglobin H

CAS Registry number
9034-79-1

Short synonyms
haemoglobin h
Hb H

hemoglobin J

WADA group
M1. ENHANCEMENT OF OXYGEN TRANSFER

MeSH descriptor
hemoglobin J

CAS Registry number
58128-48-6

Short synonyms
haemoglobin j
Hb J

hemoglobin M

WADA group
M1. ENHANCEMENT OF OXYGEN TRANSFER

MeSH descriptor
hemoglobin M

CAS Registry number
9083-28-7

Short synonyms
haemoglobin m
Hb M
hemoglobinose m

hemoglobin S

WADA group
M1. ENHANCEMENT OF OXYGEN TRANSFER

MeSH descriptor
hemoglobin, sickle

CAS Registry number
9035-22-7

Short synonyms
haemoglobin s
Hb S
hemoglobin, sickle
hemoglobin,sickle cell
s hemoglobin
sickle cell haemoglobin
sickle cell hemoglobin
sickle hemoglobin

hemoglobin variant

WADA group
M1. ENHANCEMENT OF OXYGEN TRANSFER

MeSH descriptor
hemoglobins, abnormal

Short synonyms
abnormal hemoglobin
hemoglobins, abnormal
variant,hemoglobin

heptaminol

WADA group
S1. STIMULANTS

MeSH descriptor
heptaminol

CAS Registry number
372-66-7
543-15-7

Trade names and research codes
eoden
coreptil
cortensor
heptamyl
heptonal
heptylon
rp 2831

Short synonyms
6 amino 2 methyl 2 heptanol
heptaminol chlorhydrate
heptaminol hydrochloride
6 methyl 2 amino 6 heptanol
2 methyl 6 amino 2 heptanol

hetastarch

WADA group
S8. MASKING AGENTS

MeSH descriptor
hetastarch

CAS Registry number
9005-27-0

Trade names and research codes
asl 607
asl-607
asl607
elohast
elohes
haes steril
hespan
hespander
hes steril
hextend
onkohaes
onkohas
pentafraction
pentaspan
plasmafusin
plasmasteril
volex

Short synonyms
amylopectin,hydroxyethyl
hetastarch 120
hetastarch 200
hetastarch 40
hydroxyethylamylopectin
hydroxy ethyl starch
hydroxyethyl starch
hydroxyethylstarch
2 hydroxyethyl starch
hydroxyethyl starch 60
ketastarch
pentastarch
polyhydroxyamylopectin
starch,hydroxyethyl

hexarelin

WADA group
S5. PEPTIDE HORMONES

CAS Registry number
140703-51-1

Trade names and research codes
ep 23905
ep23905

Short synonyms
examorelin

Long synonyms
histidyl dextro 2 methyltryptophylalanyltryptophyl dextro phenylalanyllysinamide

hexoprenaline

WADA group
S6. BETA-2 AGONISTS

MeSH descriptor
hexoprenaline

CAS Registry number
3215-70-1
32266-10-7

Trade names and research codes
broncholysin
byk 1512
byk1512
delaprem
etoscol
gynepral
gynipral
ipradol
st 1512
st1512

Short synonyms
hexaprenaline
hexoprenaline sulfate

Long synonyms
alpha,alpha'[hexamethylenebis(iminomethylene)bis(3, 4 dihydroxybenzylalcohol)

Terms and Synonyms

n,n'hexamethylene dinoradrenalin
n,n'hexamethylenedinoradrenaline

histidyl dextro tryptophylalanyltryptophyl dextro phenylalanyllysinamide

WADA group
S5. PEPTIDE HORMONES

CAS Registry number
87616-84-0

Trade names and research codes
skf 110679
u 75799e

Short synonyms
GHRP 6

Long synonyms
growth hormone releasing peptide 6

histrelin

WADA group
S5. PEPTIDE HORMONES

CAS Registry number
76712-82-8

Trade names and research codes
orf 17070
orf17070
rwj 17070
rwj17070
supprelin

Short synonyms
histerelin
histrelin acetate

Long synonyms
gonadorelin[1-9] ethylamide[6 (n benzyl dextro histidine)]

homococaine

WADA group
S1. STIMULANTS

CAS Registry number
529-38-4

Short synonyms
cocaethylene
cocaethylin
cocethyline
ethylcocaine
homocaine

Long synonyms
ecgonine 3 benzoate 2 ethyl ester

human growth hormone

WADA group
S5. PEPTIDE HORMONES

MeSH descriptor
human growth hormone

CAS Registry number
12629-01-5

Trade names and research codes
biotropin
cb 311
cb311
corpormon
crescormon
genotropin
humatrop
humatrope
neutropin
norditropin
novotropin
nutropin
nutropin aq
nutropin depot
prolease
saizen
salzen
scitropin
serostim
serotim
sj 0011
somatropin
umatrope
zomacton

Short synonyms
asellacrin
growth hormone,human
h.g.h.
hGH
hormone,human growth
human somatotropin
recombinant somatropin
somatotropin,human
w 752 a

Long synonyms
biosynthetic human growth hormone
growth hormone,recombinant human
recombinant human growth hormone

human insulin

WADA group
S5. PEPTIDE HORMONES

CAS Registry number
11061-68-0

Trade names and research codes
h tronin
humulin
humulin regular
nazlin

Short synonyms
insulin,human

human menopausal gonadotropin

WADA group
S5. PEPTIDE HORMONES

MeSH descriptor
menotropins

CAS Registry number
61489-71-2

Trade names and research codes
gonadoryl
homogonal
humegon
humergon
menogon

neopergonal
normegon
pergonal
pergonal 500
pregova

Short synonyms
gonadotrophin,menopause
gonadotropin,menopausal
HMG
human menopausal gonadotrophin
human menopause gonadotropin
menopausal gonadotrophin
menopausal gonadotropin
menopausal human gonadotropin
menopause gonadotrophin
menopause gonadotropin
menotropin
menotropins

hydralazine plus hydrochlorothiazide

WADA group
S8. MASKING AGENTS
P3. DIURETICS

Trade names and research codes
apresazide
apresoline esidrex
apresoline plus esidrex
esidrex apresoline
esidrex plus apresoline

Long synonyms
hydrochlorothiazide plus hydralazine

hydralazine plus hydrochlorothiazide plus reserpine

WADA group
S8. MASKING AGENTS
P3. DIURETICS

Trade names and research codes
esidri
ser ap es
serapes
serpasil apresoline esidrex

Long synonyms
reserpine plus hydralazine plus hydrochlorothiazide

hydrallostane

WADA group
S9. GLUCOCORTICOSTEROIDS

CAS Registry number
516-41-6

Short synonyms
allodihydrocortisol
allodihydro f
allodihydrohydrocortisone
4,5alpha dihydrocortisol
5alpha dihydrocortisol
5alpha dihydrohydrocortisone
cortisol,5alpha dihydro
dihydrocortisol

Long synonyms
allopregnane 11beta,17alpha,21 triol 3,20 dione
5alpha pregnane 11beta,17alpha,21 triol 3,20 dione
11beta,17alpha,21 trihydroxy 5alpha pregnane 3,20 dione
11beta,17alpha,21 trihydroxyallopregnane 3,20 dione

hydrochlorothiazide

WADA group
S8. MASKING AGENTS
P3. DIURETICS

MeSH descriptor
hydrochlorothiazide

CAS Registry number
58-93-5

Trade names and research codes
aquazide h
behyd ra
diaqua
dichlotride
disalunil
diu melusin
diu-melusin
diumelusin
esidrex
esidrex k
esidrex k forte
esidrix
fluvin
hydrochlor
hydro diuril
hydrodiuril
hydromal
hydro t
hydro z 50
hydrozide 50
hypothiazide
microzide
mictrin
oretic
urozide

Short synonyms
aquarius
bisalunil
bremil
chlorosulthiadil
cidrex
dehydratin neo
dichlorosal
dichlotride k
diclotride
dihydrochlorothiazide
dihydrodiuril
direma
disaluril
hidril
hudorex
hydril
hydro aquil
hydroaquil
hydrochlorothiamide
hydrochlorothiazid
hydro chlorothiazide
hydrochloro thiazide
hydrochlorothiazine
hydrochlorthiazide
hydrochlothiazide
hydroronol
hydro saluric
hydrosaluric
hydro saluric k
hydrosaluric k
hydrothide
hydro tonuron

hypothiazid
ivaugan
nefrix
neo codema
neo flumen
neoflumen
niagar
thiadril
thiaretic
thiuretic
urodiazin
urodiazine
vetidrex

Long synonyms
6 chloro 3,4 dihydro 2h 1,2,4 benzothiadiazine 7 sulfonamide 1,1 dioxide
6 chloro 3,4 dihydro 7 sulfamoyl 1,2,4 benzothiadiazine 1,1 dioxide
chloro 3,4 dihydro 7 sulfamoyl 2h
6 chloro 3,4 dihydro 7 sulfamoyl 2h 1,2,4 benzothiadiazine 1,1 dioxide
6 chloro 3,4 dihydroxy 7 sulfamoyl 2 h 1,2,4 benzothiadiazine
chlorsulfonamidodihydrobenzothiadiazine dioxide

hydrochlorothiazide plus irbesartan

WADA group
S8. MASKING AGENTS
P3. DIURETICS

Trade names and research codes
co aprovel
coaprovel
karvezide

Long synonyms
irbesartan plus hydrochlorothiazide

hydrochlorothiazide plus lisinopril

WADA group
S8. MASKING AGENTS
P3. DIURETICS

Trade names and research codes
novazyd
prinzide
vivazid
zestoretic

Long synonyms
lisinopril plus hydrochlorothiazide

hydrochlorothiazide plus losartan

WADA group
S8. MASKING AGENTS
P3. DIURETICS

Trade names and research codes
hizaar
hyzaar
lorzaar plus

Long synonyms
losartan plus hydrochlorothiazide

hydrochlorothiazide plus metoprolol

WADA group
S8. MASKING AGENTS
P2. BETA-BLOCKERS
P3. DIURETICS

Trade names and research codes
lopresside
lopressor hct
selopres
selopress

Long synonyms
hydrochlorothiazide with metoprolol
metoprolol plus hydrochlorothiazide

hydrochlorothiazide plus metoprolol tartrate

WADA group
S8. MASKING AGENTS
P2. BETA-BLOCKERS
P3. DIURETICS

CAS Registry number
71307-50-1

Trade names and research codes
beloc comp
cobeloc
co betaloc
cobetaloc
selokomb
selozide
zok zid

hydrochlorothiazide plus propranolol

WADA group
S8. MASKING AGENTS
P2. BETA-BLOCKERS
P3. DIURETICS

CAS Registry number
81719-07-5

Trade names and research codes
inderide
invamed

Long synonyms
hydrochlorothiazide with propranolol
propranolol plus hydrochlorothiazide
propranolol with hydrochlorothiazide

hydrochlorothiazide plus quinapril

WADA group
S8. MASKING AGENTS
P3. DIURETICS

Trade names and research codes
accuretic
accuzide

Long synonyms
quinapril plus hydrochlorothiazide

hydrochlorothiazide plus telmisartan

WADA group
S8. MASKING AGENTS
P3. DIURETICS

Trade names and research codes
bolusacplus
micardisplus
pritor plus
pritorplus

Long synonyms
telmisartan plus hydrochlorothiazide

hydrochlorothiazide plus triamterene

WADA group
S8. MASKING AGENTS
P3. DIURETICS

CAS Registry number
14124-50-6

Trade names and research codes
diutensat
diu tonolytril
diutonolytril
duradiuret
dyazide
dytenzide
dytide h
esiteren
maxide
maxzide
nephral
slimin
triampur
turfa

Short synonyms
co triamterzide
cotriamterzide
novotriamzide
prestole
sali puren
triamthiazid
trithiazid

Long synonyms
hydrochlorothiazide with triamterene
triamterene plus hydrochlorothiazide
triamterene with hydrochlorothiazide

hydrochlorothiazide plus valsartan

WADA group
S8. MASKING AGENTS
P3. DIURETICS

Trade names and research codes
co diovan
co-diovan
codiovan
cotareg
diovan comp
diovan d
diovan hct
miten plus
nisisco
tareg d

Long synonyms
valsartan plus hydrochlorothiazide

hydrocortisone

WADA group
S9. GLUCOCORTICOSTEROIDS

MeSH descriptor
hydrocortisone, topical
hydrocortisone

CAS Registry number
50-23-7

Trade names and research codes
cort dome
cortef
dioderm
duomedihaler
egocort
eksalb
ficortril
hycort
hydracort
hydrocort
hydrocortone
hydroderm
hysone
hytone
mildison lipocream
munitren
novohydrocort
nsc 10483
nsc10483
proctocort
proctosone
rectocort
schericur
scherosone f
synacort

Short synonyms
aeroseb hc
alphaderm
barseb hc
cetacort
cobadex
compound f
cortenema
cortibel
cortifan
cortifoam
cortiment
cortiphate
cortisol
cortisole
cortispray
cortoderm
cortril
dermolate
ef cortelan
efcortelan
eldecort
hebcort
hebcort v
hydrasson
hydrocorticosteroid
hydrocortisate
hydrocortison
hydrocortisone acetonide
hydrocortisone ointment
hydrocortisone plus saline
hydrocortisone steroid
hydrocortisone, topical
hydrocortisyl
hydro ricortex
17 hydroxycorticosterone
incortin h
medihaler cort

Terms and Synonyms

medihaler duo
neo cortef
neocortef
nsc 741
nutracort
otosone f
penecort
prepcort
pro cort
procort
solu cortef mix o vial
substance m
vasocort

Long synonyms
11beta,17,21 trihydroxypregn 4 ene 3,20 dione
11beta,17alpha,21 trihydroxypregn 4 ene 3,20 dione
4 pregnene 11beta,17alpha,21 triol 3,20 dione
4 pregnene 3,20 dione n beta,17alpha,21 triol

hydrocortisone 17 butyrate 21 propionate

WADA group
S9. GLUCOCORTICOSTEROIDS

CAS Registry number
72590-77-3

Trade names and research codes
pandel
ts 408

Short synonyms
hydrocortisone buteprate
hydrocortisone probutate

Long synonyms
hydrocortisone 21 propionate 17 butyrate

hydrocortisone acetate

WADA group
S9. GLUCOCORTICOSTEROIDS

CAS Registry number
50-03-3

Trade names and research codes
colifoam
cordes h
cortaid
cortef acetate
epifoam
ficortil
hydrocortal
hydrocortisone dorsch
hydrocortone acetate
litraderm
retef

Short synonyms
anusol hc
barseb
caldecort
clear aid
cortisol 21 acetate
cortisol acetate
cortril acetate as
dermacort
hydrocortisone 21 acetate
hydrocortistab
hydrosone
hysone a
komed hc
pabracort
servicort topical
sigmacort
squibb hc
wellcortin

hydrocortisone butyrate

WADA group
S9. GLUCOCORTICOSTEROIDS

CAS Registry number
13609-67-1

Trade names and research codes
alfason
bukorti
laticort
locoid
ts 1020

Short synonyms
cortisol 17 butyrate
hydrocortisone 17 butyrate

hydrocortisone derivative

WADA group
S9. GLUCOCORTICOSTEROIDS

Short synonyms
cortisol derivative

hydrocortisone plus urea

WADA group
S9. GLUCOCORTICOSTEROIDS

CAS Registry number
65272-39-1

Trade names and research codes
calmurid hc
hydrodexan

Short synonyms
hydrocortisone with urea
urea plus hydrocortisone

hydrocortisone sodium phosphate

WADA group
S9. GLUCOCORTICOSTEROIDS

CAS Registry number
315-33-3
3863-59-0
6000-74-4

Short synonyms
actocortin
cortisol 21 phosphate
cortisol phosphate
efcortesol
hydrocortisone 21 phosphate
hydrocortisone phosphate
hydrocortison sodium phosphate

Long synonyms
hydrocortisone 21 phosphate sodium
hydrocortisone 21 sodium phosphate
hydrocortisone disodium phosphate
hydrocortisone phosphate disodium
21 hydrocortisonephosphoric acid

hydrocortisone sodium succinate

WADA group
S9. GLUCOCORTICOSTEROIDS

CAS Registry number
125-04-2
2203-97-6

Trade names and research codes
a hydrocort
corlan
efcorlin
flebocortid
hydro adreson
hydroadreson
hydrocortisone 21 sodium succinate
solu cortef
solucortef
suxizon

Short synonyms
ahydrocort
buccalsone
cortisol 21 hemisuccinate
cortisol 21 succinate
cortisol hemisuccinate
cortisol sodium succinate
cortisol succinate
ef cortelan soluble
efcortelan soluble
emi corlin
hycorace
hydrocortisone 21 succinate
hydrocortisone hemisuccinate
hydrocortisone intraveineux
hydrocortisone succinate
hydrocortistab soluble
intracort
nordicort
saxizon
solu glyc
soluglyc
soly glyc

Long synonyms
hydrocortisone 21 hemisuccinate
hydrocortisone 21 hemisuccinate sodium
hydrocortisone 21 succinate sodium
hydrocortisone hemisuccinate sodium
hydrocortisone hemisuccinate sodium salt
hydrocortisone succinate sodium
sodium 17 hydroxycorticosterone 21 succinate

hydrocortisone valerate

WADA group
S9. GLUCOCORTICOSTEROIDS

CAS Registry number
57524-89-7

Trade names and research codes
westcort

Short synonyms
hydrocortisone 17 valerate

hydroflumethiazide

WADA group
S8. MASKING AGENTS
P3. DIURETICS

MeSH descriptor
hydroflumethiazide

CAS Registry number
135-09-1

Trade names and research codes
bristab
di ademil
di-ademil
diademil
diraudixin
diucardin
hiserpin
hydrenox
leodrin
leodrine
naclex
naclex glaxo
rontyl
saluron
sisuril

Short synonyms
dihydroflumethiazide
metflorylthiadiazine
trifluoromethylhydrothiazide

Long synonyms
3,4 dihydro 7 sulfamoyl 6 trifluoromethyl 1,2,4 benzothiadiazine 1,1 dioxide

hydromorphone

WADA group
S2. NARCOTICS

MeSH descriptor
hydromorphone

CAS Registry number
466-99-9
71-68-1

Trade names and research codes
biomorphyl
cofalaudid
dilaudid
dimorphone
hymorphan
laudaconum
novolaudon
palladon
palladone
palladone xl
semcox

Short synonyms
dihydromorphinone
7,8 dihydromorphinone hcl
dihydromorphone
hydromorphinone hydrochloride
hydromorphone hydrochloride

17 hydroxy 15beta,16beta methylene 7alpha methylthio 3 oxo 17alpha pregna 1,4 diene 21 carboxylic acid gamma lactone

WADA group
S8. MASKING AGENTS
P3. DIURETICS

CAS Registry number
97870-25-2

Trade names and research codes
zk 97894

6 hydroxy 2 (4 hydroxyphenyl) 3 [4 [2 (1 pyrrolidinyl)ethoxy]benzoyl]benzo[b] thiophene

WADA group
S7. AGENTS WITH ANTI-OESTROGENIC ACTIVITY

CAS Registry number
63676-25-5

Trade names and research codes
ly 10074
ly 117018

Long synonyms
6 hydroxy 2 (4 hydroxyphenyl)benzo[b]thien 3 yl 4 [2 (1 pyrrolidinyl)ethoxy]phenyl ketone
[6 hydroxy 2 (4 hydroxyphenyl)benzo[b]thien 3 yl][4 [2 (1 pyrrolidinyl)ethoxy]phenyl]methanone

4 [2 [(2 hydroxy 2 phenylethyl)amino]ethoxy]phenylacetic acid

WADA group
S6. BETA-2 AGONISTS

CAS Registry number
178600-17-4

Trade names and research codes
zd 2079

4 [2 [(2 hydroxy 2 phenylethyl)amino]propyl]benzoic acid

WADA group
S6. BETA-2 AGONISTS

CAS Registry number
90730-94-2

Trade names and research codes
brl 28410
brl28410

Long synonyms
4 [2 [(2 hydroxy 2 phenylethyl)amino]propyl]benzoate

4 [2 [(2 hydroxy 2 phenylethyl)amino]propyl]benzoic acid methyl ester

WADA group
S6. BETA-2 AGONISTS

CAS Registry number
77955-41-0

Trade names and research codes
brl 26830
brl26830

Long synonyms
methyl 4 [2 [(2 hydroxy 2 phenylethyl)amino]propyl]benzoate

4 [2 [(2 hydroxy 2 phenylethyl)amino]propyl]benzoic acid methyl ester hydrogen maleate

WADA group
S6. BETA-2 AGONISTS

CAS Registry number
87857-42-9

Trade names and research codes
brl 26830a
brl26830a

Long synonyms
4 [2 [(2 hydroxy 2 phenylethyl)amino]propyl]benzoic acid methyl ester hemimaleate
methyl 4 [2 [(2 hydroxy 2 phenylethyl)amino]propyl]benzoate hemimaleate

4 [2 hydroxy 3 [(1 methyl 3 phenylpropyl)amino]propoxy]benzeneacetamide

WADA group
P2. BETA-BLOCKERS

CAS Registry number
76805-48-6

Trade names and research codes
kf 4317

5 [2 [[2 hydroxy 3 [4 (1 methyl 4 trifluoromethyl 2 imidazolyl)phenoxy]propyl]amino]ethoxy]salicylamide

WADA group
P2. BETA-BLOCKERS

CAS Registry number
81015-67-0

Trade names and research codes
cgp 20712
cgp20712
cgp 20712 a
cgp 20712a
cgp20712a

Long synonyms
1 [[2 (3 carbamoyl 4 hydroxyphenoxy)ethyl]amino] 3 [4 (1 methyl 4 trifluoromethyl 2 imidazolyl)phenoxy] 2 propanol
2 hydroxy 5 [2 [[2 hydroxy 3 [4 (1 methyl 4 trifluoromethyl 2 imidazolyl)phenoxy]propyl]amino]ethoxy]benzamide

n [2 [2 hydroxy 3 [4 (2 isobutoxyethoxy)phenoxy]propylamino]ethyl] 4 morpholinecarboxamide

WADA group
S6. BETA-2 AGONISTS
P2. BETA-BLOCKERS

CAS Registry number
88017-05-4

Trade names and research codes
h 142 08

n [4 [2 [[2 hydroxy 3 (4 hydroxyphenoxy)propyl]amino]ethyl] phenyl]benzenesulfonamide

WADA group
S6. BETA-2 AGONISTS

Trade names and research codes
l 739574

n hydroxy 3,4 methylenedioxyamphetamine

WADA group
S1. STIMULANTS

CAS Registry number
74698-47-8

Long synonyms
amphetamine,n hydroxy 3,4 methylenedioxy
3,4 methylenedioxy n hydroxyamphetamine

4 (2 hydroxy 3 isopropylaminopropoxy)carbanilic acid propyl ester

WADA group
P2. BETA-BLOCKERS

CAS Registry number
83263-77-8

Trade names and research codes
bl 343
bl343
bl 343 ac
bl 343ac
bl343 ac

3 [4 (2 hydroxy 3 isopropylaminopropoxy)phenyl]propionic acid

WADA group
P2. BETA-BLOCKERS

CAS Registry number
81148-15-4

Trade names and research codes
asl 8123
asl8123

Long synonyms
4 (2 hydroxy 3 isopropylaminopropoxy)hydrocinnamic acid
3 [4 [2 hydroxy 3 (isopropylamino)propoxy]phenyl]propionic acid
para (2 hydroxy 3 isopropylaminopropoxy)hydrocinnamic acid

4 [2 [(2 hydroxy 3 phenoxypropyl)amino]ethoxy] n (2 methoxyethyl)phenoxyacetamide

WADA group
S6. BETA-2 AGONISTS

CAS Registry number
129689-30-1

Trade names and research codes
ici 201651
ici d 7114
ici d7114
zd 7114

4 [2 [(2 hydroxy 3 phenoxypropyl)amino]ethoxy]phenoxyacetic acid

WADA group
S6. BETA-2 AGONISTS

CAS Registry number
141269-99-0

Trade names and research codes
ici 215001
zm 215001

8 hydroxy 5 [1 hydroxy 2 [n [2 (4 methoxyphenyl) 1 methylethyl]amino]ethyl]carbostyril

WADA group
S6. BETA-2 AGONISTS

CAS Registry number
137888-11-0

Trade names and research codes
ta 2005
ta2005

4 hydroxy 7 [2 [2 [3 (2 phenylethoxy)propylsulfonyl]ethylamino]ethyl]benzothiazol 2(3h) one

WADA group
S6. BETA-2 AGONISTS

CAS Registry number
154189-24-9
154189-40-9

Trade names and research codes
ar c68397aa
arc 68397aa
arc68397aa
ar c68397xx
arc68397xx
fpl 68397
fpl68397
viozan

hydroxyamphetamine

WADA group
S1. STIMULANTS
S6. BETA-2 AGONISTS

MeSH descriptor
p-hydroxyamphetamine

CAS Registry number
103-86-6
1518-86-1
306-21-8

Trade names and research codes
h 66 37
h 66-37
paradrine
paredrine
paredrinea
paredrinex
pedrolone
pulsoton

Short synonyms
alpha methyl para tyramine
alpha methyl tyramine
alpha methyltyramine
4 (2 aminopropyl)phenol
4 hydroxyamphetamine
hydroxyamphetamine bromide
norpholedrine
oxamphetamine
p (2 aminopropyl)phenol
para (2 aminopropyl)phenol
para hydroxyamphetamine
parahydroxyamphetamine
p-hydroxyamphetamine

Long synonyms
dl 1 para hydroxyphenyl 2 propylamine
dl 1 p hydroxyphenyl 2 propylamine
dl para hydroxy alpha methylphenethylamine
dl p hydroxy alpha methylphenethylamine
hydroxyamphetamine hydrobromide
para (2 aminopropyl)phenol hydrobromide
para hydroxy alpha methylphenethylamine
para hydroxyamphetamine hydrobromide
1 para hydroxyphenyl 2 propylamine

n hydroxyamphetamine

WADA group
S1. STIMULANTS

CAS Registry number
63-90-1

Short synonyms
amphetamine,n hydroxy

Long synonyms
2 hydroxylamino 1 phenylpropane
n (1 phenyl 2 propyl)hydroxylamine
n hydroxy 1 phenyl 2 propylamine

11beta hydroxyandrostenedione

WADA group
S4. ANABOLIC AGENTS

CAS Registry number
382-44-5

Short synonyms
androsten 11beta ol dione
4 androsten 11 ol 3,17 dione
11 beta hydroxyandrostenedione
11beta hydroxy androstenedione
11 beta oh androstenedione

Long synonyms
androst 4 en 11beta ol 3,17 dione
4 androsten 11beta ol 3,17 dione
11beta hydroxy 4 androstene 3,17 dione
11beta hydroxyandrost 4 ene 3,17 dione
11 beta hydroxy androstenedione
11 beta hydroxy delta 4 androstene 3,17 dione
11 beta hydroxy delta4 androstene 3,17 dione
11beta hydroxy delta 4 androstene 3,17 dione
delta4 androsten 11beta ol 3,17 dione

19 hydroxyandrostenedione

WADA group
S4. ANABOLIC AGENTS

CAS Registry number
510-64-5

Short synonyms
androst 4 en 19 ol 3,17 dione
androst 4 en 19 ole 3,17 dione
4 androstene 19 ol 3,17 dione

Long synonyms
19 hydroxy 4 androstene 3,17 dione
19 hydroxyandrost 4 ene 3,17 dione
19 hydroxyandrostene 3,17 dione
19 hydroxy delta 4 androstene 8,17 dione

hydroxybenzylisoprenaline

WADA group
S6. BETA-2 AGONISTS

CAS Registry number
55283-70-0

Short synonyms
hydroxybenzylisoproterenol
isoprenaline,hydroxybenzyl

hydroxybenzylpindolol

WADA group
P2. BETA-BLOCKERS

CAS Registry number
69925-27-5

Short synonyms
pindolol,hydroxybenzyl

8 hydroxycarteolol

WADA group
P2. BETA-BLOCKERS

CAS Registry number
59826-22-1

Short synonyms
carteolol,8 hydroxy

Long synonyms
5 [3 (tert butylamino) 2 hydroxypropoxy] 3,4 dihydro 8 hydroxycarbostyril

3' hydroxy delta9 tetrahydrocannabinol

WADA group
S3. CANNABINOIDS

Long synonyms
3' hydroxy delta1 tetrahydrocannabinol

3 hydroxydenopamine

WADA group
S6. BETA-2 AGONISTS

Trade names and research codes
t 0509

Short synonyms
denopamine, 3 hydroxy

Long synonyms
alpha (3,4 dimethoxyphenethylaminomethyl) 3,4 dihydroxybenzyl alcohol
1 (3,4 dihydroxyphenyl) 2 (3',4' dimethoxyphenethylamino)ethanol
1 (3,4 dihydroxyphenyl) 2 [(3,4 dimethoxyphenethyl)amino]ethanol

11 hydroxydronabinol

WADA group
S3. CANNABINOIDS

CAS Registry number
26108-40-7

Short synonyms
dronabinol,11 hydroxy

Long synonyms
delta9 tetrahydrocannabinol,11 hydroxy
11 hydroxy delta 1 tetrahydrocannabinol
7 hydroxy delta 1 tetrahydrocannabinol
7 hydroxy delta1 tetrahydrocannabinol
11 hydroxy delta9 6a,10a tetrahydrocannabinol
11 hydroxy delta9 6a,10a trans tetrahydrocannabinol
11 hydroxy delta 9 tetrahydrocannabinol
11 hydroxy delta9 tetrahydrocannabinol

18 hydroxyhydrocortisone

WADA group
S9. GLUCOCORTICOSTEROIDS

CAS Registry number
81705-06-8
86002-90-6

Short synonyms
18 hydroxycortisol

Long synonyms
11beta,17alpha,18,21 tetrahydroxypregn 4 ene 3,20 dione
pregn 4 ene 11beta,17alpha,18,21 tetrol 3,20 dione

6beta hydroxyhydrocortisone

WADA group
S9. GLUCOCORTICOSTEROIDS

CAS Registry number
53-35-0

Short synonyms
6 beta hydroxycortisol
6beta hydroxycortisol
hydrocortisone,6beta hydroxy

Long synonyms
6beta,11beta,17,21 tetrahydroxypregn 4 ene 3,20 dione

alpha hydroxymetoprolol

WADA group
P2. BETA-BLOCKERS

CAS Registry number
56392-16-6

Trade names and research codes
h 119-66

Short synonyms
metoprolol,alpha hydroxy

Long synonyms
3 [4 (1 hydroxy 2 methoxyethyl)phenoxy] 1 isopropylamino 2 propanol

4 hydroxy n [2 [2 hydroxy 3 [4 [2 (isobutoxy)ethoxy]phenoxy]propylamino]ethyl] 1 piperidinecarboxamide

WADA group
S6. BETA-2 AGONISTS

CAS Registry number
108495-00-7

Trade names and research codes
h 201 70

3 (4 hydroxyphenyl) 4 methyl 2 [4 [2 (1 piperidinyl)ethoxy]phenyl] 2h 1 benzopyran 7 ol

WADA group
S7. AGENTS WITH ANTI-OESTROGENIC ACTIVITY

CAS Registry number
151533-34-5
182167-02-8
182167-58-4

Trade names and research codes
em 343
em343
em 651
em651
em 652
em652

16alpha hydroxyprednisolone

WADA group
S9. GLUCOCORTICOSTEROIDS

Short synonyms
prednisolone,16alpha hydroxy

Long synonyms
11beta,16alpha,17alpha,21 tetrahydroxypregna 1,4 diene 3,20 dione

Terms and Synonyms

3 (2 hydroxypropylamino) 3 methyl n [2,3,4,5 tetrahydro 2 oxo 1 [[2' (1h tetrazol 5 yl) 1,1' biphenyl 4 yl]methyl] 1h 1 benzazepin 3 yl]butanamide

WADA group
S5. PEPTIDE HORMONES

CAS Registry number
145455-35-2

Trade names and research codes
1 692585

hydroxytamoxifen

WADA group
S7. AGENTS WITH ANTI-OESTROGENIC ACTIVITY

CAS Registry number
68047-06-3

Short synonyms
monohydroxytamoxifen
tamoxifen,hydroxy
tamoxiphen,monohydroxy

4 hydroxytamoxifen

WADA group
S7. AGENTS WITH ANTI-OESTROGENIC ACTIVITY

CAS Registry number
65213-48-1
68392-35-8

Trade names and research codes
ici 79280

Short synonyms
4 monohydroxytamoxifen
tamoxyfen,4 hydroxy

4 hydroxytestosterone

WADA group
S4. ANABOLIC AGENTS

Short synonyms
testosterone,4 hydroxy

Long synonyms
4,17beta dihydroxy 4 androsten 3 one
4,17beta dihydroxyandrost 4 en 3 one

4 hydroxytoremifene

WADA group
S7. AGENTS WITH ANTI-OESTROGENIC ACTIVITY

CAS Registry number
110503-62-3

hypothalamus releasing factor

WADA group
S5. PEPTIDE HORMONES

MeSH descriptor
pituitary hormone-releasing hormones

Short synonyms
hypothalamic releasing factor
hypothalamus release factor

Long synonyms
pituitary hormone-releasing hormones

ibogaine

WADA group
S1. STIMULANTS

MeSH descriptor
ibogaine

CAS Registry number
83-74-9

Trade names and research codes
bogadin tm
endabuse
nih 10567
nih10567

Short synonyms
iboga
ibogine
12 methoxyibogamine

ibopamine

WADA group
S6. BETA-2 AGONISTS
S8. MASKING AGENTS
P3. DIURETICS

CAS Registry number
66195-31-1
75011-65-3

Trade names and research codes
inopamil
sb 7505
scandine
skf 100168
skf 100168 a

Short synonyms
ibopamine hydrochloride
n methyldopamine diisobutyrate

Long synonyms
diisobutyric n methyldopamine ester
3,4 diisobutyryloxy n methylphenethylamine
4 [2 (methylamino)ethyl] 1,2 phenylene diisobutyrate
4 [2 (methylamino)ethyl] ortho phenylene diisobutyrate
4 [2 (methylamino)ethyl]pyrocatechol diisobutyrate

ibutamoren

WADA group
S5. PEPTIDE HORMONES

CAS Registry number
159752-10-0

Terms and Synonyms

Trade names and research codes
mk 0677
mk 677

Short synonyms
ibutamoren mesylate

Long synonyms
2 amino n [2 benzyloxy 1 [[1,2 dihydro 1 (methylsulfonyl)spiro[3h indole 3,4' piperidin] 1' yl]carbonyl]ethyl] 2 methylpropionamide

ibuterol

WADA group
S6. BETA-2 AGONISTS

CAS Registry number
53034-85-8

Long synonyms
1 (3',5' diisobutyryloxyphenyl) 2 (tert butylamino)ethanol hydrochloride

idoxifene

WADA group
S7. AGENTS WITH ANTI-OESTROGENIC ACTIVITY

CAS Registry number
116057-75-1

Trade names and research codes
cb 7432
cb7432
sb 223030
sb223030

Short synonyms
pyrrolidino 4 iodotamoxifen

Long synonyms
1 (4 iodophenyl) 2 phenyl 1 [4 [2 (1 pyrrolidinyl)ethoxy]phenyl] 1 butene
1 [2 [4 [1 (4 iodophenyl) 2 phenyl 1 butenyl]phenoxy]ethyl]pyrrolidine

immunocortin

WADA group
S5. PEPTIDE HORMONES

CAS Registry number
150035-99-7

Short synonyms
immunocorticotropin

Long synonyms
immunoglobulin G1 heavy chain variable region[11-20]
val lys lys pro gly ser ser val lys val
valyllysyllysylprolylglycylserylserylvalyllysylvaline

immunoreactive insulin

WADA group
S5. PEPTIDE HORMONES

Short synonyms
immune reactive insulin
insulin,immunoreactive
IRI
serum immunoreactive insulin

imoxiterol

WADA group
S6. BETA-2 AGONISTS

CAS Registry number
88578-07-8

indacrinone

WADA group
S8. MASKING AGENTS
P3. DIURETICS

CAS Registry number
56049-88-8
57296-63-6

Trade names and research codes
mk 196

Short synonyms
indacrinic acid
indacrynic acid

Long synonyms
5 carboxymethoxy 6,7 dichloro 2 methyl 2 phenylindan 1 one
[(6,7 dichloro 2,3 dihydro 2 methyl 1 oxo 2 phenyl 1h inden 5 yl)oxy]acetic acid
(6,7 dichloro 2 methyl 1 oxo 2 phenyl 5 indanyloxy)acetic acid
6,7 dichloro 2 methyl 1 oxo 2 phenyl 5 indanyloxyacetic acid
[(6,7 dichloro 2 methyl 1 oxo 2 phenyl 5 indanyl)oxy]acetic acid
(6,7 dichloro 2 methyl 1 oxo 2 phenylindan 5 yloxy)acetic acid
6,7 dichloro 2 methyl 2 phenyl 1 oxoindanyloxylacetic acid

indapamide

WADA group
S8. MASKING AGENTS
P3. DIURETICS

MeSH descriptor
indapamide

CAS Registry number
26807-65-8

Trade names and research codes
arifon
fludex
fluidema
lorvas
lozol
'millibar'
natrilix
noranat
pressural
s 1520
s1520
se 1520
se1520
tandix
tertensif
usv 2555
usv2555
veroxil

Short synonyms
indopamide

Long synonyms
1 (4 chloro 3 sulfamoylbenzamido) 2 methylindoline
4 chloro n (2 methyl 1 indolinyl) 3 sulfamoylbenzamide
4 chloro n (2 methylindolin 1 yl) 3 sulfamoylbenzamide
indoline,1 (4 chloro 3 sulfamoylbenzamido) 2 methyl
3 (sulfamoyl) 4 chloro n (2,3 dihydro 2 methyl 1h indol 1 yl)benzamide

indenolol

WADA group
P2. BETA-BLOCKERS

CAS Registry number
30190-87-5
60607-68-3
68906-88-7
81789-85-7

Trade names and research codes
pulsan
yb 2
28316z

Short synonyms
indenolol hydrochloride

Long synonyms
4 (2 hydroxy 3 isopropylaminopropoxy)indene
1 (inden 4 yloxy) 3 isopropylamino 2 propanol

insulin

WADA group
S5. PEPTIDE HORMONES

MeSH descriptor
insulin

CAS Registry number
8-10-9004

Trade names and research codes
actrapid insulin
actrapid mc
humilin
iletin ii
initard
insulin actrapid
insulina pronta lilly
insulin hnc
insulin novo actrapid
insulin snc
insulinum
iszilin
maxirapid
monotard human
monotard insulin
neusulin
novolin
oralin
oro insulin

Short synonyms
cross linked insulin
destripeptide insulin
fish insulin
immunoinsulin
insuline
iodinated insulin
teleost insulin

insulin aspart

WADA group
S5. PEPTIDE HORMONES

CAS Registry number
116094-23-6

Trade names and research codes
novolog
novomix
novomix 30
novorapid
novorapide

Short synonyms
insulin, Asp(B28)
insulin[B28 aspartic acid]

insulin[B28 lysine B29 proline]

WADA group
S5. PEPTIDE HORMONES

CAS Registry number
133107-64-9

Trade names and research codes
humalog
humalog mix npl
liprolog
ly 275585
ly275585

Short synonyms
insulin lispro
insulin lyspro
lispro
lispro insulin
lyspro
lyspro insulin

Long synonyms
insulin [b28 lysine b29 proline]

insulin deoctapeptide

WADA group
S5. PEPTIDE HORMONES

CAS Registry number
39416-70-1

Short synonyms
desoctapeptide insulin
desoctapeptideinsulin
insulin desoctapeptide

insulin derivative

WADA group
S5. PEPTIDE HORMONES

Short synonyms
carbamoylinsulin
carbamylinsulin
carbonyl bis methionyl insulin
diacetoacetyl insulin
diacetylinsulin
diaminosuberoyl insulin
insulin analog
insulin analogue
methylthiocarbamoylinsulin
methylthiocarbamylinsulin

mononitroinsulin
polyalanylinsulin series
suberoyl insulin
succinyl insulin
triacetylinsulin
tricarbamylinsulin

insulin detemir

WADA group
S5. PEPTIDE HORMONES

CAS Registry number
169148-63-4
201305-44-4
270588-25-5

Trade names and research codes
nn 304
nn304

Long synonyms
insulin[B29 (6 n tetradecanoyllysine) B30 dethreonine]
insulin[B29 (n epsilon myristoyllysine) B30 dethreonine]

insulin glargine

WADA group
S5. PEPTIDE HORMONES

CAS Registry number
160337-95-1

Trade names and research codes
hoe 901
hoe901
lantus
optisulin

Short synonyms
glargine insulin

Long synonyms
insulin[A21 glycine B31 arginine B32 arginine]

insulin glulisine

WADA group
S5. PEPTIDE HORMONES

CAS Registry number
207748-29-6

Trade names and research codes
apidra
hmr 1964
hmr1964

Long synonyms
insulin [B3 lysine B29 glutamic acid]
insulin[B3 lysine B29 glutamic acid]

insulin zinc suspension

WADA group
S5. PEPTIDE HORMONES

MeSH descriptor
insulin, lente

CAS Registry number
8049-62-5

Trade names and research codes
iletin
insulin lente
insulin novo lente
insulin novolente
insulin semilente
insulin subtardum
insulin ultralente
lentard
lentard mc
lente iletin
lente insulin
monotard
monotard hm
novo lente
novolente
novolin l
novolin lente
semilente iletin
semilente insulin
semitard
subtardum
ultralente
ultralente insulin
ultratard
ultratard hm
ultratard mc

Short synonyms
crystalline zinc insulin
insulin, lente
insulin zinc
zinc insulin
zinc insulin crystalline
zinc insuline

Long synonyms
amorphous insulin zinc suspension
crystalline insulin zinc suspension
crystalline,insulin zinc suspension
insulin zinc suspension amorphous
insulin zinc suspension crystalline
insulin zinc suspension,crystalline

4 iodo 2,5 dimethoxyamphetamine

WADA group
S1. STIMULANTS

CAS Registry number
64584-34-5

Short synonyms
DOI

Long synonyms
2 amino 1 (4 iodo 2,5 dimethoxyphenyl)propane
amphetamine,4 iodo 2,5 dimethoxy
2,5 dimethoxy 4 iodoamphetamine
1 (2,5 dimethoxy 4 iodophenyl) 2 aminopropane
1 (4 iodo 2,5 dimethoxyphenyl) 2 propanamine
4 iodo 2,5 dimethoxyphenylisopropylamine

4 iodoamphetamine

WADA group
S1. STIMULANTS

CAS Registry number
21894-72-4

Short synonyms
para iodoamphetamine

Long synonyms
2 amino 1 (4 iodophenyl)propane

iodopindolol

WADA group
P2. BETA-BLOCKERS

CAS Registry number
76875-00-8

iofetamine

WADA group
S1. STIMULANTS

MeSH descriptor
iofetamine

CAS Registry number
95896-48-3

Short synonyms
4 iodo n isopropylamphetamine
n isopropyl 4 iodoamphetamine

Long synonyms
n isopropyl para iodoamphetamine

ipamorelin

WADA group
S5. PEPTIDE HORMONES

CAS Registry number
170851-70-4

Trade names and research codes
nnc 26 0161

Long synonyms
2 amino 2 methylpropionylhistidyl 3 (2 naphthyl) dextro alanyl dextro phenylalanyllysinamide

iprocrolol

WADA group
P2. BETA-BLOCKERS

CAS Registry number
37855-80-4

Long synonyms
1 [(4 hydroxy 7 methyl 5 oxo 5h furo[3,2 g][1]benzopyran 9 yl)oxy] 3 isopropylamino 2 propanol
4 hydroxy 9 (2 hydroxy 3 isopropylaminopropoxy) 7 methyl 5h furo[3,2 g][1]benzopyran 5 one

isamoltane

WADA group
P2. BETA-BLOCKERS

CAS Registry number
99740-06-4

Trade names and research codes
cgp 361 a
cgp 361a
cgp361a

Short synonyms
isazotane

Long synonyms
1 isopropylamino 3 [2 (1 pyrrolyl)phenoxy] 2 propanol

isoetarine

WADA group
S6. BETA-2 AGONISTS

MeSH descriptor
isoetharine

CAS Registry number
50-96-4
530-08-5
63550-80-1

Trade names and research codes
asthmalitan
asthmolytan
bronchosol
broncosol
bronkometer
bronkosol
dilabron
neoisuprel
numotac
numotac tablets
win 3046

Short synonyms
etyprenaline
isoarinehydrochloride
isoetharine
isoetharine hydrochloride

Long synonyms
alpha ethyl n isopropylnoradrenaline
1 (3,4 dihydroxyphenyl) 2 isopropylamino 1 butanol
4 [1 hydroxy 2 [(1 methylethyl)amino]butyl] 1,2 benzenediol

isoflupredone

WADA group
S9. GLUCOCORTICOSTEROIDS

CAS Registry number
338-95-4

Short synonyms
9 alpha fluoroprednisolone
9alpha fluoroprednisolone
9alpha fluprednisolone
9 fluoroprednisolone

isoflupredone acetate

WADA group
S9. GLUCOCORTICOSTEROIDS

CAS Registry number
338-98-7

Trade names and research codes
menaderm
predef
rectomenaderm
u 6013

Short synonyms
isoflupredone 21 acetate

Long synonyms
9alpha fluoroprednisolone 21 acetate
9alpha fluoroprednisolone acetate

isophane insulin

WADA group
S5. PEPTIDE HORMONES

MeSH descriptor
insulin, isophane
insulin, protamine zinc

CAS Registry number
9004-17-5

Trade names and research codes
actraphane
humulin i
humulin n
humulin r
insulatard
insulatard nph
mixtard
novolin n
novolin nph
nph iletin
nph insulin
nph umuline
orgasuline nph
protaphan
protaphane
protophane
protophane hm

Short synonyms
insulin, isophane
insulin plus protamine sulfate
insulin, protamine zinc
insulin zinc protamine
isofane insulin
isophane insulin suspension
isophane zinc insulin
isophan insulin
isophone insulin
nph
protamine insulin
protamine zinc insulin
zinc protamine insulin

Long synonyms
neutral protamine hagedorn insulin

isoprenaline

WADA group
S6. BETA-2 AGONISTS

MeSH descriptor
isoproterenol

CAS Registry number
299-95-6
51-30-9
6700-39-6
7683-59-2

Trade names and research codes
a 21
a 21 hf
aerolone
aerotrol
aleudrin
aleudrine
aleudrin ingelheim
alidril
alotex
aludrin
aludrine
antasthmin kwizda
antiasmatico serpero
arsiprenol
asiprenol
asmadren
asmalar
asmalidrina
asmanor
asmolidrina
asmolon
asmonor
assiprenol
asthmatermine
astmo
bellasthma medihaler
bellasthman
bronchodilatin
bronchomister
dispnoesan
dolomit
duraludrin
dyspnoesan
erydin
euspiran
iludrin
iludrina
iludrine
ingelan
iomupren
iprenol
isadren
isadrin
isadrine
iso autohaler
iso bronchisan
isobronchisan
iso glycirenan
isoglycirenan
isolin
isoprel
isoprenol
isopro
isopropidin
isopropydrin
isopropydrine
isopropydrinum
ispranil
isuprel
isoprel iso
isupren
izadrin
luf iso
medihaler iso
medihaler isoforte
meterdos iso
meterdos iso forte
mistaprel
neoasman
neodrenal
neodrenol
norisedrin
norisodine
norisodrine
norisodrine aerotrol
novadren
novodrin
novodrine
praedil
prenasma
prenomiser
prenomiser forte
protanol
proterenol
proternol
proternol l
respifral
salvasma

Terms and Synonyms

sanasma
saventrine
solvasma
vapo n iso
win 5162

Short synonyms
dextro isoprenaline
d isoprenaline
dl isoprenaline
dl isoprenaline hydrochloride
dl isoproterenol sulfate
epinephrine isopropyl homolog
ipa
isonorin
isonorin sulfate
isoprenalin
isoprenaline hydrochloride
isoprenaline sulfate
isoprenalin hydrochloride
isoprenalinum
isopropylarterenol
isopropyl noradrenalin
isopropylnoradrenalin>
isopropyl noradrenaline
isopropylnoradrenaline
isopropyl noradrenalin sulfate
isopropylnorepinephrin
isopropylnorepinephrine
isopropylnorphenylephrine
isoprotenol hydrochloride
isoproterenol
isoproterenol hydrochloride
isoproterenol sulfate
isoproterenol sulfate dihydrate
isoproterol
levo isoprenaline
levoisoprenaline
levo isoprenaline sulfate
levo isoproterenol sulfate
l isoprenaline
l isoproterenol
l isoproterenol sulfate
neoepine
neoepinephrine
neo epinine
neoepinine
neofanal
nephenal
nephenalin
n isopropylnoradrenalin
n isopropylnoradrenaline
ossiprenol
pafadrin
propylon
propynalin

Long synonyms
alpha (isopropylaminomethyl)protocatechuyl alcohol
3,4 dihydroxy alpha [(isopropylamino)methyl]benzyl alcohol
3,4 dihydroxy alpha [isopropylaminomethyl]benzyl alcohol
levo isoprenaline hydrochloride
levo isoproterenol hydrochloride

2 isopropylamino 1 (4 tolyl)propanol

WADA group
P2. BETA-BLOCKERS

CAS Registry number
13549-60-5

Trade names and research codes
h 35 25
h35 25

Short synonyms
h 35-25

Long synonyms
alpha (1 isopropylaminoethyl) 4 methylbenzyl alcohol
alpha (1 isopropylaminoethyl) 4 methylbenzyl alcohol hydrochloride
alpha (1 isopropylaminoethyl) para methylbenzyl alcohol
beta hydroxy n isopropyl 4,alpha dimethylphenethylamine
2 isopropylamino 1 (4 methylphenyl)propanol
2 isopropylamino 1 (4 tolyl)propan 1 ol
2 isopropylamino 1 (para tolyl) 1 propanol
2 isopropylamino 1 (para tolyl)propanol
2 isopropylamino 1 (para tolyl)propyl alcohol
4 methyl alpha (1 isopropylaminoethyl)benzyl alcohol
4' methyl alpha (1 isopropylaminoethyl)benzylalcohol
1 (4 methylphenyl) 2 isopropylamino propanol
1 (4 methylphenyl) 2 isopropylaminopropanol
n [1 hydroxy 1 (para tolyl)prop 2 yl] n isopropylamine
n isopropyl n (1 hydroxy 1 para tolylprop 2 yl)amine
1 (para tolyl) 2 isopropylamino 1 propanol

3 isopropylamino 1 (7 methyl 4 indanyloxy) 2 butanol

WADA group
P2. BETA-BLOCKERS

CAS Registry number
72795-19-8

Trade names and research codes
ici 118,551
ici 118551

Short synonyms
ici 188551

Long synonyms
1 [(2,3 dihydro 7 methyl 1h inden 4 yl)oxy] 3 [(1 methylethyl)amino] 2 butanol
erythro 1 (7 methylindan 4 yloxy) 3 isopropylaminobutan 2 ol
1 (7 methylindan 4 yloxy) 3 isopropylaminobutan 2 ol

1 isopropylamino 3 [4 (2 methoxyethoxy)phenoxy] 2 propanol

WADA group
P2. BETA-BLOCKERS

CAS Registry number
30311-37-6

Trade names and research codes
h 87-07

Long synonyms
1 isopropylamino 3 [4 (2 methoxyethoxy)phenoxy]propan 2 ol

isosorbide

WADA group
S8. MASKING AGENTS
P3. DIURETICS

MeSH descriptor
isosorbide

CAS Registry number
652-67-5

Trade names and research codes
at 101
at101
beta isoket
conovliss
hydronol
ismotic
isobide
iso puren
isopuren

Short synonyms
1,4:3,6 dianhydro d glucitol
1,4:3,6 dianhydrosorbitol
disodium isosorbide
isosorbide disodium
isosorbine

isoxaprolol

WADA group
P2. BETA-BLOCKERS

CAS Registry number
75949-60-9

Long synonyms
1 (tert butylamino) 3 [2 [2 (3 methylisoxazol 5 yl)vinyl]phenoxy] 2 propanol

isoxsuprine

WADA group
S6. BETA-2 AGONISTS

MeSH descriptor
isoxsuprine

CAS Registry number
395-28-8
579-56-6

Trade names and research codes
caa 40
caa40
defencin
defencin cp
dilavase
dilovasan
duvadilan
duvadilan retard
fenam
gr 62
gr62
suprilent
vasodilan
vasodilian
vasoplex
vasosuprine
vasotran
venam
xuprin

Short synonyms
isoxsuprin
isoxsuprine hydrochloride
isoxuprine
phenoxyisopropylnorsuprifen

Long synonyms
para hydroxy alpha [1 [(1 methyl 2 phenoxyethyl)amino]ethyl]benzyl alcohol
para hydroxy n (1 methyl 2 phenoxyethyl)norephedrine
para hydroxy n (2 phenoxyisopropyl)norephedrine
1 (para hydroxyphenyl) 2 (1 methyl 2 phenoxyethylamino) 1 propanol
para hydroxyphenyl ethyl para hydroxynorephedrine
2 (2 phenoxy 1 methylethylamino) 1 (4 hydroxyphenyl) 1 propanol
2 (3 phenoxy 2 propylamino) 1 (para hydroxyphenyl) 1 propanol

kadiur

WADA group
S8. MASKING AGENTS
P3. DIURETICS

Trade names and research codes
kadiur

Long synonyms
butizide plus canrenoate potassium
canrenoate potassium plus butizide

labetalol

WADA group
P2. BETA-BLOCKERS

MeSH descriptor
labetalol

CAS Registry number
32780-64-6
36894-69-6

Trade names and research codes
ah 5158
ah5158
ah 5158a
ah5158a
albetol
lamitol
normodyne
presdate
sch 15719w
sch15719w
trandate

Short synonyms
ibidomide

Long synonyms
5 [1 hydroxy 2 (1 methyl 3 phenylpropylamino)ethyl]salicylamide
5 [1 hydroxy 2 [(1 methyl 3 phenylpropyl)amino]ethyl]salicylamide

landiolol

WADA group
P2. BETA-BLOCKERS

CAS Registry number
133242-30-5

Trade names and research codes
ono 1101
ono1101
onoact

Short synonyms
landiolol hydrochloride

Long synonyms
[(2,2 dimethyl 1,3 dioxolan 4 yl)methyl] 3 [4 [2 hydroxy 3 [2 (morpholinocarbonylamino)ethylamino]propoxy]phenyl]propionate
3 [4 [2 hydroxy 3 (2 morpholinocarbonylaminoethylamino)propoxy]phenyl]propionic acid 2,2 dimethyl 1,3 dioxolan 4 ylmethyl ester

lasofoxifene

WADA group
S7. AGENTS WITH ANTI-OESTROGENIC ACTIVITY

CAS Registry number
180915-85-9
180916-16-9
190791-29-8

Trade names and research codes
cp 336156
cp336156

Short synonyms
lasofoxifene tartrate

Long synonyms
1 [4 (2 pyrrolidinoethoxy)phenyl] 2 phenyl 6 hydroxy 1,2,3,4 tetrahydronaphthalene
5,6,7,8 tetrahydro 6 phenyl 5 [4 [2 (1 pyrrolidinyl)ethoxy]phenyl] 2 naphthol

lefetamine

WADA group
S1. STIMULANTS

CAS Registry number
7262-75-1

Trade names and research codes
santenol

Short synonyms
lephetamine
n,n dimethylstilbylamine

Long synonyms
1,2 diphenyl 1 dimethylaminoethane
n,n dimethyl 1,2 diphenylethylamine
n,n dimethyl alpha phenylphenethylamine

leghemoglobin

WADA group
M1. ENHANCEMENT OF OXYGEN TRANSFER

MeSH descriptor
leghemoglobin

CAS Registry number
52365-25-0
53096-11-0

Short synonyms
legoglobin
leguminous hemoglobin

letrozole

WADA group
S7. AGENTS WITH ANTI-OESTROGENIC ACTIVITY

CAS Registry number
112809-51-5

Trade names and research codes
cgs 20267
cgs20267
femar
femara

Long synonyms
1 (4,4' dicyanobenzhydryl) 1,2,4 triazole
4,4' (1h 1,2,4 triazol 1 ylmethylene)bis(benzonitrile)

leuprorelin

WADA group
S5. PEPTIDE HORMONES

MeSH descriptor
leuprolide

CAS Registry number
53714-56-0
74381-53-6

Trade names and research codes
a 43818
a43818
abbott 43818
carcinil
depo lupron
eligard
enanton
enantone
ginecrin
ginecrin depot
leuplin
leuprogel
leupron
lucrin
lupron
lupron depot
procrin
prostap
prostap sr
tap 144
tap144
tap 144 sr
tap144 sr
trenantone
viadur

Short synonyms
leuprolid
leuprolide
leuprolide acetate
leuprorelin acetate

Long synonyms
gonadorelin[6 dextro leucine 9 (n ethylprolinamide) 10 deglycinamide]
gonadorelin ethylamide [6 dextro leucine 10 deglycine]
gonadorelin ethylamide[6 dextro leucine 10 deglycine]
5 oxoprolylhistidyltryptophylseryltyrosyl dextro leucylleucylarginyl n ethylprolinamide

levalbuterol

WADA group
S6. BETA-2 AGONISTS

CAS Registry number
50293-90-8

Trade names and research codes
xopenex

Short synonyms
levalbuterol hydrochloride

levobunolol

WADA group
P2. BETA-BLOCKERS

MeSH descriptor
levobunolol

CAS Registry number
47141-42-4

Trade names and research codes
ak beta
betagan
betasite
vistagan
w 7000a

Short synonyms
l bunolol hydrochloride
levo bunolol

levofacetoperane

WADA group
S1. STIMULANTS

CAS Registry number
24558-01-8

Trade names and research codes
lidepran
rp 8228

Short synonyms
levophacetoperan
levophacetoperane

Long synonyms
threo 1 acetoxy 1 phenyl 1 (2 piperidyl)methane

levomethadone

WADA group
S2. NARCOTICS

CAS Registry number
125-58-6

Trade names and research codes
l polamidon

Short synonyms
levadone
levo methadone
l methadone

Long synonyms
(r) 6 (dimethylamino) 4,4 diphenyl 3 heptanone

levomoprolol

WADA group
P2. BETA-BLOCKERS

CAS Registry number
77164-20-6

Trade names and research codes
levotensin

Short synonyms
levo moprolol
l moprolol
moprolol,levo

levonantradol

WADA group
S3. CANNABINOIDS

CAS Registry number
71048-87-8

Trade names and research codes
cp 50556
cp50556
cp 50,556 1
cp 50556 1
cp 505561
cp50,556 1
cp50556 1
cp505561

Short synonyms
levo nantradol
levonantradol hydrochloride
l nantradol
nantradol,levo

Long synonyms
levo 5,6,6a,7,8,9,10,10a octahydro 6 methyl 3 (1 methyl 4 phenylbutoxy) 1,9 phenanthridinediol 1 acetate

liarozole

WADA group
S7. AGENTS WITH ANTI-OESTROGENIC ACTIVITY

CAS Registry number
115575-11-6

Trade names and research codes
r 75251

Short synonyms
liarozole hydrochloride

Long synonyms
5 [(3 chlorophenyl)(1h imidazol 1 yl)methyl] 1h benzimidazole

liarozole fumarate

WADA group
S7. AGENTS WITH ANTI-OESTROGENIC ACTIVITY

CAS Registry number
145858-52-2

Trade names and research codes
liazal

Terms and Synonyms

liazol
r 85246

lobeline

WADA group
S1. STIMULANTS

MeSH descriptor
lobeline

CAS Registry number
134-63-4
134-64-5
134-65-6
90-69-7

Trade names and research codes
bantron
inflatine
lobatox
lobelidine
lobeline sandoz
lobeton
lobidan
nicerase
nikoban
no kotin
unilobin
zoolobelin

Short synonyms
alpha lobeline
labeline
levo lobeline
lobelin
lobeline hydrochloride
lobeline sulfate

Long synonyms
2 [6 (beta hydroxyphenethyl) 1 methyl 2 piperidyl]acetophenone

loop diuretic agent

WADA group
S8. MASKING AGENTS
P3. DIURETICS

Short synonyms
diuretic agent,loop
high ceiling diuretic
high ceiling diuretic agent
loop diuretic

lorinden a

WADA group
S9. GLUCOCORTICOSTEROIDS

Trade names and research codes
lorinden a

lorinden t

WADA group
S9. GLUCOCORTICOSTEROIDS

Trade names and research codes
lorinden t

loteprednol etabonate

WADA group
S9. GLUCOCORTICOSTEROIDS

CAS Registry number
82034-46-6

Trade names and research codes
alrex
cddd 5604
cddd5604
hgp 1
hgp1
lotemax
loterox
p 5604
p5604

Long synonyms
chloromethyl 17alpha ethoxycarbonyloxy 11beta hydroxy 3 oxoandrosta 1,4 diene 17 carboxylate

lotricomb

WADA group
S9. GLUCOCORTICOSTEROIDS

Trade names and research codes
lotricomb

luteinizing hormone

WADA group
S5. PEPTIDE HORMONES

MeSH descriptor
luteinizing hormone

CAS Registry number
39341-83-8
9002-67-9

Short synonyms
bovine icsh
human luteinizing hormone
icsh
LH
luteinising hormone
lutotropin
lutropin
ovine icsh
ovulating hormone

Long synonyms
hormone,interstitial cell stimulating
interstitial cell stimulating hormone
interstitial stimulating hormone

luteinizing hormone beta subunit

WADA group
S5. PEPTIDE HORMONES

MeSH descriptor
luteinizing hormone, beta subunit

Short synonyms
LH beta subunit
lutropin beta subunit

Long synonyms
luteinizing hormone, beta subunit

luteinizing hormone derivative

WADA group
S5. PEPTIDE HORMONES

Short synonyms
lh derivative
lutropin derivative

lutrelin

WADA group
S5. PEPTIDE HORMONES

CAS Registry number
66866-63-5

Trade names and research codes
wy 40972

Long synonyms
gonadorelin[6 dextro tryptophan 7 (n methylleucine) 9 (n ethylprolinamide) 10 deglycinamide]

mabuterol

WADA group
S6. BETA-2 AGONISTS

CAS Registry number
56341-08-3

Trade names and research codes
kf 868
pb 868 cl

Short synonyms
mabuterol hydrochloride

Long synonyms
4 amino 3 chloro 5 trifluoromethyl alpha [(tert butylamino)methyl]benzyl alcohol
1 (4 amino 3 chloro 5 trifluoromethylphenyl) 2 tert butylaminoethanol
4 amino alpha [(tert butylamino)methyl] 3 chloro 5 (trifluoromethyl)benzyl alcohol

mannitol

WADA group
S8. MASKING AGENTS
P3. DIURETICS

MeSH descriptor
mannitol

CAS Registry number
69-65-8
87-78-5

Trade names and research codes
osmitrol
osmofundin
osmosal
resectisol

Short synonyms
dextro mannitol
d mannitol
manitol
mannit
mannite
mannitol hydrochloride
osmosteril

mazindol

WADA group
S1. STIMULANTS

MeSH descriptor
mazindol

CAS Registry number
22232-71-9

Trade names and research codes
an 448
an-448
an448
dasten
degonan
drinamyl
fagolipo
mazanor
pento adiparthrol
sanorex
slankosan
teronac

Short synonyms
manzindol
mazindole

Long synonyms
5 (4 chlorophenyl) 2,3 dihydro 5 hydroxy 5h imidazo[2,1 a]isoindole
5 hydroxy 5 para chlorophenyl 2,3 dihydro 5h imidazo[2,1 a]isoindole

mazipredone

WADA group
S9. GLUCOCORTICOSTEROIDS

CAS Registry number
13085-08-0
60-39-9

Trade names and research codes
depersolon
depersolone

Long synonyms
11beta,17alpha dihydroxy 21 (4 methyl 1 piperazinyl) 1,4 pregnadiene 3,20 dione
11beta,17alpha dihydroxy 21 n (n methylpiperazinyl)pregna 1,4 diene 3,20 dione
11beta 17alpha dihydroxy 3,20 dioxo 21 (4 methyl 1 piperazinyl)pregna 14 diene
11beta 17alpha dihydroxy 3,20 dioxo 21 (4 methyl 1 piperazyl)pregna 1,4 diene
11 beta,17 alpha dihydroxy 3,20 dioxo 21 n (n' methylpiperazinyl) 1,4 pregnadione
11beta,17alpha dihydroxy 3,20 dioxo 21 n (n' methylpiperazinyl) 1,4 pregnadione
11 beta,17 dihydroxy 21 (4 methyl 1 piperazinyl)pregna 1,4 diene 3,20 dione hydrochloride
11beta, 17 dihydroxy 21 (4 methyl 1 piperazinyl)pregna 1,4 diene 3,20 dione hydrochloride
21 deoxy 21 n (n' methyl n piperazinyl)prednisolone
21 deoxy 21 n(n' methyl)piperazinyl prednisolone hydrochloride
21 deoxy 21 n (n' methyl) piperazinylprednisolone hydrogen chloride
21 deoxy 21 n(n' methyl)piperazinylprednisolone hydrogenchloride
21 (desoxy n methyl n piperazinyl)prednisolone hydrochloride

pregna 1,4 diene 11beta,17alpha diol 3,20 dione,21 n (n methyl piperazinyl)

meclofenoxate

WADA group
S1. STIMULANTS

MeSH descriptor
meclofenoxate

CAS Registry number
3685-84-5
51-68-3

Trade names and research codes
cerutil
helfergin

Short synonyms
anp 235
centrophenoxin
centrophenoxine
centrophenoxine hydrochloride
deanol p chlorophenoxyacetate
lucidril
meclofenoxate hydrochloride
meclophenoxate
para chlorophenoxyacetate 235

Long synonyms
(4 chlorophenoxy)acetic acid 2 (dimethylamino)ethyl ester
deanol para chlorophenoxyacetate 2989
dimethylaminoethyl 4 chlorophenoxyacetate hydrochloride
dimethylaminoethyl ester of chlorphenoxyacetic acid
dimethylaminoethyl para chlorophenoxy acetate
dimethylaminoethyl parachlorophenoxy acetate
2 dimethylaminoethyl para chlorophenoxyacetate
dimethylaminoethyl para chlorophenoxyacetate hydrochloride
para chlorophenoxyacetylcholine

medroxalol

WADA group
P2. BETA-BLOCKERS

CAS Registry number
56290-94-9

Trade names and research codes
mdl 17330 a
mdl 17330a
rmi 81,968 a
rmi 81968 a

Short synonyms
medroxalol hydrochloride

Long synonyms
5 [2 [[3 (1,3 benzodioxol 5 yl) 1 methylpropyl]amino] 1 hydroxyethyl]salicylamide
5 [1 hydroxy 2 [[1 methyl 3 [3,4 (methyllenedioxy)phenyl]propyl]amino]ethyl] 2 hydroxybenzamide

medrysone

WADA group
S9. GLUCOCORTICOSTEROIDS

CAS Registry number
2668-66-8

Trade names and research codes
hms liquifilm
medrocort
nsc 63278
ophthocort
ophthocortin
ophtocortin
spectramedryn

Short synonyms
hydroxymesteron
hydroxymesterone
hydroxymethyl progesterone
hydroxymethylprogesterone
medrisone

Long synonyms
11 beta hydroxy 6 alpha methylpregn 4 ene 3,20 dione
11beta hydroxy 6alpha methyl progesterone
11beta hydroxy 6alpha methylprogesterone

mefenorex

WADA group
S1. STIMULANTS

CAS Registry number
17243-57-1
5586-87-8

Trade names and research codes
doracil
pondinil
ro 4 5282
ro 4-5282
rondimen

Short synonyms
amphetamine,n (3 chloropropyl)
mefenorex hydrochloride
n (3 chloropropyl)amphetamine

Long synonyms
n (3 chloropropyl) 1 methyl 2 phenyl ethylamine
n (3 chloropropyl) 1 methyl 2 phenylethylamine
n 3 chloropropyl 1 methyl 2 phenylethylamine
n (3 chloropropyl) 1 methyl 2 phenylethylamine hydrochloride
n (3 chloropropyl) alpha methylphenethylamine
n (3 chloropropyl) alpha methylphenethylamine hydrochloride

mefexamide

WADA group
S1. STIMULANTS

CAS Registry number
1227-61-8

Trade names and research codes
timodyne

Short synonyms
anp 297

Long synonyms
n (2 diethylaminoethyl) 2 (4 methoxyphenoxy)acetamide
n (2 diethylaminoethyl) 2 (para methoxyphenoxy)acetamide

mefruside

WADA group
S8. MASKING AGENTS
P3. DIURETICS

MeSH descriptor
mefruside

CAS Registry number
7195-27-9

Trade names and research codes
b 1500
b1500
bay 1500
bay1500
bay caron
baycaron
baycarone
fba 1500
fba1500

Short synonyms
dl mefruside
d mefruside
l mefruside

Long synonyms
2 [(4 chloro n1 methyl 3 sulfamoylbenzene sulfonamido)methyl] 2 methyltetrahydrofuran
2 [(4 chloro n1 methyl 3 sulfamoylbenzenesulfonamido)methyl] 2 methyltetrahydrofuran
4 chloro n1 methyl n1 (tetrahydro 2 methyl furfur 2 yl) meta benzenedisulfonamide
4 chloro n1 methyl n1 (tetrahydro 2 methylfurfur 2 yl) meta benzenedisulfonamide
2 [(4 chloro n' methyl 3 sulfamoylbenzenesulfonamido)methyl] 2 methyltetrahydrofuran
4 chloro n' methyl n' (tetrahydro 2 methylfurfur 2 yl) meta benzenedisulfonamide
n (4 chloro 3 sulfamoylbenzenesulfonyl) n methyl 2 furfurylamine

mephentermine

WADA group
S1. STIMULANTS

MeSH descriptor
mephentermine

CAS Registry number
100-92-5
1212-72-2

Trade names and research codes
mephine
vialin
wyamin
wyamine

Short synonyms
hephentermine
mefentermine
mephentermine sulfate
mephetedrine

Long synonyms
n,alpha,alpha trimethylphenethylamine

mepindolol

WADA group
P2. BETA-BLOCKERS

CAS Registry number
23694-81-7
56396-94-2

Trade names and research codes
betagon
caridian
corindolan
she 222

Short synonyms
mepindolol sulfate
pindolol,methyl

Long synonyms
4 (2 hydroxy 3 isopropylaminopropoxy) 2 methylindole
1 isopropylamino 3 (2 methylindol 4 yloxy)propan 2 ol

mepitiostane

WADA group
S4. ANABOLIC AGENTS
S7. AGENTS WITH ANTI-OESTROGENIC ACTIVITY

CAS Registry number
21362-69-6

Long synonyms
2alpha,3alpha epithio 5alpha androstan 17beta yl 1 methoxycyclopentyl ether

meprednisone

WADA group
S9. GLUCOCORTICOSTEROIDS

CAS Registry number
1247-42-3

Trade names and research codes
betalone
betapar
betapred
delta cortene beta
deltisone b
sch 4358

Short synonyms
16 beta methylprednisone
16beta methylprednisone
methylprednisone

mercuderamide

WADA group
P2. BETA-BLOCKERS

CAS Registry number
525-30-4

Trade names and research codes
neptal
unephral

Long synonyms
2 [o [n (3 hydroxymercuri 2 hydroxypropyl)carbamyl]phenoxy]acetic acid

Terms and Synonyms

mersalyl

WADA group
S8. MASKING AGENTS
P3. DIURETICS

MeSH descriptor
mersalyl

CAS Registry number
486-67-9
492-18-2

Trade names and research codes
diuregan
diurgan
diursal
hydrargan
mercugan
mercusal
merphilin
merphyllin
mersalin
mersalyn
neomersyl
salurin
salyrgan
uragan

Short synonyms
mercuramide
mercurosalyl
mersalic acid
mersalyl acid

Long synonyms
mersalyl barbital complex of merethoxylline with procaine
n (gamma hydroxymercuri beta methoxypropyl)salicylamide o acetic acid sodium salt
o [[3 (hydroxymercuri) 2 methoxypropyl]carbamoyl]phenoxyacetic acid sodium salt
sodium o [(3 hydroxymercuri 2 methoxypropyl)carbamoyl]phenoxyacetate

mespirenone

WADA group
S8. MASKING AGENTS
P3. DIURETICS

CAS Registry number
87952-98-5

Trade names and research codes
sh 467
zk 94679

Long synonyms
7alpha acetylthio 17 hydroxy 15beta,16beta methylene 3 oxo 17alpha pregna 1,4 diene 21 carboxylic acid gamma lactone

mestanolone

WADA group
S4. ANABOLIC AGENTS

CAS Registry number
521-11-9

Trade names and research codes
ermalone
hermalone gloset
methybol
protergine

Short synonyms
androstalone
mestalonone
17 methylandrostanolone

Long synonyms
17alpha methyl 5alpha androstan 17beta ol 3 one
17alpha methylandrostan 17beta ol 3 one
androstan 17beta ol 3 one,17 methyl
17beta hydroxy 17alpha methyl 5alpha androstan 3 one
17beta hydroxy 17alpha methylandrostan 3 one

mesterolone

WADA group
S4. ANABOLIC AGENTS

MeSH descriptor
mesterolone

CAS Registry number
1424-00-6

Trade names and research codes
androviron
mestoranum
nsc 75054
proviron
sh 723
vistimon

Long synonyms
5alpha androstane 1alpha methyl 17 beta ol 3 one
1 alpha methyl 5 alpha androstan 17 beta ol 3 one
1alpha methyl 5alpha androstan 17beta ol 3 one
1alpha methyl 5alpha dihydrotestosterone
17beta hydroxy 1alpha methyl 5alpha androstan 3 one
1 methylandrostane 17beta ol 3 one

metandienone

WADA group
S4. ANABOLIC AGENTS

MeSH descriptor
methandrostenolone

CAS Registry number
72-63-9

Trade names and research codes
abirol
c 17309
c17309
danabol
dianabol
geabol
metabolina
nabolin
nbl
nerabol
nerobol
neroboletta
nsc 42722
stenolon
vanabol
verobol

Short synonyms
metadienone
metandienon
metandrostenolone
methandienone

methandrostenolone

Long synonyms
17alpha methyl 1,2 dehydrotestosterone
17alpha methyl 17beta hydroxy 1,4 androstadien 3 one
17alpha methyl 17beta hydroxy androsta 1,4 dien 3 one
17alpha methyl 17beta hydroxyandrosta 1,4 dien 3 one
17beta hydroxy 17alpha methylandrosta 1,4 dien 3 one
17beta hydroxy 17 methyl 1,4 androstadien 3 one
1 dehydro 17alpha methyltestosterone
delta1 dehydro 17alpha methyltestosterone
testosterone,1 dehydro 17alpha methyl

metaraminol

WADA group
S1. STIMULANTS

MeSH descriptor
metaraminol

CAS Registry number
33402-03-8
54-49-9

Trade names and research codes
aramine
araminum
icoralb
levicor
metaril
pressonex
pressonex bitartrate
pressonol

Short synonyms
dextro metaraminol
dextro metaraminol bitartrate
isophenylephrine
levo metaraminol
levo metaraminol bitartrate
l metaraminol bitartrate
meta hydroxynorephedrine
metaradrine
metaraminol bitartrate
metharaminol

Long synonyms
alpha (1 aminoethyl) meta hydroxybenzylalcohol
2 amino 1 (meta hydroxyphenyl) 1 propanol bitartarte

metenolone

WADA group
S4. ANABOLIC AGENTS

MeSH descriptor
methenolone

CAS Registry number
153-00-4

Short synonyms
methenolon
methenolone
methylandrostenolone
1 methyl delta1 androstenolone

Long synonyms
androst 1 en 3 one,17beta hydroxy 1alpha methyl
17beta hydroxy 1alpha methyl 5alpha androst 1 en 3 one
17beta hydroxy 1 methyl 5alpha androst 1 en 3 one
1 methyl delta1 androsten 17beta ol 3 one

metenolone acetate

WADA group
S4. ANABOLIC AGENTS

CAS Registry number
434-05-9

Trade names and research codes
nibal
nsc 74226
primobolan
primobolan s

Short synonyms
methenolone acetate

metenolone enantate

WADA group
S4. ANABOLIC AGENTS

CAS Registry number
303-42-4

Trade names and research codes
nibal injection
nsc 64967
primobolan depot
sq 16374

Short synonyms
metenolone enanthate
metenolone heptanoate
metenolone heptanonate
methenolone enanthate
methenolone oenanthate

methadone

WADA group
S2. NARCOTICS

MeSH descriptor
methadone

CAS Registry number
1095-90-5
125-56-4
23142-53-2
297-88-1
76-99-3

Trade names and research codes
algolysin
an 148
an148
depridol
dolophine
hoe 10820
hoe10820
ketalgin
mephenon
metasedin
methadose
polamidon

Short synonyms
adanon
adanon hydrochloride
algidon
algoxale
althose
althose hydrochloride
amidon
amidone

Terms and Synonyms

amidosan
anadon
butalgin
deamin
diaminon
dianone
dolafin
dolamid
dolesone
dolophine hydrochloride
dorex
dorexol
fenadon
heptadon
heptanon
mecodin
mepecton
methadon
methadone base
methadone hydrobromide
methadone hydrochloride
miadone
moheptan
phenadon
physepton
physeptone
polamivet
polamivit
sinalgin
symoron
win

Long synonyms
6 dimethylamino 4,4 diphenyl 3 heptanone
1,1 diphenyl 1 (2 dimethylaminopropyl) 2 butanone
4,4 diphenyl 6 dimethylamino 3 heptanone

methallibure

WADA group
S5. PEPTIDE HORMONES

MeSH descriptor
methallibure

CAS Registry number
926-93-2

Trade names and research codes
aimax
ay 61122
ay61122
ici 33,828
ici 33828
ici33,828
ici33828
ici compound 33828
nsc 69536
nsc69536

Short synonyms
metallibure

Long synonyms
1 methyl 6 (1 methylallyl) 2,5 dithiobiurea
1 (methylallylthiocarbamoyl) 2 (methylthiocarbamoyl)hydrazine
1 (1 methylallylthiocarbamoyl) 2 (methylthiocarbamoyl)hydrazine
n methylthiocarbamoyl n' [(1 methylallyl)thiocarbamoyl]hydrazine

methamphetamine

WADA group
S1. STIMULANTS

MeSH descriptor
methamphetamine

CAS Registry number
28297-73-6
51-57-0
537-46-2
2-10-7632

Trade names and research codes
adipex
desoxyn
methampex
methedrine
norodin
pervitin
philopon

Short synonyms
ambar
amphedroxyn
corvitin
daropervamin
deofed
deoxyephedrine
desamine
desfedrin
desoxo 5
desoxyephedrine
desoxyfed
destim
desyphed
detrex
dextrim
dextro desoxyephedrine
dextrolevo deoxyephedrine
dextro methylamphetamine
dexyfed
dl methamphetamine
d methamphetamine
doe
doxephrin
doxyfed
drinalfa
effroxine
efroxin
efroxine
esophan
estimulex
eufodrin
eufodrinal
gerovit
hiropon
isophan
isophen
kemodrin
l methamphetamine
metamphetamine
methamine
methamphetamin
methamphetamine hcl
methamphetamine hydrochloride
methamphetamine sulfate
methamphetaminium chloride
methamphin
methoxyn
2 methylamino 1 phenylpropane
methyl amphetamine
methylamphetamine
methylbenzedrine
methylisamin
methylisomyn

methylpropamine
neopharmedrine
n methyl amphetamine
n methylamphetamine
normadrine
norodrin
oxydess
oxydrene
oxyfed
philipon
premodrin
psykoton
semoxydrine
soxysympamine
syndrox
tonedron

Long synonyms
d desoxyephedrine hydrochloride
dextro 1 phenyl 2 methylaminopropane hydrochloride
dextro desoxyephedrine hydrochloride
d methamphetamine hydrochloride
d n,alpha dimethylphenethylamine
d n alpha methyl beta phenylisopropylamine hydrochloride
d n methylamphetamine hydrochloride
methylamphetamine hydrochloride
o desoxyephedrine hydrochloride
phenylisopropylmethylamine hydrochloride
phenylmethylaminopropane hydrochloride

methanandamide

WADA group
S3. CANNABINOIDS

CAS Registry number
157182-49-5
157182-50-8

Trade names and research codes
am 356
am356

Long synonyms
arachidonoyl 1' hydroxy 2' propylamide
n (2 hydroxy 1 methylethyl) 5,8,11,14 eicosatetraenamide

methandriol

WADA group
S4. ANABOLIC AGENTS

MeSH descriptor
methandriol

CAS Registry number
521-10-8

Short synonyms
17 alpha methylandrostenediol
17alpha methylandrostenediol
androdiol
androteston m
diolandrone
diolostene
esjaydiol
madiol
masdiol
megabion
mestenediol
metanabol
metandiol
metandrostenediol
metendiol
methanabol
methandiol
methocryst
methostan
methylandrostendiole
methylandrostenediol
methylandrostenediole
methyldihydrotestosterone
metidione
metildiolo
metocryst
nabadial
neostene
neosteron
neosterone
neutrormone
neutrosteron
notandron
protandren
reviron
stenediol
stenesium

Long synonyms
17alpha methyl 5 androstene 3beta,17beta diol
17alpha methylandrost 5 ene 3beta,17beta diol
17 methyl 5 androstene 3beta,17beta diol

methandriol dipropionate

WADA group
S4. ANABOLIC AGENTS

CAS Registry number
3593-85-9

Trade names and research codes
durabolic
probolin
therabolin
therobolin

methazolamide

WADA group
S8. MASKING AGENTS
P3. DIURETICS

MeSH descriptor
methazolamide

CAS Registry number
554-57-4

Trade names and research codes
cl 8490
cl8490
neptazane

Short synonyms
metazolamide

Long synonyms
5 acetamido 4 methyl 1,3,4 thiadiazole 2 sulfonamide
5 acetylimino 4 methyl 2 sulfamoyl 1,3,4 thiadiazoline

methcathinone

WADA group
S1. STIMULANTS

CAS Registry number
5650-44-2

Short synonyms
ephedrone
2 methylaminopropiophenone
methylpropion

methemoglobin

WADA group
M1. ENHANCEMENT OF OXYGEN TRANSFER

MeSH descriptor
methemoglobin

Short synonyms
ferric hemoglobin
ferrihemoglobin
haemiglobin
hemiglobin
metahaemoglobin
metahemoglobin
methaemoglobin
oxymethemoglobin

methoxamine

WADA group
S6. BETA-2 AGONISTS

MeSH descriptor
methoxamine

CAS Registry number
390-28-3
61-16-5

Trade names and research codes
mexan
mexane
pressomin
pressomin hydrochloride
vasoxine
vasoxine hydrochloride
vasoxyl
vasoxyl hydrochloride
vasylox
vasylox hydrochloride

Short synonyms
methoxamedrine
methoxamine hydrochloride
metoxamine

Long synonyms
alpha (1 aminoethyl) 2,5 dimethoxybenzyl alcohol
alpha (1 aminoethyl) 2,5 dimethoxybenzyl alcohol hydrochloride
2 amino 1 (2,5 dimethoxyphenyl) 1 propanol
2 amino 1 (2,5 dimethoxyphenyl) 1 propanol hydrochloride
beta (2,5 dimethoxyphenyl) beta hydroxyisopropylamine hydrochloride
beta hydroxy beta (2,5 dimethoxyphenyl)isopropylamine hydrochloride
2,5 dimethoxynorephedrine hydrochloride

4 methoxyamphetamine

WADA group
S1. STIMULANTS

CAS Registry number
23239-32-9

Short synonyms
amphetamine,4 methoxy
para methoxyamphetamine

Long synonyms
2 amino 1 (4 methoxyphenyl)propane
1 (4 methoxyphenyl) 2 aminopropane
1 (4 methoxyphenyl)isopropylamine
(4 methoxyphenyl)isopropylamine

2 methoxymethamphetamine

WADA group
S1. STIMULANTS

Short synonyms
amphetamine,2 methoxy n methyl
methamphetamine,2 methoxy
2 methoxy n methylamphetamine

3 methoxymethamphetamine

WADA group
S1. STIMULANTS

Short synonyms
amphetamine,3 methoxy n methyl
methamphetamine,3 methoxy
3 methoxy n methylamphetamine

4 methoxymethamphetamine

WADA group
S1. STIMULANTS

CAS Registry number
22331-70-0

Short synonyms
amphetamine,4 methoxy n methyl
methamphetamine,4 methoxy
4 methoxy n methylamphetamine

methoxyphenamine

WADA group
S1. STIMULANTS
S6. BETA-2 AGONISTS

CAS Registry number
3-10-5588
93-30-1

Trade names and research codes
orthoxine
ortodrinex
u 433

Short synonyms
methoxiphenadrin
methoxyphenamine hydrochloride
mexyphamine

Long synonyms
1 (ortho methoxyphenyl) n methyl 2 propylamine
phenethylamine,n,alpha dimethyl ortho methoxy

methyclothiazide

WADA group
S8. MASKING AGENTS
P3. DIURETICS

MeSH descriptor
methyclothiazide

CAS Registry number
135-07-9

Trade names and research codes
aquatensen
enduron
enduronum
thiazidil

Short synonyms
methiclothiazide
methylchlorothiazide
methylclothiazide

Long synonyms
6 chloro 3 chloromethyl 3,4 dihydro 2 methyl 2h 1,2,4 benzothiadiazine 7 sulfonamide 1,1 dioxide
6 chloro 3 chloromethyl 3,4 dihydro 2 methyl 7 sulfamoyl 1,2,4 benzothiadiazine 1,1 dioxide

4 [4 methyl 2 [4 [2 (1 piperidinyl)ethoxy]phenyl] 7 pivaloyloxy 2h 1 benzopyran 3 ylphenyl] pivalate

WADA group
S7. AGENTS WITH ANTI-OESTROGENIC ACTIVITY

CAS Registry number
182167-03-9
182167-49-3

Trade names and research codes
em 776
em776
em 800
em800
sc 5705
sc5705

Long synonyms
4 [7 (2,2 dimethyl 1 oxopropoxy) 4 methyl 2 [4 [2 (1 piperidinyl)ethoxy]phenyl] 2h 1 benzopyran 3 ylphenyl] 2,2 dimethylpropanoate

4 methylaminorex

WADA group
S1. STIMULANTS

Trade names and research codes
mcm 822

Short synonyms
aminorex,4 methyl

Long synonyms
2 amino 4 methyl 5 phenyl 2 oxazoline
4,5 dihydro 4 methyl 5 phenyl 2 oxazolamine

4 methylamphetamine

WADA group
S1. STIMULANTS

CAS Registry number
64-11-9

Short synonyms
aptrol
(4 methylphenyl)isopropylamine
para methylamphetamine
1 para tolyl 2 propylamine
1 (p tolyl) 2 propylamine

Long synonyms
2 amino 1 (para methylphenyl)propane
para,alpha dimethylphenethylamine

methyldienolone

WADA group
S4. ANABOLIC AGENTS

Trade names and research codes
methyl d
methyl dien
methyldien

Long synonyms
17alpha methyl 17beta hydroxyestra 4,9(10)dien 3 one
17beta hydroxy 17alpha methylestra 4,9(10)dien 3 one
17beta hydroxy 17 methylestra 4,9(10)dien 3 one

3,4 methylenedioxyamphetamine

WADA group
S1. STIMULANTS

MeSH descriptor
3,4-methylenedioxyamphetamine

CAS Registry number
4764-17-4

Short synonyms
mda
methylene dioxyamphetamine
methylenedioxyamphetamine
3,4-methylenedioxyamphetamine
tenamfetamine

Long synonyms
1 (3,4 methylenedioxyphenyl) 2 aminopropane
3,4 methylenedioxyphenylisopropylamine

3,4 methylenedioxyamphetamine derivative

WADA group
S1. STIMULANTS

Long synonyms
amphetamine,3,4 methylenedioxy derivative
3,4 methylenedioxyphenylisopropylamine derivative

3,4 methylenedioxymethamphetamine

WADA group
S1. STIMULANTS

MeSH descriptor
n-methyl-3,4-methylenedioxyamphetamine

CAS Registry number
42542-10-9

Short synonyms
'ecstasy'
MDMA
methylenedioxymethamphetamine

Long synonyms
1 (1,3 benzodioxol 5 yl) n methyl 2 propanamine
1 (1,3 benzodioxol 5 yl) n methyl 2 propylamine

Terms and Synonyms

methamphetamine,3,4 methylenedioxy
2 methylamino 1 (3,4 methylenedioxyphenyl)propane
5 (2 methylaminopropyl) 1,3 benzodioxole
1 (3,4 methylenedioxyphenyl) 2 methylaminopropane
n,alpha dimethyl 3,4 methylenedioxyphenethylamine
n,alpha dimethyl beta (3,4 methylenedioxyphenyl)ethylamine
n,alpha dimethylhomopiperonylamine
n methyl 1 (3,4 methylenedioxyphenyl) 2 aminopropane
n methyl 3,4 methylenedioxyamphetamine
n-methyl-3,4-methylenedioxyamphetamine

15beta,16beta methylenemexrenone

WADA group
S8. MASKING AGENTS
P3. DIURETICS

CAS Registry number
84542-26-7

Trade names and research codes
sh d515
zk 91587

Long synonyms
7alpha methoxycarbonyl 15beta,16beta methylene 3 oxo 17alpha pregn 4 ene 21,17 carbolactone
mexrenone,15beta,16beta methylene

methylephedrine

WADA group
S1. STIMULANTS

CAS Registry number
552-79-4
69671-02-9

Short synonyms
methephedrine
n methyl ephedrine
n methylephedrine

3 methylnaringenin

WADA group
S7. AGENTS WITH ANTI-OESTROGENIC ACTIVITY

CAS Registry number
132147-69-4

Trade names and research codes
be 14348b
be14348b
be 14348c
be14348c
ws 7528
ws7528

methylphenidate

WADA group
S1. STIMULANTS

MeSH descriptor
methylphenidate

CAS Registry number
113-45-1
298-59-9

Trade names and research codes
c 4311-b
c4311-b
c4311b
centedrin
concerta
concerta xl
metadate
methylin
methypatch
phenidylate
ritalin
ritalin hydrochloride
ritalin la
ritalin sr
sr 20

Short synonyms
dl threo methylphenidate
methylfenidate
methyl phenidate
methylphenidate hydrochloride
methylphenidylacetate
methylphenindate
methylphenydate
phenidyl hydrochloride

Long synonyms
alpha phenyl 2 piperidineacetic acid methyl ester
alpha phenyl alpha (2 piperidyl)acetic acid methyl ester
d erythro methyl phenidylacetate
dl erythro methyl phenidylacetate
methyl 2 phenyl 2 piperid 2 ylacetate

methylprednisolone

WADA group
S9. GLUCOCORTICOSTEROIDS

MeSH descriptor
methylprednisolone

CAS Registry number
6923-42-8
83-43-2

Trade names and research codes
medrol
medrol adt pak
medrol compositum
medrol dosepak
medrone
mesopren
metrisone
metypresol
neomedrone
nsc 19987
prednol
solomet
solu decortin
urbason

Short synonyms
6 alpha methylprednisolone
6alpha methylprednisolone
beta methylprednisolone
meprednisolone
methyl prednisolone
2 methylprednisolone
5 methylprednisolone
6 methyl prednisolone
6 methylprednisolone
methylsterolone

Long synonyms
6alpha methyl delta1 hydrocortisone

11beta,17alpha,21 trihydroxy 6alpha methyl 1,4 pregnadiene 3,20 dione
6 methyl delta 1 hydrocortisone

16beta methylprednisolone

WADA group
S9. GLUCOCORTICOSTEROIDS

CAS Registry number
79645-29-7

Trade names and research codes
betanison
betanisone

Short synonyms
16beta methylprednisolene
16 methylprednisolone

methylprednisolone aceponate

WADA group
S9. GLUCOCORTICOSTEROIDS

CAS Registry number
86401-95-8

Trade names and research codes
advantan
adventan
sh 440
zk 91588

methylprednisolone acetate

WADA group
S9. GLUCOCORTICOSTEROIDS

CAS Registry number
53-36-1

Trade names and research codes
depo medrol
depomedrol
depomedron
depo medrone
depomedrone
depot medrate
urbason retard
veriderm medrol

Short synonyms
depmedalone 40
depmedalone 80
depo medrate
medrol enpak
mepred
methyl prednisolon acetate
methyl prednisolone acetate
6 methylprednisolone acetate

Long synonyms
6alpha methylprednisolone (21 acetate)
6alpha methylprednisolone 21 acetate
6 alpha methylprednisolone acetate
6alpha methylprednisolone acetate
methyl 6 delta hydrocortisone acetate

methylprednisolone sodium succinate

WADA group
S9. GLUCOCORTICOSTEROIDS

MeSH descriptor
methylprednisolone hemisuccinate

CAS Registry number
3-3-2375
2921-57-5

Trade names and research codes
a methopred
amethopred
solu medrol
solumedrol
solumedrone
urbason solubile

Short synonyms
methylprednisolone succinate

Long synonyms
6alpha methylprednisolone 21 sodium succinate
6alpha methylprednisolone 21 succinate
6 alpha methylprednisolone 21 succinate sodium
methylprednisolone 21 hemisuccinate
methylprednisolone hemisuccinate
methylprednisolone hemisuccinate hydrochloride
6 methyl prednisolon hemisuccinate sodium

methylprednisolone suleptanate

WADA group
S9. GLUCOCORTICOSTEROIDS

CAS Registry number
90350-40-6

Trade names and research codes
medrosol
promedrol
u 67590a

Long synonyms
methylprednisolone 21 [8 [(2 sulfoethyl)methylamino] 8 oxooctanoate]
methylprednisolone 21 [8 [methyl(2 sulfoethyl)amino] 8 oxooctanoate]

methyltestosterone

WADA group
S4. ANABOLIC AGENTS

MeSH descriptor
methyltestosterone

CAS Registry number
58-18-4

Trade names and research codes
agovirin
agovirin depot
'android'
testoviron
testred

Short synonyms
17 alpha methyltestosterone
17alpha methyltestosterone
andrhormone
andrometh
andronex
androral
androsan
androsten
androxil oral
anertan
anertan perlingual
entestil m

glosso sterandryl
glossosterandryl
homan
homandren
hormale
malestrone
malogen
malogene
masenone
menandron
mesteron
mesterone
metandren
metandrene
metestine
metexterona
methylets
methyltesterone
methyltestosteron
methyl testosterone
17 methyl testosterone
17 methyltestosterone
nadosterone
neo hambreol m
neo hombreol m
neohombreol m
nsc 9701
nu man
numan
oraviron
oravirone
orchisteron
orchisterone m
oreon methyl
oreton m
oreton methyl
pantestin oral
suprasteron
synandrets
synandrotabs
syndren
telipex
testahomen
testhormone
testin
testin tabletter
testipron
testobase
testoform
testogenina
testogenine
testonorpon
testora
testore
testorex
testovis
testovis compresse
testoxyl perlinguale
testral
testrina m
tostrina m
virex oral
virormolo
virormone oral

Long synonyms
17alpha methyl 4 androsten 17beta ol 3 on
17beta hydroxy 17alpha methyl 4 androsten 3 on

4' methylthiopropranolol

WADA group
P2. BETA-BLOCKERS

Short synonyms
propranolol,4' methylthio

Long synonyms
1 isopropylamino 3 (4 methylthio 1 naphthyloxy) 2 propanol

metipranolol

WADA group
P2. BETA-BLOCKERS

MeSH descriptor
metipranolol

CAS Registry number
22664-55-7

Trade names and research codes
betamann
betamet
betanol
beta ophtiole
disorat
glauline
ophtiole
optipranolol
trimepranol

Short synonyms
betanolol
methypranol
metipranolol hydrochloride

Long synonyms
1 (4 hydroxy 2,3,5 trimethylphenoxy) 3 (isopropylamino) 2 propanol 4 acetate
4 [2 hydroxy 3 (isopropylamino)propoxy] 2,3,6 trimethylphenyl acetate

metolazone

WADA group
S8. MASKING AGENTS
P3. DIURETICS

MeSH descriptor
metolazone

CAS Registry number
17560-51-9

Trade names and research codes
diulo
metenix
miclox
microx
mykrox
sr 720 22
sr 72022
zaroxolyn

Short synonyms
metalazone
metolazon

Long synonyms
7 chloro 1,2,3,4 tetrahydro 2 methyl 3 (2 methylphenyl) 4 oxo 6 quinazolinesulfonamide
7 chloro 1,2,3,4 tetrahydro 2 methyl 4 oxo 3 ortho tolyl 6 quinazolinesulfonamide

metoprolol

WADA group
P2. BETA-BLOCKERS

MeSH descriptor
metoprolol

CAS Registry number
37350-58-6

Trade names and research codes
beloc duriles
belok zok
betaloc
h 93-26
metoprolol durules
metoprolol oros

Short synonyms
metropolol

Long synonyms
1 isopropylamino 3 [4 (2 methoxyethyl)phenoxy] 2 propanol

metoprolol fumarate

WADA group
P2. BETA-BLOCKERS

CAS Registry number
80274-67-5

Trade names and research codes
lopresor oros
metoros

metoprolol succinate

WADA group
P2. BETA-BLOCKERS

CAS Registry number
98418-47-4

Trade names and research codes
toprol
toprol xl

metoprolol tartrate

WADA group
P2. BETA-BLOCKERS

CAS Registry number
56392-17-7

Trade names and research codes
beloc
bloxan
cgp 2175e
cgp2175e
kapodine
lopresor
lopresor sr
lopressor
lopressor retard
prelis
selokeen
seloken
seloken zoc
selozok
slow lopresor

metribolone

WADA group
S4. ANABOLIC AGENTS

MeSH descriptor
metribolone

CAS Registry number
965-93-5

Trade names and research codes
r 1881
ru 1881

Short synonyms
methyltrienolone

Long synonyms
17alpha methyl 4,9,11 estratrien 17beta ol 3 one
17alpha methylestra 4,9,11 trien 17beta ol 3 one
17beta hydroxy 17alpha methyl estra 4,9,11 trien 3 one
17beta hydroxy 17 methyl 19 norandrosta 4,9,11 trien 3 one
17beta hydroxy 17 methylestra 4,9,11 trien 3 one
estra 4,9,11 trien 17beta ol 3 one,17alpha methyl

metyrapone

WADA group
S8. MASKING AGENTS

MeSH descriptor
metyrapone

CAS Registry number
22752-91-6
2405-72-3
54-36-4
908-35-0

Trade names and research codes
methopyrone
metopiron
metopirone
metopyrone
metroprione
su 4885
su 8874
su4885
su8874

Short synonyms
mepyrapone
metapiron
metapirone
metapyrone
methbipyranone
methbipyrapone
methopyrapone
methyrapone
metopirone ditartrate
metyrapon
metyrapone 637
metyrapone hydrochloride
metyrapone tartrate

Long synonyms
1,2 bis(pyrid 3 yl) 2 methyl 1 propanone
2 methyl 1,2 bis(3 pyridyl) 1 propanone
2 methyl 1,2 dipyrid 3 yl 1 oxopropane
2 methyl 1,2 dipyridyl(3') 1 oxo propane
2 methyl 1,2 di 3 pyridyl 1 propanone

Terms and Synonyms

mexrenoate potassium

WADA group
S8. MASKING AGENTS
P3. DIURETICS

CAS Registry number
41020-67-1

Trade names and research codes
sc 26714

Short synonyms
potassium mexrenoate

Long synonyms
17 hydroxy 3 oxo 17alpha pregn 4 ene 7alpha,21 dicarboxylic acid 7 methyl ester 21 potassium salt
17 hydroxy 7alpha methoxycarbonyl 3 oxo 17alpha pregn 4 ene 21 carboxylate potassium

mexrenoic acid

WADA group
S8. MASKING AGENTS
P3. DIURETICS

CAS Registry number
41020-68-2

Short synonyms
mexrenoate

mexrenone

WADA group
S8. MASKING AGENTS
P3. DIURETICS

CAS Registry number
41020-65-9

Trade names and research codes
sc 25152
zk 32055

Short synonyms
mexrenoic acid lactone

Long synonyms
7alpha methoxycarbonyl 3 oxo 17alpha pregn 4 ene 21,17 carbolactone

mibolerone

WADA group
S4. ANABOLIC AGENTS

CAS Registry number
4-9-3704

Trade names and research codes
'cheque'
matenon
u 10997
u10997

Short synonyms
7alpha,17 dimethylnandrolone
nandrolone,7alpha,17 dimethyl

Long synonyms
7alpha,17alpha dimethyl 19 nortestosterone
7alpha,17alpha dimethylnandrolone
7alpha,17 dimethyl 19 nortestosterone

midodrine

WADA group
S1. STIMULANTS

MeSH descriptor
midodrine

CAS Registry number
3092-17-9
42794-76-3

Trade names and research codes
a 4020 linz
a4020 linz
alphamine
gutron
midon
proamatine
st 1085
st1085

Short synonyms
midodrin
misodrine
mitodrine

Long synonyms
alpha (2,5 dimethoxyphenyl) beta glycinamidoethanol
alpha glycinamidomethyl 2,5 dimethoxybenzyl alcohol
1 (2',5' dimethoxyphenyl) 2 glycinamidoethan 1 ol hydrochloride
1 (2,5 dimethoxyphenyl) 2 glycinamidoethanol
1 (2',5' dimethoxyphenyl) 2 glycinamidoethanol hydrochloride
dl 1 (2',5' dimethoxyphenyl) 2 glucinamidoethan 1 ol hydrochloride
dl 1 (2',5' dimethoxyphenyl) 2 glycinamidoethan 1 ol hcl
dl 1 (2',5' dimethoxyphenyl) 2 glycinamidoethan 1 ol hydrochloride
2 glycinamido 1 (2,5 dimethoxyphenyl)ethanol

minamestane

WADA group
S7. AGENTS WITH ANTI-OESTROGENIC ACTIVITY

CAS Registry number
105051-87-4

Trade names and research codes
fce 24928
fce24928

Long synonyms
4 aminoandrosta 1,4,6 triene 3,17 dione

miproxifene phosphate

WADA group
S7. AGENTS WITH ANTI-OESTROGENIC ACTIVITY

CAS Registry number
115767-74-3

Trade names and research codes
tat 59

Long synonyms
4 [1 [4 [2 (dimethylamino)ethoxy]phenyl] 2 (4 isopropylphenyl) 1 butenyl]phenyl phosphate

modafinil

WADA group
S1. STIMULANTS

CAS Registry number
68693-11-8

Trade names and research codes
alertec
crl 40476
crl40476
modasomil
modiodal
provigil
vigil

Short synonyms
benzhydrylsulfinylacetamide

Long synonyms
2 [(diphenylmethyl)sulfinyl]acetamide

mometasone furoate

WADA group
S9. GLUCOCORTICOSTEROIDS

CAS Registry number
83919-23-7

Trade names and research codes
asmanex
ecural
elocom
elocon
nasonex
sch 32088
sch32088

Short synonyms
mometasone 17 (2 furoate)
mometasone 17 furoate

Long synonyms
9,21 dichloro 11,17 dihydroxy 16 methylpregna 1,4 diene 3,20 dione 17 (2 furoate)

monocomponent insulin

WADA group
S5. PEPTIDE HORMONES

Trade names and research codes
actrapid hm
insulin lente mc

Short synonyms
human monocomponent insulin
insulin,monocomponent
monocomponent human insulin

moprolol

WADA group
P2. BETA-BLOCKERS

CAS Registry number
27058-84-0
5741-22-0

Trade names and research codes
s.d. 1601
sd 1601

Long synonyms
1 isopropylamino 3 (2 methoxyphenoxy) 2 propanol

morazone

WADA group
S1. STIMULANTS

CAS Registry number
6536-18-1

Trade names and research codes
delimon
novartrina
rosimon neu
tarugan

morphine

WADA group
S2. NARCOTICS

MeSH descriptor
morphine

CAS Registry number
52-26-6
57-27-2

Trade names and research codes
anpec
duromorph
epimorph
miro
morfin
morfine
opso
skenan

Short synonyms
cis morphine
morphia
morphin
morphine alkaloid
morphine chlorhydrate
morphine chloride
morphine hydrochloride
morphine suspension
morphinium
morphium
trans morphine

Long synonyms
3,6 dihydroxy n methyl 4,5 epoxy 7 morphinene
microcrystalline morphine suspension

morphine 6 acetate

WADA group
S2. NARCOTICS

CAS Registry number
2784-73-8

Short synonyms
6 acetylmorphine
6 monoacetylmorphine
6 o acetylmorphine
6 o monoacetylmorphine

morphine sulfate

WADA group
S2. NARCOTICS

CAS Registry number
23095-84-3
35764-55-7
64-31-3

Trade names and research codes
astramorph
avinza
depomorphine
dolcontin
duramorph
duramorple
kadian
kapanol
moraxen
moscontin
ms contin
msir
mst
mst 100
mst 60
mst continus
mst mundipharma
mxl
noceptin
oblioser
oramorph
'rms'
roxanol
roxanol sr
sevredol
skenan lp

Short synonyms
morphine 3 ethereal sulfate
morphine 3 sulfate
morphine 6 sulfate
morphinesulfate
morphine sulfate pentahydrate

muzolimine

WADA group
S8. MASKING AGENTS
P3. DIURETICS

MeSH descriptor
muzolimine

CAS Registry number
55294-15-0

Trade names and research codes
bayer g 2821
bayer g2821
bay g 2821
bay g2821
edrul

Short synonyms
musolimino

Long synonyms
3 amino 1 [1 (3,4 dichlorophenyl)ethyl] 2 pyrazolin 5 one
3 amino 1 (3,4 dichloro alpha methylbenzyl) 2 pyrazolin 5 one
3 amino 1 (dichloro alpha methylbenzyl) 2 pyrazolin 5 one
2 pyrazolin 5 one,3 amino 1 (3,4 dichloro alpha methylbenzyl)

mycolog

WADA group
S9. GLUCOCORTICOSTEROIDS

CAS Registry number
53262-75-2

Trade names and research codes
kenacomb
kenacombin
mycolog
mytrex
triadcortyl

Long synonyms
gramicidin with neomycin,nystatin and triamcinolone acetonide

nadolol

WADA group
P2. BETA-BLOCKERS

MeSH descriptor
nadolol

CAS Registry number
42200-33-9

Trade names and research codes
betadol
corgard
solgol
solgol mite
sq 11725

Long synonyms
5 (3 tert butylamino 2 hydroxypropoxy) 1,2,3,4 tetrahydronaphthalene 2,3 diol
1 (tert butylamino) 3 [(5,6,7,8 tetrahydro 6,7 dihydroxynaphth 1 yl)oxy] 2 propanol

nafarelin

WADA group
S5. PEPTIDE HORMONES

MeSH descriptor
nafarelin

CAS Registry number
76932-56-4

Trade names and research codes
rs 94991

Long synonyms
gonadorelin[6 [3 (2 naphthyl) dextro alanine]]
gonadorelin[6 dextro [3 (2 naphthyl)alanine]]
5 oxoprolylhistidyltryptophylseryltyrosyl[3 (2 naphthyl) dextro alanyl]leucylarginylprolylglycinamide
pyroglutamylhistidyltryptophylseryltyrosyl[3 (2 naphthyl) dextro alanyl]leucylarginylprolylglycinamide

nafarelin acetate

WADA group
S5. PEPTIDE HORMONES

CAS Registry number
76932-60-0

Trade names and research codes
rs 94991 298
synarel

Short synonyms
napharelin acetate

nafoxidine

WADA group
S7. AGENTS WITH ANTI-OESTROGENIC ACTIVITY

MeSH descriptor
nafoxidine

CAS Registry number
1845-11-0
1847-63-8

Trade names and research codes
nsc 70735
u 11 100 a
u 11100 a
u 11100a

Short synonyms
nafoxidine hydrochloride

Long synonyms
3,4 dihydro 6 methoxy 2 phenyl 1 [4 (2 pyrrolidinoethoxy)phenyl]naphthalene
1 [2 [4 (3,4 dihydro 6 methoxy 2 phenyl 1 naphthyl)phenoxy]ethyl]pyrrolidine
1 [2 [4 (6 methoxy 2 phenyl 3,4 dihydro 1 naphthyl)phenoxy]ethyl]pyrrolidine
1 [2 [para (3,4 dihydro 6 methoxy 2 phenyl 1 naphthyl)phenoxy]ethyl]pyrrolidine
1 [2 [para (3,4 dihydro 6 methoxy 2 phenyl 1 naphthyl)phenoxy]ethyl]pyrrolidine hydrochloride
1 [2 [para (6 methoxy 2 phenyl 3,4 dihydronaphth 1 yl)phenoxy]ethyl]pyrrolidine
1 [4 (2 pyrrolidinoethoxy)phenyl] 2 phenyl 6 methoxy 3,4 dihydronaphthalene

naminterol

WADA group
S6. BETA-2 AGONISTS

CAS Registry number
93047-40-6

nandrolone

WADA group
S4. ANABOLIC AGENTS

MeSH descriptor
nandrolone

CAS Registry number
434-22-0

Short synonyms
17alpha 19 nortestosterone
beta 19 nortestosterone
17beta hydroxy 4 estren 3 one
17beta hydroxyestr 4 en 3 one
beta nortestosterone
17beta nortestosterone
estr 4 en 17beta ol 3 one
estr 4 en 3 one,17beta hydroxy
4 estren 17beta ol 3 one
norandrostenolone
19 norandrostenolone
19 nor d homosterone
19 nortesterone
nortestonate
nortestosterone
17 nortestosterone
19 nortestosterone
19 nortestosterone enantiomer
nortestosterone ester
3 oxo 4 estren 17beta ol

Long synonyms
17beta hydroxy 19 nor 4 androsten 3 one
17beta hydroxy 19 norandrost 4 en 3 one

nandrolone 4 hexyloxyhydrocinnamate

WADA group
S4. ANABOLIC AGENTS

CAS Registry number
52279-57-9

Trade names and research codes
anadur

Long synonyms
17beta hydroxy 4 estren 3 on 17beta [3 (para hexyloxyphenyl)propionate]
nandrolone 3 (4 hexyloxyphenyl)propionate
nandrolone para hexyloxyhydrocinnamate
nortestosterone 3 (4 hexyloxyphenyl)propionate
19 nortestosterone 3 (para hexyloxyphenyl)propionate
nortestosterone beta (para hexyloxyphenyl)propionate
19 nortestosterone beta (para hexyloxyphenyl)propionate

nandrolone cyclohexylpropionate

WADA group
S4. ANABOLIC AGENTS

CAS Registry number
912-57-2

Trade names and research codes
andol
retarbolin
sanabolicum

Long synonyms
nortestosterone cyclohexyl propionate
19 nortestosterone cyclohexylpropionate

nandrolone decanoate

WADA group
S4. ANABOLIC AGENTS

CAS Registry number
360-70-3

Trade names and research codes
anabolin la
analone
deca durabolin
decadurabolin
hybolin decanoate
kabolin
nandrobolic la
neo durabolic
retabolil

Short synonyms
nandrolondecanoate

Terms and Synonyms

nandrolone 17 decanoate
norandrostenolonedecanoate
norandrostenolone decanoate
nortestosterone decanoate
19 nortestosterone decanoate

Long synonyms
17beta hydroxestr 4 en 3 one 17beta decanoate
17beta hydroxy 19 norandrost 4 en 3 one decanoate
17beta hydroxy 4 estren 3 one 17 decanoate
17beta hydroxyestr 4 en 3 one 17 decanoate
17beta hydroxyestr 4 en 3 one decanoate
17beta hydroxygon 4 en 3 one decanoate
gon 4 en 17beta ol 3 one decanoate
19 nortestosterone 17 decanoate

nandrolone derivative

WADA group
S4. ANABOLIC AGENTS

Short synonyms
norandrostenolone derivative
nortesterone derivative
19 nortesterone derivative
nortestosterone derivative
19 nortestosterone derivative

Long synonyms
19 norandrostenolone derivative
nortestosterone adamantane carboxylate

nandrolone furylpropionate

WADA group
S4. ANABOLIC AGENTS

CAS Registry number
7642-64-0

Trade names and research codes
demelon

nandrolone laurate

WADA group
S4. ANABOLIC AGENTS

CAS Registry number
26490-31-3

Trade names and research codes
fortadex
laurabolin
laurobolin

Short synonyms
nandrolone dodecanoate
nandrolone laurinate
norandrostenolone laurinate
nortestosterone laurate
19 nortestosterone laurate
nortestosterone laurinate
19 nortestosterone laurinate

Long synonyms
17 beta hydroxy 19 norandrost 4 en 3 one laurinate
17 beta hydroxyestr 4 en 3 one laurinate

nandrolone phenpropionate

WADA group
S4. ANABOLIC AGENTS

CAS Registry number
62-90-8

Trade names and research codes
anticatabolin
durabolin
ft 19
ft19
hormonabol
hybolin
hybolin improved
nandrobolic
nandrolin
nerobolil
nerobolyl
norabol
norandrol
norbalin
norstenol
nsc 23162
nsc23162
sintabolin
strabolene
superanabolon
superanabolone
superbolin

Short synonyms
nandrolone phenylpropionate
nandrolonephenylpropionate
nortestosterone hydrocinnamate
nor tpp

Long synonyms
17beta hydroxy 4 estren 3 one hydrocinnamate
17beta hydroxyestr 4 en 3 one 3 phenylpropionate
19 nor 17beta hydroxy 3 ketoandrostene 17 phenylpropionate
nor androstenolone phenyl propionate
norandrostenolone phenylpropionate
norandrostenolonphenylpropionate
19 nor delta 4 androsten 17beta ol 3 one beta phenylpropionate
17 nortestosterone 3 phenylpropionate
19 nortestosterone beta phenylpropionate
nortestosterone phenylpropionate
nortestosteronephenylpropionate
19 nor testosterone phenylpropionate
19 nortestosterone phenylpropionate
19 nortestosteronephenylpropionate

nandrolone undecanoate

WADA group
S4. ANABOLIC AGENTS

CAS Registry number
862-89-5

Trade names and research codes
dynabolon

Short synonyms
nandrolone 17beta undecanoate
nandrolone 17beta undecylate
nandrolone undecylate
nortestosterone undecanoate
nortestosterone undecylate
nortestosterone undecylenate
undecyloyl norandrostenolone
undecyloylnorandrostenolone

Long synonyms
17beta hydroxy 19 nor 4 androsten 3 one 17alpha n decanoate
17beta undecylol 19 nor 4 androsten 3 one
17beta undecyloyl 19 nor 4 androstene 3 one

19 norandrostenolone undecylate

nantradol

WADA group
S3. CANNABINOIDS

CAS Registry number
72028-54-7

Trade names and research codes
cp 44001
cp44001
cp 44,001 1
cp 44001 1
cp 440011
cp44,001 1
cp44001 1
cp440011

Short synonyms
nantradol hydrochloride

Long synonyms
5,6,6a,7,8,9,10,10a octahydro 6 methyl 3 (1 methyl 4 phenylbutoxy) 1,9 phenanthridinediol 1 acetate
5,6,6abeta,7,8,9alpha,10,10aalpha octahydro 6beta methyl 3 (1 methyl 4 phenylbutoxy) 1,9 phenanthridinediol 1 acetate

1 (1 naphthyloxy) 3 [6 [2 (2 pyridyl)ethoxy]hexylamino] 2 propanol

WADA group
P2. BETA-BLOCKERS

Trade names and research codes
gr 81706

nebivolol

WADA group
P2. BETA-BLOCKERS

CAS Registry number
99200-09-6

Trade names and research codes
lobivon
nebilet
nebilox
r 067555
r 65824
r 67138
r 67145
r 67555

Short synonyms
narbivolol
nebivolol hydrochloride

Long synonyms
bis[2 (6 fluoro 1,2,3,4 tetrahydrobenzo[b]pyran 2 yl) 2 hydroxyethyl]amine

neutral insulin

WADA group
S5. PEPTIDE HORMONES

CAS Registry number
9004-14-2

Trade names and research codes
actrapid
berlinsulin
endopancrine
hoe 21 gh
hoe 21 ph
humulin s
novo actrapid
novopen
nuralin
orgasuline
umuline
velasulin
velosulin

Short synonyms
novoactrapid insulin

nicocortonide

WADA group
S9. GLUCOCORTICOSTEROIDS

CAS Registry number
65415-41-0

Long synonyms
11beta,14,17,21 tetrahydroxypregn 4 ene 3,20 dione cyclic 14,17 acetal with crotonaldehyde 21 isonicotinate

nicomorphine

WADA group
S2. NARCOTICS

CAS Registry number
12040-41-4
35055-78-8
639-48-5

Trade names and research codes
vilan

Short synonyms
3,6 dinicotinoylmorphine
morphine 3,6 dinicotinate
nicomorphine hydrochloride

nifenalol

WADA group
P2. BETA-BLOCKERS

CAS Registry number
5054-57-9
5704-60-9
7413-36-7

Short synonyms
dextro inpea
dextro levo inpea
d inpea
dl inpea
INPEA
inpea hydrochloride
isophenethanol
isophenethyl alcohol
levo inpea
l inpea
nefenalol

Long synonyms
alpha [[(1 methylethyl)amino]methyl] 4 nitrobenzenemethanol

alpha isopropylaminomethyl para nitrobenzyl alcohol
alpha isopropylaminomethyl para nitrophenylbenzyl alcohol
dextro n isopropyl 4 nitrophenylethanolamine
dextro n isopropyl para nitrophenylethanolamine
dl n isopropyl para nitrophenyl ethanolamine
2 isopropylamino 1 (4 nitrophenyl)ethanol
2 (isopropylamino) 1 (para nitrophenyl)ethanol
2 isopropylamino 1 (para nitrophenyl)ethanol
isopropylamino 2 (4 nitrophenyl)ethan 2 ol hydrochloride
isopropylamino 2 para nitrophenyl 1 ethanol hydrochloride
isopropylaminomethyl para nitrobenzyl alcohol
isopropylaminomethyl para nitrobenzylalcohol
isopropylaminomethyl p nitrobenzyl alcohol
isopropylaminonitrophenylethanol
levo n isopropyl para nitrophenylethanolamine
n isopropyl(4 nitrophenyl)ethanolamine
n isopropylamino 1 (4 nitrophenyl)ethanol
n isopropyl para nitrophenyl ethanolamine
n isopropyl para nitrophenylethanolamine
n isopropyl para nitrophenyl ethanolamine hydrochloride
n isopropyl para nitrophenylethanolamine hydrochloride
1 (4 nitrophenyl) 2 isopropylaminoethanol
1 (4' nitrophenyl) 2 isopropylaminoethanol
1 (4 nitrophenyl) 2 isopropylaminoethanol hydrochloride
1 (4' nitrophenyl) 2 isopropylaminoethanol hydrochloride
1 (para nitrophenyl) 2 isopropylaminoethanol
1 para nitrophenyl 2 isopropylaminoethanol
1 (para nitrophenyl) 2 isopropylaminoethanol hydrochloride

nikethamide

WADA group
S1. STIMULANTS

MeSH descriptor
nikethamide

CAS Registry number
59-26-7

Short synonyms
aminocordin
anacardone
anacordone
astrocar
betapyrimidum
camphozone
carbamidal
cardamin
cardiagen
cardiamid
cardiamin
cardiamina
cardiamine
cardimon
cardiopiridina
citocor
coracon
coraethamide
coraethamidum
coralept
coramine
coravita
corazone
cordiamid
cordiamin
cordiamine
cordin
corditon
cordynil
corediol
coreopsin
corespin
corethamide
corethamidum
coretone
cormed
cormid
cormotyl
corotonin
corvin
corvitan
corvotone
corywas
danamine
diethylnicotinamide
dinacoryl
dynacoryl
dynamicarde
elitone
eucoran
inicardio
kardonyl
kordiamin
leptamin
mediamid
miocardina
nekethamide
neocordial
nicaethamidum
nicamide
nicardin
nicetamid
nicetamide
nicethamide
nickethamide
ni cor
nicor
nicordamin
nicorine
nicorine latema
nicoryl
nicotinic acid diethylamide
nikardin
nikethamine
niketharol
nikethyl
nikorin
n,n diethylnicotinamide
percoral
procardin(e)
procorman
pyricardyl
pyrocardyl
saluacard
salvacard
salvacerin
stellamine
stiminol
stimulin
tonazol
vasazol kwisda
ventramine

Long synonyms
pyridine 3 carboxylic acid diethylamide

nipradilol

WADA group
P2. BETA-BLOCKERS

CAS Registry number
81486-22-8

Trade names and research codes
hypadil
k 351
kt 210

Short synonyms
nipradolol

Long synonyms
1 (3,4 dihydro 3 nitroxy 2h 1 benzopyran 8 yl) 3 isopropylamino 2 propanol
3,4 dihydro 8 (2 hydroxy 3 isopropylaminopropoxy) 3 nitroxy 2h 1 benzopyran
8 [2 hydroxy 3 (isopropylamino)propoxy] 3 chromanol 3 nitrate

niravoline

WADA group
S8. MASKING AGENTS
P3. DIURETICS

CAS Registry number
130610-93-4

Trade names and research codes
ru 51599

Long synonyms
n [2,3 dihydro 2 (1 pyrrolidinyl) 1h inden 1 yl] n methyl 3 nitrobenzeneacetamide
n methyl 2 (3 nitrophenyl) n [2 (1 pyrrolidinyl) 1 indanyl]acetamide

nitromifene

WADA group
S7. AGENTS WITH ANTI-OESTROGENIC ACTIVITY

MeSH descriptor
nitromifene

CAS Registry number
5863-35-4

Trade names and research codes
c 1628
c1628
ci 628
ci628
cl 628
cl628
cn 55,945
cn 55945
cn55,945
cn55945
cn 55 945 27
cn 55945 27
cn 5594527
cn55945 27
cn5594527

Short synonyms
nitromiphene

Long synonyms
alpha [4 (2 pyrrolidinoethoxy)phenyl] 4 methoxy alpha' nitrostilbene
alpha (4 pyrrolidinoethoxy)phenyl 4 methoxy alpha' nitrostilbene
alpha [para [2 (1 pyrrolidino)ethoxy]phenyl] 4 methoxy alpha' nitrostilbene
4 methoxy alpha' nitro alpha [4 (2 pyrrolidinoethoxy)phenyl]stilbene
4' methoxy alpha nitro alpha [para (2 pyrrolidin 1 ylethoxy)phenyl]stilbene

nivacortol

WADA group
S9. GLUCOCORTICOSTEROIDS

CAS Registry number
24358-76-7

Trade names and research codes
win 27914

Short synonyms
nivazol

Long synonyms
2' (4 fluorophenyl) 2'h 17alpha pregna 2,4 dien 20 yno[3,2 c]pyrazol 17 ol

noradrenalin

WADA group
S1. STIMULANTS
S6. BETA-2 AGONISTS

MeSH descriptor
norepinephrine

CAS Registry number
1407-84-7
51-41-2

Trade names and research codes
adrenor
alginodia
arterenal
arterenol
dl arterenol
levarterenol
levonor
levophed
neomelubrin
noradrec
noradrine
norexadrin
revarterenol
sympathin
sympathin e

Short synonyms
baycain green
dextro noradrenalin
dextro noradrenaline
dl noradrenalin
dl noradrenalin hydrochloride
d noradrenalin
levo noradrenalin
levo noradrenaline
levo norepinephrine
l noradrenalin
l noradrenaline
l noradrenalin hydrochloride
l norepinephrine
neurogenic noradrenalin
noradrenaline
noradrenalin hydrochloride
norepinephrin
norepinephrine
norepinephrine hydrochloride

Long synonyms
l alpha aminomethyl 3,4 dihydroxybenzyl alcohol

Terms and Synonyms

noradrenalin bitartrate

WADA group
S6. BETA-2 AGONISTS

CAS Registry number
51-40-1

Trade names and research codes
aktamin
binodrenal
norartrinal
noratrinal
nordrin

Short synonyms
d noradrenalin bitartrate
levarterenol bitartrate
levo noradrenalin bitartrate
l noradrenalin bitartrate
l noradrenaline acid tartrate
l noradrenaline bitartrate
noradrenalin acid tartrate
noradrenaline bitartrate
noradrenalin hydrotartrate
noradrenalin tartrate
norepinephrine bitartrate

Long synonyms
noradrenalin bitartrate hydrate
noradrenalin bitartrate monohydrate

norboletone

WADA group
S4. ANABOLIC AGENTS

CAS Registry number
1235-15-0

Trade names and research codes
genabol
wy 3475
wy3475

Short synonyms
norbolethane
norbolethone

Long synonyms
13 ethyl 17 hydroxy 18,19 dinor 17alpha pregn 4 en 3 one

norclostebol

WADA group
S4. ANABOLIC AGENTS

Trade names and research codes
skf 6611

Short synonyms
4 chloronandrolone
4 chloro 19 nortestosterone
4 chloronortestosterone

norclostebol acetate

WADA group
S4. ANABOLIC AGENTS

Trade names and research codes
cp 73

Short synonyms
4 chloronandrolone acetate
4 chloro 19 nortestosterone acetate
4 chloronortestosterone acetate

norcocaine

WADA group
S1. STIMULANTS

CAS Registry number
18717-72-1

Short synonyms
psi norcocaine

norethandrolone

WADA group
S4. ANABOLIC AGENTS

MeSH descriptor
norethandrolone

CAS Registry number
52-78-8

Trade names and research codes
nilevar
u 6817

Short synonyms
17alpha ethylnortestosterone
17 ethyl 19 nor testosterone
17 ethyl 19 nortestosterone
19 ethyl 19 nortestosterone
norethandrolon

Long synonyms
17alpha ethyl 17 hydroxy 19 norandrost 4 en 3 one
17 alpha ethyl 19 nortestosterone
17alpha ethyl 19 nortestosterone
17beta hydroxy 19 nor 17alpha pregn 4 en 3 one
17 hydroxy 19 nor 17alpha pregn 4 en 3 one
17 hydroxy 19 norpregn 4 en 3 one
19 norpregn 4 en 3 one,17 hydroxy

norfenfluramine

WADA group
S1. STIMULANTS

MeSH descriptor
norfenfluramine

CAS Registry number
1886-26-6

Short synonyms
dextro norfenfluramine

Long synonyms
alpha methyl meta (trifluoromethyl)phenethylamine
alpha methyl [3 (trifluoromethyl)benzene]ethaneamine
2 amino 1 [3 (trifluoromethyl)phenyl]propane
amphetamine,meta trifluoromethyl
meta trifluoromethylamphetamine

norpseudoephedrine

WADA group
S1. STIMULANTS

CAS Registry number
2153-98-2
36393-56-3
492-39-7

Trade names and research codes
adiposetten
adiposettin
amorphan depot
exponcit

Short synonyms
cathin
cathine
kathine
katine
levo norpseudoephedrine
l norpseudoephedrine
norisoephedrine
norisophedrine
pseudonorephedrine

Long synonyms
alpha (1 aminoethyl) benzyl alcohol
norpseudoephedrine hydrochloride
threo alpha (1 aminoethyl)benzyl alcohol

nortamoxifen

WADA group
S7. AGENTS WITH ANTI-OESTROGENIC ACTIVITY

CAS Registry number
31750-48-8

Short synonyms
demethyltamoxifen
desmethyltamoxifen
ici 55548
n demethyltamoxifen
n desmethyltamoxifen
n nortamoxifen
tamoxifen,nor

novel erythropoiesis stimulating protein

WADA group
S5. PEPTIDE HORMONES
M1. ENHANCEMENT OF OXYGEN TRANSFER

Trade names and research codes
aranesp
nespo

Short synonyms
darbepoetin alfa
NESP

orciprenaline

WADA group
S6. BETA-2 AGONISTS

MeSH descriptor
orciprenaline

CAS Registry number
586-06-1
5874-97-5

Trade names and research codes
alotec
alupent
arm a med
asthmopent
astmopent
metaprel
th 152
tranquo alupent

Short synonyms
meta proterenol
metaproterenol
metaproterenol sulfate
oceprenalin
ociprenaline
orchiprenaline sulfate
orciprenalin
orciprenaline sulfate

Long synonyms
3,5 dihydroxy (alpha isopropylaminomethyl)benzyl alcohol
1 (3,5 dihydroxyphenyl) 1 hydroxy 2 isopropylaminoethane
1 (3,5 dihydroxyphenyl) 1 hydroxy 2 isopropylaminoethane sulfate
1 (3,5 dihydroxyphenyl) 2 isopropylaminoethanol
1 (3,5 dihydroxyphenyl) 2 isopropylaminoethanol sulfate

oropivalone

WADA group
S9. GLUCOCORTICOSTEROIDS

Trade names and research codes
oropivalone

Short synonyms
bacitracin oropivalone
oropivalone bacitracin
oropivalone bacitracine

Long synonyms
bacitracin zinc plus tixocortol pivalate
tixocortol pivalate plus bacitracin zinc

osmotic diuretic agent

WADA group
S8. MASKING AGENTS
P3. DIURETICS

MeSH descriptor
diuretics, osmotic

Short synonyms
diuretics, osmotic
osmotic diuretic

ospemifene

WADA group
S7. AGENTS WITH ANTI-OESTROGENIC ACTIVITY

Trade names and research codes
fc 1271a
fc1271a

Long synonyms
2 [4 (4 chloro 1,2 diphenyl 1 butenyl)phenoxy]ethanol
2 [4 (4 chloro 1,2 diphenylbut 1 enyl)phenoxy]ethanol

ovurelin

WADA group
S5. PEPTIDE HORMONES

CAS Registry number
115803-96-8

Long synonyms
gonadorelin[1-9] ethylamide[6 dextro phenylalanine]

oxabolone

WADA group
S4. ANABOLIC AGENTS

Short synonyms
4 hydroxy 19 nortestosterone
oxabol

Long synonyms
4,17beta dihydroxyestr 4 en 3 one

oxabolone cipionate

WADA group
S4. ANABOLIC AGENTS

CAS Registry number
1254-35-9

Trade names and research codes
fi 5852
fi5852

Short synonyms
oxabolone cypionate
steranabol depot

oxandrolone

WADA group
S4. ANABOLIC AGENTS

MeSH descriptor
oxandrolone

CAS Registry number
53-39-4

Trade names and research codes
anavar
hepandrin
lonovar
omnisterin
oxandrine
sc 11585

Long synonyms
17beta hydroxy 17alpha methyl 2 oxa 5alpha androstan 3 one
17beta hydroxy 17 methyl 2 oxa 5alpha androstan 3 one

oxilofrine

WADA group
S1. STIMULANTS

CAS Registry number
365-26-4
52671-39-3
8053-65-4

Trade names and research codes
carnigen

Short synonyms
carnigen forte
ephedrine,4 hydroxy
4 hydroxyephedrine
hydroxyfedrine
methylsympathol
oxilofrin
para hydroxyephedrine
suprifen

Long synonyms
1 (4 hydroxyphenyl) 2 methylamino 1 propanol
para hydroxyephedrine hydrochloride
1 (para hydroxyphenyl) 2 methylamino 1 propanol
1 para hydroxyphenyl 2 methylamino propane 1 ol
1 para oxyphenyl 2 methylaminopropane 1 ol

19 oxoandrostenedione

WADA group
S4. ANABOLIC AGENTS

CAS Registry number
968-49-0

Short synonyms
4 androstene 3,17 dion 19 al
androstenedion 19 al
3,17 dioxoandrost 4 en 19 al
19 formylandrostenedione

18 oxohydrocortisone

WADA group
S9. GLUCOCORTICOSTEROIDS

CAS Registry number
2410-60-8

Short synonyms
hydrocortisone,18 oxo
18 oxocortisol

Long synonyms
11beta,17alpha,21 trihydroxy 3,20 dioxopregn 4 en 18 al

11 oxotestosterone

WADA group
S4. ANABOLIC AGENTS

CAS Registry number
564-35-2

Short synonyms
11 ketotestosterone
testosterone,11 oxo

Long synonyms
17beta hydroxyandrost 4 ene 3,11 dione

oxprenoate potassium

WADA group
S8. MASKING AGENTS
P3. DIURETICS

CAS Registry number
76676-34-1

probably not prohibited

Trade names and research codes
ru 28318

oxprenolol

WADA group
P2. BETA-BLOCKERS

MeSH descriptor
oxprenolol

CAS Registry number
22972-97-0
6452-71-7
6452-73-9

Trade names and research codes
39089 ba
39089ba
ba 39,089
ba 39089
ba39,089
ba39089
ciba 39089
ciba39089
ciba 39 089 b
ciba 39089 b
ciba 39089b
ciba39089b
ciba 39 089 ba
ciba 39 089ba
ciba 39,089 ba
ciba 39,089ba
ciba 39.089 ba
ciba 39.089ba
ciba 39089 ba
ciba 39089ba
ciba39,089 ba
ciba39.089 ba
ciba39089ba
ciba 42.244 ba
ciba 42.244ba
ciba42.244ba
cordexol
coretal
skf uk 52
slow trasicor
tevacor
trasacor
trasicor
trasicor retard

Short synonyms
dextro oxyprenolol
d oxyprenolol
levo oxprenolol
levo oxyprenolol
l oxyprenolol
oxprenol
oxprenolol hydrochloride
oxtrenolol
oxyprenolol
oxyprenolol hydrochloride

Long synonyms
1 (2 allyloxyphenoxy) 3 isopropylamino 2 propanol
1 (2 allyloxyphenoxy) 3 isopropylamino 2 propanol hydrochloride
2 hydroxy 1 isopropylamino 3 (2 allyloxyphenoxy)propane
2 hydroxy 1 isopropylamino 3 (ortho allyloxyphenoxy)propane
1 isopropylamine 2 hydroxy 3 (ortho allyloxyphenoxy)propane
1 isopropylamino 2 hydroxy 3 (o allyloxyphenoxy)propane hydrochloride
1 isopropylamino 2 hydroxy 3 (ortho allyloxyphenoxy)propane
1 isopropylamino 2 hydroxy 3 (ortho allyloxyphenoxy)propane hydrochloride
1 isopropylamino 3 (2 allyloxyphenoxy) 2 propanol hydrochloride
1 isopropyl amino 3 (ortho allyl oxyphenoxy) 2 propanol hydrochloride
1 isopropylamino 3 (ortho allyloxy phenoxy) 2 propanol hydrochloride
1 isopropylamino 3 (ortho allyloxyphenoxy) 2 propanol hydrochloride
levo 1 [ortho (allyloxy)phenoxy] 3 (isopropylamino) 2 propanol
1 (ortho allyloxyphenoxy) 3 isopropylamino 2 propanol
1 (ortho allyloxyphenoxy) 3 isopropylamino 2 propanol hydrochloride
1 (ortho allyloxyphenoxy) 3 isopropylaminopropan 2 ol

oxyamal

WADA group
S8. MASKING AGENTS

CAS Registry number
127068-75-1

oxycodone

WADA group
S2. NARCOTICS

MeSH descriptor
oxycodone

CAS Registry number
124-90-3
76-42-6

Trade names and research codes
eukodal
oxycontin
oxygesic
roxicodone
roxycodone
tylox

Short synonyms
bionine
bionone
bolodorm
broncodal
bucodal
cafacodal
cardanon
codenon
dihydrohydroxycodeinone
dihydrohydroxydodeinone
dihydrone
dinarkon
endone
eubine
eucodal
eucodale
eudin
eukdin
eumorphal
eurodamine
eutagen
hydrocodal
hydroxycodeinoma
14 hydroxydihydrocodeinone
ludonal

Terms and Synonyms

medicodal
narcobasina
narcobasine
narcosin
nargenol
narodal
nsc 19043
nucodan
opton
ossicodone
oxanest
oxicone
oxiconum
oxikon
oxycodeinonhydrochloride
oxycodone hydrochloride
oxycodonhydrochlorid
oxycodyl
oxycone
oxykon
pancodine
pavinal
pronarcin
sinthiodal
stupenal
tebodal
tekodin
thecodin

oxyfedrine

WADA group
S1. STIMULANTS
S6. BETA-2 AGONISTS

MeSH descriptor
oxyfedrine

CAS Registry number
15687-41-9
16777-42-7

Trade names and research codes
d 563
d563
ildamen

Short synonyms
dextro,levo oxyfedrine
dl oxyfedrine
oxyfedrin
oxyfedrine hydrochloride
oxyphedrin
oxyphedrine
oxyphedrine hydrochloride

Long synonyms
3 [(beta hydroxy alpha methylphenethyl)amino] 3' methoxypropiophenone
(1 hydroxy 1 phenyl 2 propylamino) 1 (meta methoxyphenyl) 1 propanone

oxyhemoglobin

WADA group
M1. ENHANCEMENT OF OXYGEN TRANSFER

MeSH descriptor
oxyhemoglobins

CAS Registry number
9061-63-6

Short synonyms
oxyhaemoglobin
oxyhemoglobin a
oxyhemoglobins

oxymesterone

WADA group
S4. ANABOLIC AGENTS

CAS Registry number
145-12-0

Trade names and research codes
anamidol
balnimax
oranabol
theranabol

Short synonyms
oxymestrone

Long synonyms
4,17beta dihydroxy 17alpha methylandrost 4 en 3 one
4 hydroxy 17alpha methyltestosterone
4 hydroxy 17 methyltestosterone

oxymetholone

WADA group
S4. ANABOLIC AGENTS

MeSH descriptor
oxymetholone

CAS Registry number
434-07-1

Trade names and research codes
adroyd
anadrol
anadrol 50
anapolon
anapolon 50
androyd f
ci 406
ci406
hmd
nastenon
nsc 26198
nsc26198
plenastril
synasteron

Short synonyms
anasterone
oxymethalone
oxymetolone

Long synonyms
17beta hydroxy 2 hydroxymethylene 17alpha methyl 5alpha androstan 3 one
2 hydroxymethylene 17alpha methyldihydrotestosterone

oxymorphone

WADA group
S2. NARCOTICS

MeSH descriptor
oxymorphone

CAS Registry number
357-07-3
76-41-5

Trade names and research codes
numorphan

Short synonyms
hydroxydihydromorphinone
oxymorphone hydrochloride

Long synonyms
7,8 dihydro 14 hydroxymorphinone
4,5 epoxy 3,14 dihydroxy 17 methylmorphinan 6 one

oxypolygelatin

WADA group
S8. MASKING AGENTS

CAS Registry number
9005-91-8

Trade names and research codes
gelifundol

Short synonyms
plazmozid

ozolinone

WADA group
S8. MASKING AGENTS
P3. DIURETICS

CAS Registry number
56784-39-5

Trade names and research codes
go 3282
go3282
goe 3282
goe3282

Short synonyms
goedecke 3282

Long synonyms
3 methyl 4 oxo 5 (1 piperidinyl) 2 thiazolidinylideneacetic acid
3 methyl 4 oxo 5 piperid 1 ylthiazolidinylidene 2 acetic acid
3 methyl 4 oxo 5 piperidino delta2,alpha thiazolidineacetic acid
3 methyl 4 oxo 5 piperidinothiazolidin 2 ylideneacetic acid

pafenolol

WADA group
P2. BETA-BLOCKERS

CAS Registry number
75949-61-0

Long synonyms
1 [4 [2 hydroxy 3 (isopropylamino)propoxy]phenethyl] 3 isopropylurea
1 (isopropylamino) 3 [4 [2 (3 isopropylureido)ethyl]phenoxy] 2 propanol

palmidrol

WADA group
S3. CANNABINOIDS

CAS Registry number
544-31-0

Trade names and research codes
impulsin

Short synonyms
n (2 hydroxyethyl)palmitamide
n palmitoylethanolamine
palmitoylethanolamide

pamatolol

WADA group
P2. BETA-BLOCKERS

CAS Registry number
59110-35-9

Trade names and research codes
h 104-08

Long synonyms
3 (isopropropylamino) 1 [4 [2 [(methoxycarbonyl)amino]ethyl]phenoxy] 2 propanol

panomifene

WADA group
S7. AGENTS WITH ANTI-OESTROGENIC ACTIVITY

CAS Registry number
77599-17-8

Trade names and research codes
egis 5650
egis5650
gyki 13504
gyki13504

Long synonyms
1,2 diphenyl 1 [4 [2 (2 hydroxyethylamino)ethoxy]phenyl] 3,3,3 trifluoropropene
2 [[2 [4 (3,3,3 trifluoro 1,2 diphenyl 1 propenyl)phenoxy]ethyl]amino]ethanol

paramethasone

WADA group
S9. GLUCOCORTICOSTEROIDS

MeSH descriptor
paramethasone

CAS Registry number
53-33-8

Trade names and research codes
alfa 6
alfa6
aloxicort
cortiden
metilar
paramesone
paramezone

Short synonyms
parametazon
paramethason
para methasone
paramethazone

Long synonyms
6alpha fluoro 11beta,17alpha,21 trihydroxy 16alpha methyl 1,4 pregnadiene 3,20 dione
6 alpha fluoro 16 alpha methylprednisolone

Terms and Synonyms

6alpha fluoro 16alpha methyl prednisolone
6alpha fluoro 16alpha methylprednisolone
16alpha methyl 6alpha fluoro prednisolone
16alpha methyl 6alpha fluoroprednisolone

paramethasone acetate

WADA group
S9. GLUCOCORTICOSTEROIDS

CAS Registry number
1597-82-6

Trade names and research codes
alondra
cortidene
depodillar
dilar
dillar
flumethone
haldrate
haldrone
monocortin
netilar
syntecort
triniol

Short synonyms
paramethasone 21 acetate
paramethasone acetat
paramethazone acetate

Long synonyms
6alpha fluoro 11beta,17alpha,21 trihydroxy 16alpha methyl 1,4 pregnadiene 3,20 dione 21 acetate
6alpha fluoro 16alpha methylprednisolone 21 acetate
6 alpha fluoro 16 alpha methylprednisolone acetate
16 alpha methyl 6 alpha fluoroprednisolone acetate

pemoline

WADA group
S1. STIMULANTS

MeSH descriptor
pemoline

CAS Registry number
2152-34-3

Trade names and research codes
abbott 31528
aturgyl delta
betanamin
cyclert
deltamine
dynalert
hyton
kethamed
la 956
nsc 25159
nsc 25259
pioxol
pw-135
ronyl
tradon
volital

Short synonyms
azoxodone
fenoxazol
pemolin
phenoxazole
phenylisohydantoin

Long synonyms
2 amino 5 phenyl 2 oxazolin 4 one
2 amino 5 phenyl 4(5h) oxazolone
2 imino 5 phenyloxazolidin 4 one
phenyl 5 imino 2 oxo 4 oxazolidine

pemoline magnesium

WADA group
S1. STIMULANTS

CAS Registry number
18968-99-5

Trade names and research codes
abbott 30400
cylert
ecylert

Short synonyms
magnesium pemolate
magnesium pemolinate
magnesium pemoline
pemolate magnesium
pemolinate magnesium
pemoline magnesiumchelate
pemoline magnesium hydroxide

Long synonyms
[2 imino 5 phenyloxazolidinonato (2)]diaquomagnesium
pemoline plus magnesium hydroxide
pemoline with magnesium hydroxide

penbutolol

WADA group
P2. BETA-BLOCKERS

MeSH descriptor
penbutolol

CAS Registry number
38363-32-5
38363-40-5

Trade names and research codes
betapressin
blocotin
hoe 39893d
hoe39893d
hoe 893d
hoe893d
levatol
paginol

Short synonyms
penbutalol
penbutolol sulfate

Long synonyms
1 (tert butylamino) 3 (2 cyclopentylphenoxy) 2 propanol

11 [4 [[5 [(4,4,5,5,5 pentafluoropentyl)sulfonyl]pentyl]oxy]phenyl]estradiol

WADA group
S7. AGENTS WITH ANTI-OESTROGENIC ACTIVITY

CAS Registry number
151555-47-4

Terms and Synonyms

Trade names and research codes
ru 58668

Long synonyms
11beta [4 [[5 [(4,4,5,5,5 pentafluoropentyl)sulfonyl]pentyl]oxy]phenyl]estra 1,3,5(10) triene 3,17beta diol

pentazocine

WADA group
S2. NARCOTICS

MeSH descriptor
pentazocine

CAS Registry number
359-83-1
64024-15-3

Trade names and research codes
dolapent
fortal
fortalgesic
fortral
fortraline
fortwin
liticon
nih 7958
nsc 107430
peltazon
pentafen
pentagin
pentalgina
perutagin
sosegon
sosigon
talioin
talwin
win 20,228
win 20228

Short synonyms
dl pentazocine
d pentazocine
l pentazocine
pentacozine
pentazocin
pentazocine hydrochloride
pentazocine isomer
pentozocine

Long synonyms
6,11 dimethyl 3 (3 methyl 2 butenyl) 1,2,3,4,5,6 hexahydro 2,6 methano 3 benzazocin 8 ol
2 (3,3 dimethylallyl) 2' hydroxy 5,9 dimethyl 6,7 benzomorphan
2 dimethylallyl 5,9 dimethyl 2' hydroxy benzomorphan
1,2,3,4,5,6 hexahydro 6,11 dimethyl 3 (3 methyl 2 butenyl) 2,6 methano 3 benzazocin 8 ol
1,2,3,4,5,6 hexahydro 6,11 dimethyl 3 (3 methyl 2 butenyl) 2,6 methano 3 benzazocin 8 ol hydrochloride
2' hydroxy 5,9 dimethyl 2 (3,3 dimethylallyl) 6,7 benzomorphan
3 (3 methyl 2 butenyl) 1,2,3,4,5,6 hexahydro 6,11 dimethyl 2,6 methano 3 benzazocin 8 ol

pentetrazole

WADA group
S1. STIMULANTS

MeSH descriptor
pentylenetetrazole

CAS Registry number
54-95-5

Trade names and research codes
cardiazol
cardiazole
cardiazolum
corasole
corazol
metrazole
pentacard

Short synonyms
angiazol
angioton
cardifortan
cardosal
cardosan
cenalene m
cenazol
centrazole
coranormol
corazole
corvasol
corvis
denmacard
deumacard
diovascole
gewazol
korazole
korazoli
leptazol
leptazole
levo tetrazol
metrazol
naurazol
neocardol
opticor
pemetesan
pentamethazol
pentamethylene 1,5 tetrazole
pentamethylenetetrazol
pentamethylene tetrazole
pentamethylenetetrazole
1,5 pentamethylenetetrazole
pentamethylenetrazol
pentazol
pentazole
pentemesan
pentetrazol
pentrozol
pentylene tetrazol
pentylenetetrazol
pentylene tetrazole
pentylenetetrazole
phrenazol
stillcardiol
tetracor
tetrazol
vasazol
ventrazol
yetrazol

Long synonyms
alpha,beta cyclopentamethylenetetrazole
1,2,3,3a tetrazacyclohepta 8a,2 cyclopentadiene
6,7,8,9 tetrahydro 5 azepotetrazole
6,7,8,9 tetrahydro 5 h tetrazoloazepine
6,7,8,9 tetrahydro 5 h tetrazolocrepine
6,7,8,9 tetrahydroazepotetrazole
7,8,9,10 tetrazabicyclo [5.3.0] 8,10 decadiene

percocet

WADA group
S2. NARCOTICS

Trade names and research codes
percocet

percodan

WADA group
S2. NARCOTICS

Trade names and research codes
percodan
percodan demi

perfluorobutyltetrahydrofuran

WADA group
M1. ENHANCEMENT OF OXYGEN TRANSFER

CAS Registry number
26446-59-3
39289-24-2

Trade names and research codes
fc 80
fc80
fx 80
fx80
rm 101
rm101

Short synonyms
fluorocarbon fc 80

Long synonyms
tetrahydro(nonafluorobutyl)furan

perfluorodecalin

WADA group
M1. ENHANCEMENT OF OXYGEN TRANSFER

CAS Registry number
306-94-5

Trade names and research codes
adato deca
dk line
flutec pp5

Short synonyms
perflunafene

Long synonyms
octadecafluorodecahydronaphthalene

perfluorooctyl bromide

WADA group
M1. ENHANCEMENT OF OXYGEN TRANSFER

CAS Registry number
423-55-2

Trade names and research codes
af 0104
af0104
liquivent
oxygent
oxygent ht

Short synonyms
bromoheptadecafluorooctane
perflubron
perfluorooctylbromide

perfluoroperhydrofluoranthene

WADA group
M1. ENHANCEMENT OF OXYGEN TRANSFER

CAS Registry number
662-28-2

perfluorotributylamine

WADA group
M1. ENHANCEMENT OF OXYGEN TRANSFER

CAS Registry number
311-89-7
94395-15-0

Trade names and research codes
fc 43
fc43
fc 47
fc47
fl 75
fl75
fl 80
fl80
fluosol 43
fluosol fc 43
fluosol fc43
oxyferol
oxypherol

Short synonyms
fluorocarbon 43
fluorocarbon fc 43
fluorocarbon fc43
heptacosafluorotributylamine
perfluorotri(n butyl)amine

perfluorotripropylamine

WADA group
M1. ENHANCEMENT OF OXYGEN TRANSFER

CAS Registry number
338-83-0

Short synonyms
heneicosafluorotripropylamine
perfluamine
tris(heptafluoropropyl)amine

perhexiline

WADA group
S8. MASKING AGENTS
P3. DIURETICS

MeSH descriptor
perhexiline

CAS Registry number
6621-47-2

Trade names and research codes
mdl 3978g

Long synonyms
2 (2,2 dicyclohexylethyl)piperidine

probably not prohibited

perhexiline maleate

WADA group
S8. MASKING AGENTS
P3. DIURETICS

CAS Registry number
6724-53-4

Trade names and research codes
corzepin
pexid

Short synonyms
perhexilene hydrogen maleate
perhexilene maleate

pethidine

WADA group
S2. NARCOTICS

MeSH descriptor
meperidine

CAS Registry number
28097-96-3
50-13-5
57-42-1

Trade names and research codes
alodan
centralgin
centralgine
demerol
dolantin
dolantine
dolargan
dolcontral
dolosal
dolsin
lydol
pethidin
petidin

Short synonyms
algil
demerol hydrochloride
dispadol
dolanquifa
dolantal
dolenal
dolestin
dolin
dolocontral
doloneurin
doloneurotrat
dolor
dolosa
dolosan
dolvanol
endolate
isonipecaine
lidol
l pethidine
mefedina
mepadin
meperiden
meperidin
meperidine
meperidine hydrobromide
meperidine hydrochloride
mephedine
mepiridine
mialgin
pantalgin
petadin
petantin
petantina
pethanol
pethedine
pethidine hydrobromide
pethidine hydrochloride
pethidine roche
phetidine
piridosal
sauteralgyl
simesalgina
supplosal
synlaudine

Long synonyms
4 ethoxycarbonyl 1 methyl 4 phenylpiperidine
1 methyl 4 phenyl 4 carbethoxypiperidine
1 methyl 4 phenylisonipecotic acid ethyl ester
methylphenylcarbethoxypiperidine hydrochloride
n methyl 4 phenyl 4 carbethoxypiperidine hydrochloride

phendimetrazine

WADA group
S1. STIMULANTS

CAS Registry number
634-03-7

Short synonyms
dextro levo phendimetrazine
fendimetrazine
phenimethoxazine

Long synonyms
d 3,4 dimethyl 2 phenylmorpholine

phendimetrazine embonate

WADA group
S1. STIMULANTS

CAS Registry number
27922-80-1

Trade names and research codes
fringanor

Short synonyms
phendimetrazine pamoate

phendimetrazine tartrate

WADA group
S1. STIMULANTS

CAS Registry number
50-58-8

Trade names and research codes
bontril
melfiat
phenzine
plegine

Short synonyms
adipost
bacarate
hyrex
metra
phendimetrazine bitartrate
slyn ll
trimcaps

Long synonyms
phendimetrazine hydrogen tartrate

phenmetrazine

WADA group
S1. STIMULANTS

MeSH descriptor
phenmetrazine

CAS Registry number
134-49-6
1707-14-8
57919-12-7

Trade names and research codes
a 66
a66
afagil
anapetol
gracidin
ikapharm
marsin
neo zine
preludin
probose p
psychamine
psychamine a 66

Short synonyms
dexfenmetrazin
dexphenmetrazine
dexphenmetrazine hydrochloride
dextro phenmetrazine
d phenmetrazine
fenmetralin
fenmetrazine
3 methyl 2 phenylmorpholine
phemetrazine
phenmetrazin
phenmetrazine hydrochloride
phenylmethyltetrahydro oxazine

Long synonyms
3 methyl 2 phenyltetrahydro 2h 1,4 oxazine
2 phenyl 3 methyltetrahydro 1,4 oxazine
2 phenyl 3 methyltetrahydro 1,4 oxazine hydrochloride

phentermine

WADA group
S1. STIMULANTS

MeSH descriptor
phentermine

CAS Registry number
1197-21-3
122-09-8

Trade names and research codes
adipex p
ex adipos
exadipos
fastin
obermine black and yellow
panbesy
phentrol
reducyl
wilpo

Short synonyms
2 benzyl 2 propylamine
beta aminoisopropylbenzene
beta phenyltert.butylamine
dimethylphenethylamine
dimethylphenetylamine
phentermide
phentermin
phentermine hydrochloride
terbutylamine

Long synonyms
alpha,alpha dimethylphenethylamine
1,1 dimethyl 2 phenylethylamine

phentermine resin

WADA group
S1. STIMULANTS

Trade names and research codes
adipex neu
duromine
ionamin
ionamine 15
ionomin
linyl
mirapront

Short synonyms
phentermine resinate

☝ phenylpropanolamine

WADA group
S1. STIMULANTS

MeSH descriptor
phenylpropanolamine

CAS Registry number
14838-15-4
154-41-6
4345-16-8
48115-38-4

Trade names and research codes
acutrim
apodrine
appedrine
descon
dexatrim
dietac premeal
diet gard
kontexin
monydrin
mydriatin
nobese
pressedrine
procol
propadrine
propagest
trimolet

Short synonyms
2 amino 1 phenyl 1 propanol
apoephedrine
apophedrine
dl norephedrine
phenylpropanolamide
phenyl propanolamine
phenylpropylolamine

Long synonyms
alpha (1 aminoethyl)benzyl alcohol
phenylpropanolamine hydrochloride

Terms and Synonyms

☝ *probably not prohibited*

pholedrine

WADA group
S1. STIMULANTS

CAS Registry number
370-14-9

Trade names and research codes
adyston
venosan

Short synonyms
4 hydroxymethamphetamine
4 hydroxy n methylamphetamine
para hydroxymethamphetamine
paredrinol
pulsotyl
veritol

Long synonyms
beta (para hydroxyphenyl)isopropylmethylamine
1 (4 hydroxyphenyl) 2 methylaminopropane
1 (4 hydroxyphenyl) n methyl 2 aminopropane

picamilon

WADA group
S1. STIMULANTS

CAS Registry number
34562-97-5

Short synonyms
4 nicotinamidobutyric acid
4 nicotinoylaminobutyric acid
pikamilon

Long synonyms
n nicotinoyl 4 aminobutyric acid
n nicotinoyl gamma aminobutyric acid

picrotoxin

WADA group
S1. STIMULANTS

MeSH descriptor
picrotoxin

CAS Registry number
124-87-8

Short synonyms
cocculin
picrotoxine

picumeterol

WADA group
S6. BETA-2 AGONISTS

CAS Registry number
112192-20-8
130641-36-0
130641-37-1
139423-79-3

Trade names and research codes
gr 114297a
gr 63411
gr 63411b

Short synonyms
picumeterol fumarate

pig insulin

WADA group
S5. PEPTIDE HORMONES

CAS Registry number
12584-58-6

Trade names and research codes
u 100

Short synonyms
insulin,pig
porcine insulin

pindolol

WADA group
P2. BETA-BLOCKERS

MeSH descriptor
pindolol

CAS Registry number
13523-86-9
21870-06-4

Trade names and research codes
betapindol
calvisken
carvisken
decreten
durapindol
glauco visken
lb 46
lb46
lb 4675
pectobloc
pectoblock mite
pinolol lb 46
viskeen
visken
visken mite
visken retard

Short synonyms
hydroxypropylaminopropoxyindol
prindolol
prinodolol

Long synonyms
dextrolevo 4 (2 hydroxy 3 isopropylaminopropoxy)indole
dl 4 (2 hydroxy 3 isopropylaminopropoxy) indol
dl 4 (2 hydroxy 3 isopropylamino propoxy)indole
dl 4 (2 hydroxy 3 isopropylaminopropoxy)indole
1 (1h indol 4 yloxy) 3 [(1 methylethyl)amino] 2 propanol
4 (2 hydroxy 3 isopropylaminopropoxy)indol
2 (4 hydroxy 3 isopropylaminopropoxy)indole
4 (2 hydroxy 3 isopropyl aminopropoxy)indole
4 (2 hydroxy 3 isopropylaminopropoxy) indole
4 (2 hydroxy 3 isopropylaminopropoxy)indole
4 [2 hydroxy 3 (isopropylamino)propoxy]indole
4 (2 hydroxy 3 isopropylpropoxy)indole
4 (2 hydroxyisopropylaminopropoxy)indole
1 (indol 4 oxy) 3 isopropylaminopropan 2 ol
1 (indol 4 oxyl) 3 isopropylaminopropan 2 ol
1 (indol 4 yl oxy) 3 isopropylamino propan 2 ol
(3 isopropylaminopropoxy)indole

pindolol derivative

WADA group
P2. BETA-BLOCKERS

Terms and Synonyms

Short synonyms
pindolol analog

pipendoxifene

WADA group
S7. AGENTS WITH ANTI-OESTROGENIC ACTIVITY

CAS Registry number
198480-55-6
245124-69-0
389125-71-7

Trade names and research codes
era 923
era923

Short synonyms
pipendoxifene hydrochloride

Long synonyms
5 hydroxy 2 (4 hydroxyphenyl) 3 methyl 1 [4 [2 (1 piperidinyl)ethoxy]benzyl]indole
2 (4 hydroxyphenyl) 3 methyl 1 [4 [2 (1 piperidinyl)ethoxy]benzyl] 1h indol 5 ol

2 [4 (2 piperidinoethoxy)phenyl] 3 phenyl 2h 1 benzopyran

WADA group
S7. AGENTS WITH ANTI-OESTROGENIC ACTIVITY

CAS Registry number
130064-18-5

Trade names and research codes
cdri 85 287
cdri 85-287
cdri 85287
cdri85 287
cdri85-287
cdri85287

Long synonyms
2 [4 (2 piperidinoethoxy)phenyl] 3 phenyl 2h benzo[b]pyran

☝ pipradol

WADA group
S1. STIMULANTS

CAS Registry number
467-60-7
71-78-3

Trade names and research codes
alertol
alertonic
leptidrol
meratan
meratonic
meratran
meretran
metadin sodium
mrd 108

Short synonyms
alpha piperid 2 ylbenzhydrol
dextro pipradol
levo pipradol
pipradol chloride
pipradol hydrochloride
pipradrol
pipradrol chloride
pipradrol hydrochloride

Long synonyms
alpha,alpha diphenyl 2 piperidinemethanol

pirbuterol

WADA group
S6. BETA-2 AGONISTS

CAS Registry number
38677-81-5

Trade names and research codes
cp 24314
cp24314
cp 24,314 1
cp 24314 1
cp 243141
cp24,314 1
cp24314 1
cp243141
exirel
zeisin

Long synonyms
2 tert butylamino 1 (5 hydroxy 6 hydroxymethyl 2 pyridyl)ethanol
2 tert butylamino 1 (5 hydroxy 6 hydroxymethylpyrid 2 yl)ethanol

pirbuterol acetate

WADA group
S6. BETA-2 AGONISTS

CAS Registry number
65652-44-0

Trade names and research codes
cp 24,314 14
cp 24314 14
cp 24314-14
cp24,314 14
cp24314 14
cp24314-14
maxair

piretanide

WADA group
S8. MASKING AGENTS
P3. DIURETICS

CAS Registry number
55837-27-9

Trade names and research codes
arelix
eurelix
hoe 118
hoe118
perbilen
s 73 4118
s 734118
s734118

Short synonyms
arlix
lafax
tauliz

☝ *probably not prohibited*

Long synonyms
3 (aminosulfonyl) 4 phenoxy 5 (1 pyrrolidinyl)benzoic acid
4 phenoxy 3 (1 pyrrolidinyl) 5 sulfamoylbenzoic acid

plasma substitute

WADA group
S8. MASKING AGENTS
M1. ENHANCEMENT OF OXYGEN TRANSFER

MeSH descriptor
plasma substitutes

Short synonyms
blood plasma substitute
blood volume expander
colloidal plasma substitute
plasma expander
plasma expanding agent
plasma expansion
plasma substituent
plasma substitute agent
plasma substitutes
plasma substitution
plasma volume expander
transfusion substitute
volume expander,plasma

plasmion

WADA group
S8. MASKING AGENTS
M1. ENHANCEMENT OF OXYGEN TRANSFER

CAS Registry number
54847-63-1

Trade names and research codes
plasmion

polygeline

WADA group
S8. MASKING AGENTS

MeSH descriptor
polygeline

CAS Registry number
66455-30-9

Trade names and research codes
haemaccel
haemaccel 35
haemacel
hemaccel
hemacel
hemacell
hemagel

Short synonyms
polygelin

polymerized hemoglobin

WADA group
S8. MASKING AGENTS
M1. ENHANCEMENT OF OXYGEN TRANSFER

CAS Registry number
197252-65-6

Trade names and research codes
hboc 201
hboc-201
hemopure
polyheme

Short synonyms
hemoglobin polymer

polythiazide

WADA group
S8. MASKING AGENTS
P3. DIURETICS

MeSH descriptor
polythiazide

CAS Registry number
346-18-9

Trade names and research codes
drenusil
nephril
nsc 108161
p 2525
renese

Short synonyms
polythiaside

Long synonyms
6 chloro 3,4 dihydro 2 methyl 7 sulfamoyl 3 (2,2,2 trifluoroethylthiomethyl) 2h 1,2,4 benzothiadiazine 1,1 dioxide

potassium sparing diuretic agent

WADA group
S8. MASKING AGENTS
P3. DIURETICS

Short synonyms
potassium sparing diuretic

practolol

WADA group
P2. BETA-BLOCKERS

MeSH descriptor
practolol

CAS Registry number
6673-35-4

Trade names and research codes
ay 21,011
ay 21011
ay21011
eraldin
eraldin inj.
hy 21011
hy21011
i.c.i. 50172
ici 50,172
ici 50172
ici50172

Short synonyms
dextro levo practolol
dl practolol
practalol
practolole
praktolol

Terms and Synonyms

proctalol

Long synonyms
4 (2 hydroxy 3 isopropylaminopropoxy) acetanilide
4 (2 hydroxy 3 isopropylaminopropoxy)acetanilide
4' (2 hydroxy 3 isopropylaminopropoxy)acetanilide
4 (2 hydroxy 3 isopropylaminopropoxy)acetanilide hydrochloride
4 (2 hydroxyisopropylaminopropoxy)acetanilide hydrochloride

pralmorelin

WADA group
S5. PEPTIDE HORMONES

CAS Registry number
158861-67-7

Trade names and research codes
kp 102

Short synonyms
GHRP 2

Long synonyms
dextro alanyl 3 (2 naphthyl) dextro alanylalanyltryptophyl dextro phenylalanyllysinamide
growth hormone releasing peptide 2

prasterone

WADA group
S4. ANABOLIC AGENTS

MeSH descriptor
prasterone

CAS Registry number
53-43-0

Trade names and research codes
anastar
aslera
astenile
diandron
diandrone
el 10
el10
gl 701
gl701
hormoformin
pb 005
pb005
prestara
psicosterone

Short synonyms
7alpha dehydro epiandrosterone
7alpha dehydroepiandrosterone
androst 5 en 3 beta ol 17 one
androst 5 en 3beta ol 17 one
androst 5 ene 3beta ol 17 one
androstane 17 one
5 androsten 3 beta 17 one
5 androsten 3 beta ol 17 one
5 androsten 3beta ol 17 one
5 androsten 3 ol 17 one
5 androstene 3 beta ol 17 one
5 androstene 3beta ol 17 one
androstene 5 3b ol 17 one
3beta hydroxy 17 androstanone
chetovis
17 chetovis
dehydroepiandrosteron
dehydro epiandrosterone
dehydroepiandrosterone
dehydroisoandrosterone
dehyroepiandrosterone
delta5 androsten 3 beta 17 one
delta5 androsten 3beta 17 one
DHEA
dihydroepiandrosterone
dihydroisoandrosterone
17 hormoforin
3 hydroxyetioallocholan 17 one
17 oxo 5 androsten 3beta ol
trans dehydroandrosterone

Long synonyms
7alpha (3h)dehydroepiandrosterone
5 alpha androstan 3 beta ol 17 one
5 alpha androstane 3 beta ol 17 one
5alpha androstane 3beta ol 17 one
5 alpha androsten 3 beta ol 17 one
5alpha androsten 3 beta ol 17 one
5alpha androsten 3beta ol 17 one
3 beta hydroxy 5 androsten 17 one
3beta hydroxy 5 androsten 17 one
3 beta hydroxyandrost 5 en 17 one
3beta hydroxyandrost 5 en 17 one
3beta hydroxyandrost 5 ene 17 one
3beta hydroxyetioallocholan 17 one
delta 5 androsten 3 beta ol 17 one
delta 5 androsten 3beta ol 17 one
delta5 androsten 3beta ol 17 one

prasterone acetate

WADA group
S4. ANABOLIC AGENTS

CAS Registry number
853-23-6

Short synonyms
dehydroepiandrosterone acetate
DHEA acetate
prasterone 3 beta acetate

Long synonyms
5 androstene 3 beta acetoxy 17 one
3beta acetoxyandrost 5 en 17 one
dehydroepiandrosterone 3beta acetate
delta5 androstan 3beta ol 17 one acetate

prasterone sulfate

WADA group
S4. ANABOLIC AGENTS

MeSH descriptor
dehydroepiandrosterone sulfate

CAS Registry number
651-48-9

Trade names and research codes
inflarest
mylis

Short synonyms
17 chetovis 3 sulfate
dehydroepiandrosterone sulfate
dehydroisoandrosterone sulfate
dheas
DHEA sulfate
diandron 3 sulfate
dihydroepiandrosterone sulfate
17 hormoforin 3 sulfate
psicosterone 3 sulfate

ro 6 62827
ro 6 6827
ro 6 6827-2
ro 66827-2

Long synonyms
5 alpha androsten 3 beta ol 17 one sulfate
5alpha androsten 3beta ol 17 one sulfate
androst 5 en 17 on 3beta ol sulfate
androst 5 en 17 on 3beta yl sulfate
5 androsten 3 beta ol 17 one sulfate
5 androsten 3beta ol 17 one sulfate
3 beta hydroxy 5 androsten 17 one 3 sulfate
dehydroepiandrosterone 3beta sulfate
dehydroepiandrosterone 3 sulfate
dehydroepiandrosterone 3 sulphate
dehydroepiandrosterone sulfate sodium
dehydroepiandrosterone sulphate
delta 5 androsten 3beta ol 17 one 3 sulfate
delta5 androsten 3beta ol 17 one sulfate
17 oxo 5 androsten 3beta ol sulfate

prednicarbate

WADA group
S9. GLUCOCORTICOSTEROIDS

CAS Registry number
73771-04-7

Trade names and research codes
dermatop
escort
hoe 777
hoe777
s 77 0777
s 770777
s77 0777
s770777

Long synonyms
prednisolone 17 (ethyl carbonate) 21 propionate

prednisolone

WADA group
S9. GLUCOCORTICOSTEROIDS

MeSH descriptor
prednisolone

CAS Registry number
50-24-8

Trade names and research codes
codelcortone
dacortin
decortin h
delta cortef
delta cortril
di adresone f
diadresone f
di adreson f
diadreson f
encortelon
encortelone
encortolon
hostacortin h vet
hydeltra
hydrocortancyl
inflanefran
meprisolon
meticortelone
mydrapred
precortalon
prednicort
prednifor drops
predni h tablinen
predniment
predniretard
predonine
prelone
prezolon
scherisolon
solone
spiricort

Short synonyms
antisolon
antisolone
aprednislon
aprednislone
benisolon
benisolone
berisolon
berisolone
caberdelta
co hydeltra
cortadeltona
cortadeltone
cortelinter
cortisolone
dacortin h
dacrotin
decortril
dehydro cortex
dehydrocortex
dehydrocortisol
dehydrocortisole
dehydro hydrocortison
dehydrohydrocortison
1,2 dehydro hydrocortison
dehydro hydrocortisone
dehydrohydrocortisone
delcortol
delta1 dehydrocortisol
delta1 dehydrohydrocortisone
delta 1 hydrocortisone
delta1 hydrocortisone
deltacortef
deltacortenolo
deltacortil
deltacortoil
deltaderm
delta ef cortelan
delta f
deltaglycortril
delta hycortol
deltahycortol
delta hydrocortison
deltahydrocortison
delta hydrocortisone
deltahydrocortisone
delta ophticor
deltaophticor
deltasolone
delta stab
deltastab
deltidrosol
deltisilone
deltisolon
deltisolone
deltolasson
deltolassone
deltosona
deltosone
dicortol
domucortone
glistelone
hostacortin h
hydeltrone
hydrelta
hydrocortidelt

Terms and Synonyms

hydrodeltalone
hydrodeltisone
hydroretrocortin
hydroretrocortine
insolone
keteocort h
leocortol
mediasolone
meprisolone
metacortalon
metacortalone
metacortandralon
metacortandralone
metacortelone
meti derm
metiderm
morlone
neo delta
nisolon
nisolone
nsc 9120
panafcortolone
panafort
paracortol
phlogex
precortancyl
pre cortisyl
precortisyl
predartrina
predartrine
predne dome
prednedome
prednelan
predni coelin
prednicoelin
prednicortelone
prednis
prednisolon
prednisolone alcohol
prednisolone h
prednisolone oleosae sr 82
prednisolone, topical
prednivet
prednorsolon
prednorsolone
predorgasolona
predorgasolone
prenolone
serilone
solupren
soluprene
spolotane
sterolone
supercortisol
supercortizol
taracortelone
wysolone

Long synonyms
11beta,17,21 trihydroxypregna 1,4 diene 3,20 dione
11beta,17alpha,21 trihydroxy 1,4 pregnadien 3,20 dion
11beta,17alpha,21 trihydroxypregna 1,4 diene 3,20 dione
delta 1 17 hydroxycorticosterone 21 acetate
3,20 dioxo 11beta,17alpha,21 trihydroxy 1,4 pregnadiene
pregna 1,4 diene 11beta,17alpha,21 triol 3,20 dione
1,4 pregnadien 11beta,17alpha,21 triol 3,20 dion
1,4 pregnadiene 11beta,17alpha,21 triol 3,20 dione
1,4 pregnadiene 3,20 dione 11beta,17alpha,21 triol

prednisolone 21 phosphate

WADA group
S9. GLUCOCORTICOSTEROIDS

CAS Registry number
302-25-0

Short synonyms
prednisolone phosphate

prednisolone 3 sulfobenzoate

WADA group
S9. GLUCOCORTICOSTEROIDS

CAS Registry number
3694-41-5
39175-74-1

Trade names and research codes
corti clyss
corty clyss
predfoam
r 812
solupred

Long synonyms
prednisolone 3 sulfobenzoate sodium ester
prednisolone meta sulfobenzoate
prednisolone metasulfobenzoate sodium ester
prednisolone sodium meta sulfobenzoate

prednisolone acetate

WADA group
S9. GLUCOCORTICOSTEROIDS

CAS Registry number
52-21-1
52628-64-5

Trade names and research codes
deppredalone
econopred
isopto cetapred
key pred
poly pred
pred forte
predforte
pred forte tm
pred mild
predni h
savacort
ultracortensol
ultracortinol

Short synonyms
meticortelone acetate
prednisolone 17 acetate
prednisolone 21 acetate

prednisolone derivative

WADA group
S9. GLUCOCORTICOSTEROIDS

prednisolone hemisuccinate

WADA group
S9. GLUCOCORTICOSTEROIDS

CAS Registry number
2920-86-7

Trade names and research codes
prednisolut

Short synonyms
prednisolone 21 hemisuccinate
prednisolone 21 succinate
prednisolone bisuccinate
prednisolone succinate

prednisolone pivalate

WADA group
S9. GLUCOCORTICOSTEROIDS

CAS Registry number
1107-99-9

Trade names and research codes
ultracortenol

Short synonyms
prednisolone trimethylacetate

Long synonyms
prednisolone 21 trimethylacetate

prednisolone sodium phosphate

WADA group
S9. GLUCOCORTICOSTEROIDS

CAS Registry number
125-02-0

Trade names and research codes
codelsol
deltelan
hydeltrasol
inflamase
metreton
phortisolone
prednesol
predsol
psp iv
solucort

Short synonyms
prednisolone phosphate sodium

Long synonyms
prednisolone 21 phosphoric acid disodium salt
prednisolone disodium 21 phosphate
prednisolone disodium phosphate
prednisolone phosphate disodium

prednisolone sodium succinate

WADA group
S9. GLUCOCORTICOSTEROIDS

CAS Registry number
1715-33-9

Trade names and research codes
hostacortin h solubile
prednisol
prednisol n
soludacortin
solu decortin h
soludecortin h
soludeltacortef

Short synonyms
prednisolone succinate sodium

Long synonyms
prednisolone 21 hemisuccinate sodium
prednisolone 21 succinate sodium
prednisolone sodium hemisuccinate

prednisolone sodium tetrahydrophthalate

WADA group
S9. GLUCOCORTICOSTEROIDS

CAS Registry number
10059-14-0

Trade names and research codes
fenicort
ultracortene h
ultracorten h

Long synonyms
prednisolone sodium 1,2,3,6 tetrahydrophthalate

prednisone

WADA group
S9. GLUCOCORTICOSTEROIDS

MeSH descriptor
prednisone

CAS Registry number
53-03-2

Trade names and research codes
decortin
deltacorten
deltacortisone
deltasone
di adreson
di-adreson
diadreson
encorton
encortone
enkorton
meprison
meticorten
nsc 10023
nsc10023
orasone
ultracorten

Short synonyms
ancortone
biocortone
colisone
cortidelt
decortancyl
decortine
decortin e merck
de cortisyl
dehydrocortisone
1,2 dehydrocortisone
dekortin
delitisone
delta 1 dehydrocortisone
delta cortelan
delta cortisone
deltacortone
delta dome
delta e
delta prenovis
deltra
hostacortin
insone
metacortandracin
meticortine
orisane
paracort
precort
precortal
prednison

Terms and Synonyms

prednisone alcohol
prednisone test
pronison
pronisone
pronizone
rectodelt
urtilone

Long synonyms
17,21 dihydroxypregna 1,4 diene 3,11,20 trione
pregna 1,4 diene 3,11,20 dione 17,21 diol

prednisone acetate

WADA group
S9. GLUCOCORTICOSTEROIDS

CAS Registry number
125-10-0

Trade names and research codes
cortancyl
delcortin
deltalone
ferrosan
nisone

prednival acetate

WADA group
S9. GLUCOCORTICOSTEROIDS

CAS Registry number
72064-79-0

Trade names and research codes
acepreval

Short synonyms
prednisolone valerate acetate

Long synonyms
prednisolone 17 valerate 21 acetate
prednisolone 21 acetate 17 valerate

prednylidene

WADA group
S9. GLUCOCORTICOSTEROIDS

CAS Registry number
599-33-7

Trade names and research codes
decortilen

Short synonyms
methylene prednisolone
methyleneprednisolone
16 methylene prednisolone
16 methyleneprednisolone
16 methylenprednisolone
prednilidene
prednylidine
st 104

pregnenolone

WADA group
S9. GLUCOCORTICOSTEROIDS

MeSH descriptor
pregnenolone

CAS Registry number
145-13-1

Trade names and research codes
natolone
prenolon
regnosone
skinostelon

Short synonyms
3beta hydroxy 5 pregnen 20 one
3beta hydroxypregn 5 en 20 one
delta5 pregnen 3beta ol 20 one
delta 5 pregnenolone
3 hydroxy 20 oxo 5 pregnene
hydroxypregnenone
pregn 5 en 3 beta ol 20 one
pregn 5 en 3beta ol 20 one
4 pregnen 20 ol 3 one
5 pregnen 3 beta ol 20 one
5 pregnen 3beta ol 20 one
5 pregnen 3 ol 20 one
pregnenalone
5 pregnenolone

Long synonyms
3beta hydroxy 20 oxo 5 pregnene
3 beta hydroxy pregn 5 en 20 one
3 beta hydroxypregn 5 en 20 one
3 beta hydroxypregn 5 en 20 one sulfate
3beta hydroxypregn 5 en 20 one sulfate
3 beta hydroxy pregn 5 ene 20 one
3beta hydroxypregn 5 ene 20 one
delta 5 pregnen 3 beta ol 20 one

pregnenolone derivative

WADA group
S9. GLUCOCORTICOSTEROIDS

MeSH descriptor
hydroxypregnenolone

Short synonyms
hydroxypregnenolone
pregnenolone 16 alpha nitrite
pregnenolone derivates

Long synonyms
17 alpha 21 hydroxy pregnenolone
pregn 5 en 3beta ol 20 one derivative

pregnenolone sulfate

WADA group
S9. GLUCOCORTICOSTEROIDS

CAS Registry number
1247-64-9

Short synonyms
hydroxypregnenone sulfate

Long synonyms
pregnenolone sulfate metabolism

prenalterol

WADA group
S6. BETA-2 AGONISTS

MeSH descriptor
prenalterol

CAS Registry number
57526-81-5

62340-37-8

Trade names and research codes
cgp 7760b
cgp7760b
h 133 22
h 133-22
h 13322
h 133-80
h 80-62
hyprenan

Long synonyms
1 (4 hydroxyphenoxy) 3 isopropylamino 2 propanol
1 (4 hydroxyphenoxy) 3 isopropylaminopropanol
1 (4' hydroxyphenoxy) 3 isopropylaminopropanol
1 isopropylamino 3 (4' hydroxyphenoxy)propan 2 ol

prenylamine

WADA group
S1. STIMULANTS

MeSH descriptor
prenylamine

CAS Registry number
390-64-7

Trade names and research codes
b 436
b436
clemodril
hostaginan
segontin
segontin 60
synadrin

Short synonyms
fpdfpa
prenyl
prenylamin

Long synonyms
amphetamine,n (3,3 diphenylpropyl)
3,3 diphenyl n (3 phenylprop 2 yl) 1 propylamine
n (3,3 diphenylpropyl) 1 phenyl 2 propylamine
n (3,3 diphenylpropyl) alpha methylphenethylamine
n (3,3 diphenylpropyl)amphetamine
n (3' phenyl 2' propyl) 1,1 diphenyl 3 propylamine

preproinsulin

WADA group
S5. PEPTIDE HORMONES

CAS Registry number
61116-24-3

Short synonyms
insulin precursor precursor

prethcamide

WADA group
S1. STIMULANTS

CAS Registry number
8015-51-8

Trade names and research codes
g 5668
g5668

Short synonyms
cropropamide plus crotetamide
crotetamide plus cropropamide
micoren
mycoren
pretcamide
prethcamine
prothecamide

primidolol

WADA group
P2. BETA-BLOCKERS

CAS Registry number
67227-55-8

Trade names and research codes
uk 11443

Long synonyms
1 [2 [[2 hydroxy 3 (2 methylphenoxy)propyl]amino]ethyl] 5 methyl 2,4(1h,3h) pyrimidinedione
1 [2 [[2 hydroxy 3 (ortho tolyloxy)propyl]amino]ethyl]thymine

prizidilol

WADA group
P2. BETA-BLOCKERS

CAS Registry number
59010-44-5
73793-66-5

Trade names and research codes
sk and f 92657
skf 92657
skf 92657 a2

Short synonyms
prezidilol
prizidilol hydrochloride

Long synonyms
dextro,levo 3 [2 (3 tert butylamino 2 hydroxypropoxy)phenyl] 6 hydrazinopyridazine
3 [2 (3 tert butylamino 2 hydroxypropoxy)phenyl] 6 hydrazinopyridazine
1 (tert butylamino) 3 [o (6 hydrazino 3 pyridazinyl)phenoxy] 2 propanol
1 (tert butylamino) 3 [o (6 hydrazinopyridazin 3 yl)phenoxy] 2 propanol

probenecid

WADA group
S8. MASKING AGENTS

MeSH descriptor
probenecid

CAS Registry number
57-66-9

Trade names and research codes
benemid
benemide
benemin
probalan
probecid
probenid
procid
prolongine
uricosid
urocid

Short synonyms
probemecid
probenecide
probenicid

Long synonyms
4 (dipropylsulfamoyl)benzoic acid
para (dipropylsulfamoyl)benzoic acid
para (dipropylsulfamyl)benzoic acid

procaterol

WADA group
S6. BETA-2 AGONISTS

MeSH descriptor
procaterol

CAS Registry number
62929-91-3
72332-33-3

Trade names and research codes
beta air
ci 888
ci888
masacin
meptin
mucodine
onsuki
onsukil
opc 2009
opc2009
proair
procadil

Short synonyms
erythroprocaterol
procaterol,erythro
procaterol hydrochloride

Long synonyms
1 (8 hydroxy 2 oxoquinolin 5 yl) 2 (isopropylamino) 1 butanol
8 hydroxy 5 [1 hydroxy 2 [(1 methylethyl)amino]butyl] 2(1h) quinolinone
8 hydroxy 5 (1 hydroxy 2 isopropylaminobutyl) 2 quinolinol
8 hydroxy 5 (1 hydroxy 2 isopropylaminobutyl) carbostyril
8 hydroxy 5 (1 hydroxy 2 isopropylaminobutyl)carbostyril
1 (quinoline 2,8 diol 5 yl) 2 isopropylamino 1 butanol

procinolol

WADA group
P2. BETA-BLOCKERS

CAS Registry number
27325-36-6

Trade names and research codes
sd 2124 01
sd 2124-01
sd2124 01
sd2124-01

Long synonyms
1 (2 cyclopropylphenoxy) 3 isopropylamino 2 propanol
1 (ortho cyclopropylphenoxy) 3 isopropylamino 2 propanol hydrochloride

procinonide

WADA group
S9. GLUCOCORTICOSTEROIDS

CAS Registry number
58497-00-0

Trade names and research codes
rs 2362
rs2362

Long synonyms
fluocinolone acetonide 21 propionate

proinsulin

WADA group
S5. PEPTIDE HORMONES

MeSH descriptor
proinsulin

CAS Registry number
11062-00-3
9035-68-1

Short synonyms
big insulin
bovine proinsulin
insulin,pro
porcine proinsulin
pro insulin
proinsulin,bovine
proinsuline

prolintane

WADA group
S1. STIMULANTS

CAS Registry number
1211-28-5
493-92-5

Trade names and research codes
catovit
katovit
promotil
vilescon
villescon

Short synonyms
1 phenyl 2 pyrrolidinopentane
phenylpyrrolidine pentane
phenylpyrrolidone pentane
prolintane hydrochloride

pronetalol

WADA group
P2. BETA-BLOCKERS

CAS Registry number
51-02-5
54-80-8

Trade names and research codes
alderlin
ay 6204
ay6204
ici 38174
ici38174
n alderlin

nethalide

Short synonyms
pronetal
pronetalol hydrochloride
pronethalol
pronethalol hydrochloride

Long synonyms
alpha (isopropylaminomethyl) 2 naphthalenemethanol
2 isopropylamino 1 naphth 2 ylethanol

10 propargylestr 4 ene 3,17 dione

WADA group
S7. AGENTS WITH ANTI-OESTROGENIC ACTIVITY

CAS Registry number
77016-85-4

Trade names and research codes
mdl 18962

Long synonyms
10beta (2 propynyl)estr 4 ene 3,17 dione
10beta propargylestr 4 ene 3,17 dione
estr 4 ene 3,17 dione,10 propargyl
10 (2 propynyl)estr 4 ene 3,17 dione

propranolol

WADA group
P2. BETA-BLOCKERS

MeSH descriptor
propranolol

CAS Registry number
13013-17-7
318-98-9
3506-09-0
1-9-4199
525-66-6

Trade names and research codes
anaprilin
anapriline
arcablock
authus
avlocardyl
ay 64043
ay64043
bedranol
beprane
betadipresan
betaryl
beta timelets
cardinol
ciplar
corbeta
deralin
dociton
efektolol
elbrol
frekven
ici 45520
inderal
inderal la
inderal retard
inderex
innopran
innopran xl
ipran
obsidan
prandol
propabloc
propal
propercuten
prophylux
propral
propranur
propra ratiopharm
sagittol
sumial

Short synonyms
anaprilinium
anapryline
arcablock retard
avlocardyl retard
bercolol
beta neg
betaneg
betaprol
betares
beta tablinen
beta tablinen retard
dextrolevo propranolol
dideral
dl propanolol hydrochloride
dl propranolol
docitone
dociton retard
durabeton
efektolol retard
ikopal
indobloc
lederpronol
levo propranolol
levopropranolol
l propranolol
napriline
nsc 91523
obsin
obzidan
prano puren
pranopuren
prolol
pronovan
propanolol hydrochloride
propranolol hydrochloride
propranolol isomer
proprasylyt
proprasylyte
stapranolol

Long synonyms
1 (2 hydroxy 3 isopropylaminopropoxy)naphthalene
1 isopropylamino 3 (1 naphthoxy) 2 propanol
1 (isopropylamino) 3 (1 naphthyloxy) 2 propanol
1 isopropylamino 3 (1 naphthyloxy)propan 2 ol

propranolol derivative

WADA group
P2. BETA-BLOCKERS

Short synonyms
propanolol derivative
propranolol analog
propranolol quaternary analog

Long synonyms
1 (alpha naphthoxy) 2,3 propyleneglycol
n,n dimethyl 1 isopropylamino 3 (1 naphthyloxy)propan 2 ol
propanolol phenylethylbarbiturate

Terms and Synonyms

propylhexedrine

WADA group
S1. STIMULANTS

CAS Registry number
101-40-6
7-11-3595
532-52-5
6192-97-8

Trade names and research codes
benzedrex
dristan inhaler
e 111
e111
eventin
obesin

Short synonyms
cyclexedrine
hexahydrodesoxyephedrine

Long synonyms
2 cyclohexyl 1 methylaminopropane
1 cyclohexyl 2 methylaminopropane
(cyclohexylisopropyl)methylamine
2 cyclohexyl n methylpropylamine
n (2 cyclohexylpropyl)methylamine
n,alpha dimethylcyclohexaneethylamine
n,alpha dimethylcyclohexylethylamine

7alpha propylspironolactone

WADA group
S8. MASKING AGENTS
P3. DIURETICS

CAS Registry number
76676-33-0

Trade names and research codes
ru 26752

Short synonyms
7alpha propylspirolactone

Long synonyms
17 hydroxy 3 oxo 7alpha propyl 17alpha pregn 4 ene 21 carboxylic acid gamma lactone

proxodolol

WADA group
P2. BETA-BLOCKERS

CAS Registry number
158446-41-4

Long synonyms
1 [(1,1 dimethylethyl)amino] 3 [2 [(3 methoxy 1,2,4 oxadiazol 5 yl)methoxy]phenoxy] 2 propanol
3 methoxy 5 [2 (3 tert butylamino 2 hydroxypropoxy)phenoxymethyl] 1,2,4 oxadiazole
5 [2 (3 tert butylamino 2 hydroxypropoxy)phenoxymethyl] 3 methoxy 1,2,4 oxadiazole

psychostimulant agent

WADA group
S1. STIMULANTS

Short synonyms
psychostimulant
psychostimulating agent

pyridoglutethimide

WADA group
S7. AGENTS WITH ANTI-OESTROGENIC ACTIVITY

CAS Registry number
92788-10-8

Short synonyms
rogletimide

Long synonyms
3 ethyl 3 (4 pyridyl) 2,6 piperidinedione
3 ethyl 3 (4 pyridyl)piperidine 2,6 dione

pyridoxylhemoglobin

WADA group
S8. MASKING AGENTS
M1. ENHANCEMENT OF OXYGEN TRANSFER

Short synonyms
hemoglobin,pyridoxylated
pyridoxylated hemoglobin

pyridoxylpolyhemoglobin

WADA group
S8. MASKING AGENTS
M1. ENHANCEMENT OF OXYGEN TRANSFER

Short synonyms
polyhemoglobin,pyridoxylated
pyridoxylated polyhemoglobin

pyrovalerone

WADA group
S1. STIMULANTS

CAS Registry number
1147-62-2
3563-49-3

Trade names and research codes
f 1983
f1983
thymergix

Short synonyms
centroton
pyrovalerone hydrochloride

Long synonyms
4' methyl 2 (1 pyrrolidinyl)valerophenone
4' methyl 2 pyrrolidin 1 ylvalerophenone
1 (4 methylphenyl) 2 (1 pyrrolidinyl) 1 pentanone
2 pyrrolidin 1 yl 1 para tolyl 1 pentanone

quinbolone

WADA group
S4. ANABOLIC AGENTS

CAS Registry number
2487-63-0

Trade names and research codes
anabolicum

Long synonyms
17beta (1 cyclopentenyloxy)androsta 1,4 dien 3 one

quinethazone

WADA group
S8. MASKING AGENTS
P3. DIURETICS

CAS Registry number
73-49-4

Trade names and research codes
aquamox
hydromox

Short synonyms
chinethazon
chinethazone
guinethazone
kinetazone
quinethazon

Long synonyms
7 chloro 2 ethyl 1,2,3,4 tetrahydro 4 oxo 6 quinazolinesulfonamide
7 chloro 2 ethyl 6 sulfamoyl 1,2,3,4 tetrahydroquinazolin 4 one

quinprenaline

WADA group
S6. BETA-2 AGONISTS

CAS Registry number
13757-97-6

Short synonyms
quinoprenaline
quinterenol
quinterenol dihydrochloride

racephedrine

WADA group
S1. STIMULANTS

CAS Registry number
134-71-4
90-81-3

Trade names and research codes
ephetonin

Short synonyms
cophedrine
ephedron
methylmydriatin
racedrine
racemic ephedrine
racephedrine hydrochloride

ractopamine

WADA group
S6. BETA-2 AGONISTS

CAS Registry number
97825-25-7

Trade names and research codes
el 737
el737
ly 031537
ly031537
ly 31537
ly31537

Short synonyms
ractopamine hydrochloride

Long synonyms
1 (4 hydroxyphenyl) 2 [[3 (4 hydroxyphenyl) 1 methylpropyl]amino]ethanol

raloxifene

WADA group
S7. AGENTS WITH ANTI-OESTROGENIC ACTIVITY

MeSH descriptor
raloxifene

CAS Registry number
82640-04-8
84449-90-1

Trade names and research codes
evista
loxifen
ly 139481
ly139481
ly 156758
ly156758
optruma

Short synonyms
keoxifene
raloxifene hydrochloride

Long synonyms
6 hydroxy 2 (4 hydroxyphenyl) 3 [4 [2 (1 piperidyl)ethoxy]benzoyl]benzo[b]thiophene
6 hydroxy 2 (4 hydroxyphenyl)benzo[b]thien 3 yl 4 [2 (1 piperidinyl)ethoxy]phenyl ketone
[6 hydroxy 2 (4 hydroxyphenyl)benzo[b]thien 3 yl][4 [2 (1 piperidinyl)ethoxy]phenyl]methanone

recombinant chorionic gonadotropin

WADA group
S5. PEPTIDE HORMONES

CAS Registry number
177073-44-8

Trade names and research codes
ovidrel
ovidrelle
ovitrelle

Long synonyms
chorionic gonadotropin,recombinant
recombinant human chorionic gonadotropin

recombinant erythropoietin

WADA group
S5. PEPTIDE HORMONES
M1. ENHANCEMENT OF OXYGEN TRANSFER

MeSH descriptor
epoetin alfa
erythropoietin, recombinant

CAS Registry number
113427-24-0
122312-54-3
130455-76-4

Trade names and research codes
dynepo
epoch
epoconn
epogen
epogin
epoietin
epoxitin
eprex
erypo
espo
exprex
globuren
hemax
krn 5702
marogen
neorecormon
procrit
recormon
recormone
snb 5001
tyb 5220

Short synonyms
biosynthetic erythropoietin
epoetin
epoetin alfa
epoetin beta
epoetin delta
epoietin alfa
epoietin alpha
epoietin beta
erantin
erythropoietin, recombinant

Long synonyms
human recombinant erythropoietin
recombinant human erythropoietin

recombinant follitropin

WADA group
S5. PEPTIDE HORMONES

Trade names and research codes
follistim
gonal f
org 32489
org32489
puregon
recagon
sj 0021
sj0021

Short synonyms
follitropin alfa
follitropin beta
recombinant fsh
recombinant human follitropin

Long synonyms
recombinant follicle stimulating hormone
recombinant human follicle stimulating hormone

recombinant growth hormone

WADA group
S5. PEPTIDE HORMONES

Short synonyms
biosynthetic growth hormone
growth hormone,biosynthetic
recombinant somatotropin
somatotropins, recombinant

recombinant hemoglobin

WADA group
M1. ENHANCEMENT OF OXYGEN TRANSFER

Trade names and research codes
optro

recombinant human insulin

WADA group
S5. PEPTIDE HORMONES

Trade names and research codes
humalin r
huminsulin
huminsulin normal
insuman
lilly 410001

Short synonyms
biosynthetic human insulin
humanized insulin
recombinant DNA insulin
recombinant insulin

Long synonyms
bacterial human insulin (biosynthetic)
human insulin,biosynthetic (recombinant dna)
insulin,human biosynthetic (recombinant dna)
synthetic insulin,bacterial (recombinant dna)

recombinant luteinizing hormone

WADA group
S5. PEPTIDE HORMONES

Trade names and research codes
lhadi
luveris

recombinant somatomedin B

WADA group
S5. PEPTIDE HORMONES

Long synonyms
recombinant insulin like growth factor ii

recombinant somatomedin C

WADA group
S5. PEPTIDE HORMONES

Trade names and research codes
myotrophin

Short synonyms
mecasermin

Long synonyms
recombinant insulin like growth factor 1
recombinant insulin like growth factor i

relefact

WADA group
S5. PEPTIDE HORMONES

Trade names and research codes
relefact

reproterol

WADA group
S6. BETA-2 AGONISTS

CAS Registry number
13055-82-8
54063-54-6

Trade names and research codes
bronchodil
bronchospasmin
d 1959
d1959
w 2946m
w2946m

Short synonyms
asmaterolo
reproterol hydrochloride

Long synonyms
beta,3,5 trihydroxy n (3 theophyllin 7 yl)propylphenethylamine
7 [3 [(beta,3,5 trihydroxyphenethyl)amino]propyl]theophylline
7 [3 [2 (3,5 dihydroxyphenyl) 2 hydroxyethylamino]propyl]theophylline

rheodextran

WADA group
S8. MASKING AGENTS

CAS Registry number
9004-54-0

Trade names and research codes
rheodextran
rheopolyglucin
rheopolyglucine

ridazolol

WADA group
P2. BETA-BLOCKERS

CAS Registry number
83395-21-5

Long synonyms
4 chloro 5 [2 [3 (2 chlorophenoxy) 2 hydroxypropylamino]ethylamino] 2,3 dihydro 3 pyridazinone
4 chloro 5 [[2 [[3 (2 chlorophenoxy) 2 hydroxypropyl]amino]ethyl]amino] 3(2h) pyridazinone

rimexolone

WADA group
S9. GLUCOCORTICOSTEROIDS

CAS Registry number
49697-38-3

Trade names and research codes
org 6216
org6216
rimexel
vexol

Short synonyms
trimexolone

Long synonyms
16alpha,17alpha,21 trimethylpregna 1,4 dien 11beta ol 3,20 dione
11beta hydroxy 16alpha,17alpha,21 trimethyl 3,20 dioxopregna 1,4 diene
11beta hydroxy 16alpha,17alpha,21 trimethylpregna 1,4 diene 3,20 dione
pregna 1,4 dien 11beta ol 3,20 dione,16alpha,17alpha,21 trimethyl

rimiterol

WADA group
S6. BETA-2 AGONISTS

CAS Registry number
31842-61-2
32953-89-2

Trade names and research codes
pulmadil
r 798
r798
wg 253
wg253

Short synonyms
rimiterol hydrobromide

Long synonyms
alpha (3,4 dihydroxyphenyl) 2 piperidinemethanol
3,4 dihydroxy alpha (2 piperidyl)benzyl alcohol
3,4 dihydroxy alpha (2 piperidyl)benzyl alcohol hydrobromide

ritodrine

WADA group
S6. BETA-2 AGONISTS

MeSH descriptor
ritodrine

CAS Registry number
23239-51-2
26652-09-5

Trade names and research codes
du 21 220
du 21220
du21220
miolene
prempar
prepar
utemerine
utopar
yutopar

Short synonyms
ritodrin
ritodrine hydrochloride

Long synonyms
erythro 1 (4 hydroxyphenyl) 2 (4 hydroxyphenethylamino)propan 1 ol

erythro para hydroxy alpha [1 [(para hydroxyphenethyl)amino]ethyl]benzylalcohol

salbutamol

WADA group
S6. BETA-2 AGONISTS

MeSH descriptor
albuterol

CAS Registry number
18559-94-9

Trade names and research codes
aero clenil
aeroclenil
aerolin
ah 3365
ah3365
asmalin
asmol
broncho spray
butovent
buventol
cibutamol
ecovent
frespire
loftan
proventil
proventil repetabs
repetabs
salamol
salbuair
salbumol fort
salbupart
salgem
saltos
sultanol
sultanol n
venetlin
ventilan
ventodisk
ventodisks
ventolin
ventoline
ventolin nebules
volmac

Short synonyms
albuterol
asmaven
proventil inhaler
respolin
salbulin
salbuvent
solbutamol
ventolin aerosol
ventolin tablets

Long synonyms
alpha (tert butylaminomethyl) 4 hydroxy 3 (hydroxymethyl)benzyl alcohol
alpha (tert butylaminomethyl) 4 hydroxy meta xylene alpha,alpha' diol
2 tert butylamino 1 (4 hydroxy 3 hydroxymethylphenyl)ethanol

salbutamol sulfate

WADA group
S6. BETA-2 AGONISTS

CAS Registry number
51022-70-9

Trade names and research codes
airomir
epaq
volmax

Short synonyms
albuterol sulfate
cobutolin
salbutax

salcardolol

WADA group
P2. BETA-BLOCKERS

CAS Registry number
106716-46-5

Trade names and research codes
cgp 17582
cgp17582
cgp 17582 b
cgp 17582b
cgp17582b

Long synonyms
1 [2 (3 carbamoyl 4 hydroxyphenoxy)ethylamino] 3 [4 (2 methoxyethoxy)phenoxy] 2 propanol methanesulfonate

sali aldopur

WADA group
S8. MASKING AGENTS
P3. DIURETICS

CAS Registry number
101660-06-4

Trade names and research codes
sali aldopur

Long synonyms
bendroflumethiazide plus spironolactone
spironolactone plus bendroflumethiazide

salmefamol

WADA group
S6. BETA-2 AGONISTS

CAS Registry number
18910-65-1

Long synonyms
1 [4 hydroxy 3 (hydroxymethyl)phenyl] 2 (4 methoxy alpha methylphenethylamino)ethanol

salmeterol

WADA group
S6. BETA-2 AGONISTS

CAS Registry number
89365-50-4

Trade names and research codes
beglan
gr 33343x

Long synonyms
1 (4 hydroxy 3 hydroxymethylphenyl) 2 [6 (4 phenylbutoxy)hexylamino]ethanol

salmeterol xinafoate

WADA group
S6. BETA-2 AGONISTS

CAS Registry number
94749-08-3

Trade names and research codes
aeromax
arial
gr 33343
salmetedur
serevent
sn 408

Short synonyms
salmeterol hydroxynaphthoate

sandoz 204545

WADA group
P2. BETA-BLOCKERS

Trade names and research codes
sandoz 204545

sauvagine

WADA group
S5. PEPTIDE HORMONES

CAS Registry number
74434-59-6

selegiline

WADA group
S1. STIMULANTS

MeSH descriptor
selegiline

CAS Registry number
14611-51-9
14611-52-0
2079-54-1
2323-36-6

Trade names and research codes
anipryl
antiparkin
atapryl
deprenyl
e 250
e250
egibren
eldeprine
eldepryl
emsam
jumex
jumexal
movergan
parkryl
plurimen
seledat
zelapar

Short synonyms
deprenaline
deprenil
l deprenyl
levo deprenyl
selegiline hydrochloride

Long synonyms
amphetamine,n methyl n (2 propynyl)
n,alpha dimethyl n 2 propynylphenethylamine
n,alpha dimethyl n prop 2 ynylphenethylamine
n isopropyl 1 methyl n phenyl 2 propynylamine
n isopropyl 1 methyl n phenylpropynylamine
n methyl n (2 phenylisopropyl)prop 2 ynylamine
n methyl n 2 propynyllevamfetamine
n methyl n prop 2 ynylamphetamine
phenylisopropylmethylpropynylamine

seric gonadotropin

WADA group
S5. PEPTIDE HORMONES

MeSH descriptor
gonadotropins, equine

CAS Registry number
9002-70-4

Trade names and research codes
anteron
antex
antostab
eleagol
equinex
equoman
folligon
gestyl
gonadin
gonadogen
gonadotraphon f.s.h.
gonadotraphon fsh
gonadyl seric
gormon
hemoantine
lobulantina
pregnacol
prelobane
priantin
primantron
seragon
serogan
serotropin
thylakentrin

Short synonyms
equine gonadotrophin
estrogen conjugated equine
gonadotropins, equine
pg 600
PMSG
pms gonadotrophin
pms gonadotropin
pregnant mare serum
seric gonadotrophin
seric gonadotropins

Long synonyms
pregnant donkey serum gonadotropin
pregnant mare serum gonadotrophin
pregnant mare serum gonadotropin

sermorelin

WADA group
S5. PEPTIDE HORMONES

MeSH descriptor
sermorelin

Terms and Synonyms

CAS Registry number
86168-78-7

Trade names and research codes
geref
groliberin
groliverin

Short synonyms
ghrh[1-29] amide

Long synonyms
growth hormone releasing factor[1-29] amide
somatotropin releasing hormone[1-29] amide

skf 105494

WADA group
S8. MASKING AGENTS
P3. DIURETICS

CAS Registry number
114923-99-8

Trade names and research codes
skf 105494
skf105494

sofradex

WADA group
S9. GLUCOCORTICOSTEROIDS

Trade names and research codes
sofradex

somatomedin

WADA group
S5. PEPTIDE HORMONES

MeSH descriptor
somatomedins

Short synonyms
growth factor,insulin
insulin growth factor
insulin like growth factor
somatomedins

somatomedin A

WADA group
S5. PEPTIDE HORMONES

CAS Registry number
62046-94-0

somatomedin B

WADA group
S5. PEPTIDE HORMONES

MeSH descriptor
insulin-like growth factor ii

CAS Registry number
63774-77-6
67763-97-7

Short synonyms
growth factor ii,insulin like
insulin like growth factor 2
insulin like growth factor II
insulin-like growth factor ii

Long synonyms
multiplication stimulating activity

somatomedin C

WADA group
S5. PEPTIDE HORMONES

MeSH descriptor
insulin-like growth factor i

CAS Registry number
67763-96-6

Short synonyms
insulin like growth factor 1
insulin like growth factor I
insulin-like growth factor i

somatrem

WADA group
S5. PEPTIDE HORMONES

CAS Registry number
82030-87-3

Trade names and research codes
genotonorm
protropin
sm 9500
sm9500
somatohorm
somatonorm
sometribove
ym 17798
ym17798

Short synonyms
growth hormone,methionyl
methionyl growth hormone
methionylgrowth hormone
methionylgrowth hormone 20k
methionylgrowth hormone 22k
methionyl somatotropin
methionylsomatotropin
somatotropin,methionyl

soquinolol

WADA group
P2. BETA-BLOCKERS

CAS Registry number
61563-18-6

Long synonyms
[5 (3 tert butylamino) 2 hydroxypropoxy] 3,4 dihydro 2(1h) isoquinolinecarbaldehyde
[5 (3 tert butylamino) 2 hydroxypropoxy] 3,4 dihydro 2(1h) isoquinolinecarboxaldehyde

soquinolol mucate

WADA group
P2. BETA-BLOCKERS

Trade names and research codes
sertum

we 704

sorbitol

WADA group
S8. MASKING AGENTS
P3. DIURETICS

MeSH descriptor
sorbitol

CAS Registry number
26566-34-7
50-70-4
53469-19-5

Trade names and research codes
sorbelite
sorbit

Short synonyms
dextro sorbitol
d glucitol
d glucohexitol
diakarmon
glucitol
glucohexitol
glycitol
gulitole
karion
neosorb
nivitin
sionon
sorbital
sorbite
sorbo
sorbol

sotalol

WADA group
P2. BETA-BLOCKERS

MeSH descriptor
sotalol

CAS Registry number
3930-20-9
80456-07-1
959-24-0

Trade names and research codes
betacardone
betades
betapace
bmy 5763 1
bmy 57631
bmy5763 1
bmy57631
bonpro
corsotalol
darob
gilucor
rentibloc
sotabeta
sotacor
sotahexal
sotalex
sotapor
sota saar
sotastad
tachytalol

Short synonyms
dexsotalol
dexsotalol hydrochloride
dextro sotalol
dextrosotalol
d sotalol
isotalol
levo sotalol
levosotalol
l sotalol
mj 1999
mj 5763 1
rotalol
satalol
satolol
sotacol
sotalol hydrochloride

Long synonyms
dl 4 (2 isopropylamino 1 hydroxyethyl) methanesulfonanilide hydrochloride
4' [1 hydroxy 2 (isopropylamine)ethyl]methanesulfonanilide hydrochloride
4 (2 isopropyl 1 hydroxyethyl)methanesulfonanilide
4 (2 isopropylamine 1 hydroxyethyl)methanesulfonanilide
4' (2 isopropylamine 1 hydroxyethyl)methane sulfonanilide
4 (2 isopropylamino 1 hydroxyethyl)methanesulfoanilide
4 (2 isopropylamino 1 hydroxyethyl)methanesulfonamide
(2 isopropylamino 1 hydroxyethyl)methane sulfonanilide
4 (2 isopropylamino 1 hydroxyethyl)methane sulfonanilide
4 (2 isopropylamino 1 hydroxyethyl)methanesulfonanilide
(2 isopropylamino 1 hydroxyethyl)methane sulfonanilide hydrochloride
(2 isopropylamino 1 hydroxyethyl)methanesulfonanilide hydrochloride
4 (isopropylamino 1 hydroxyethyl) methanesulfonanilide hydrochloride
4 (2 isopropylamino 1 hydroxyethyl)methanesulfonanilide hydrochloride
4 (2 isopropylamino) 1 hydroxyethylmethanesulfonilide hydrochloride
l 4 (2 isopropylamino 1 hydroxyethyl)methanesulfonamide
levo 4' [1 hydroxy 2 (isopropylamino)ethyl]methanesulfonanilide

soterenol

WADA group
S6. BETA-2 AGONISTS

CAS Registry number
13642-52-9
14816-67-2

Short synonyms
mj 1992
my 1997
soterenol hydrochloride

spirendolol

WADA group
P2. BETA-BLOCKERS

CAS Registry number
65429-87-0

Trade names and research codes
li 32 468

li 32-468
li 32468
sandoz li 32468

Long synonyms
4' [3 (tert butylamino) 2 hydroxypropoxy]spiro[cyclohexane 1,2' indan] 1' one

spironolactone

WADA group
S8. MASKING AGENTS
P3. DIURETICS

MeSH descriptor
spironolactone

CAS Registry number
52-01-7

Trade names and research codes
alaton
alatone
aldactone
crl 635
crl635
osiren
osyrol
sas 1060
sas1060
sc 9420
sc9420
spiridon
spiroctan
spirolang
uractone
verospiron
xenalon

Short synonyms
abbolactone
acelat
aldace
aldactone 50
aldactone a
aldactone diurapid
aldopur
aquareduct
beta aldopur
duraspiron
dyta urese
dytaurese
osyrol 50 100
practon
spiroctan m
spirolactone
spirone
spironolacton
spironone
spirothiobarbiturate 03620
spirotone
supra puren
suprapuren
verospirone

Long synonyms
7alpha acetylthio 3 oxo 4 androsten 17 spiro 2' tetrahydrofuran 5' one
17 hydroxy 7 mercapto 3 oxo 17alpha pregn 4 ene 21 carboxylic acid gamma lactone 7 acetate
3 (3 oxo 7alpha acetylthio 17beta hydroxy 4 androsten 17alpha yl)propionic acid gamma lactone

spiroxasone

WADA group
S8. MASKING AGENTS
P3. DIURETICS

CAS Registry number
6673-97-8

Long synonyms
7alpha acetylthio 20 spirox 4 en 3 one
7alpha (acetylthio) 4',5' dihydrospiro[androst 4 ene 17,2'(3'h)furan] 3 one
7alpha acetylthio 4',5' dihydrospiro[androst 4 ene 17,2'(3'h) furan] 3 one
2',3' alpha tetrahydrofuran 2' spiro 17 (7 acetylthio 4 androsten) 3 one
2',3'alpha tetrahydrofuran 2' spiro 17 [7 (acetylthio) 4 androsten 3 one]
4',5' dihydro 7alpha mercaptospiro[androst 4 ene 17,2'(3'h) furan] 3 one acetate
4,5 dihydro 7alpha mercaptospiro[androst 4 ene 17,2'(3'h)furan] 3 one acetate
20 spirox 4 en 3 one,7alpha acetylthio

stanozolol

WADA group
S4. ANABOLIC AGENTS

MeSH descriptor
stanozolol

CAS Registry number
10418-03-8
302-96-5

Trade names and research codes
anabol
strombaject
winstrol

Short synonyms
androstanasol
androstanazole
androstanopyrazole
methylandrostanopyrazole
methylstanazole
nsc 43193
stanazolol
stanozol
stanozole
stromba
win 14833

Long synonyms
17alpha methyl 17beta hydroxyandrostano[3,2 c]pyrazole
17alpha methylandrostano[3,2 c]pyrazol 17beta ol
17 beta hydroxy 17 alpha methylandrostano [3,2 c] pyrazole
17beta hydroxy 17alpha methylandrostano(3,2 c)pyrazole
17beta hydroxy 17alpha methylandrostano[3,2 c]pyrazole

stenbolone

WADA group
S4. ANABOLIC AGENTS

CAS Registry number
5197-58-0

Terms and Synonyms

Short synonyms
stenobolone

Long synonyms
17beta hydroxy 2 methyl 5alpha androst 1 en 3 one

stenbolone acetate

WADA group
S4. ANABOLIC AGENTS

CAS Registry number
1242-56-4

Trade names and research codes
anatrofin

Short synonyms
stenobolone acetate

Long synonyms
17beta hydroxy 2 methyl 5alpha androst 1 en 3 one acetate

strychnine

WADA group
S1. STIMULANTS

MeSH descriptor
strychnine

CAS Registry number
1421-86-9
57-24-9

Short synonyms
strichnine
strychnidin 10 one
strychnine hydrochloride

sulfhemoglobin

WADA group
M1. ENHANCEMENT OF OXYGEN TRANSFER

MeSH descriptor
sulfhemoglobin

Short synonyms
sulfemoglobin
sulfohemoglobin

sydnocarb

WADA group
S1. STIMULANTS

CAS Registry number
34262-84-5

Trade names and research codes
pharmanocarb

Short synonyms
mesocarb
sidnocarb

Long synonyms
3 (alpha methylphenethyl) n (phenylcarbamoyl)sydnoneimine
3 (1 methyl 2 phenylethyl) 1 (n phenylcarbamoylimino)sydnone
3 (2 phenylisopropyl)sydnone imine n phenylcarbamoyl derivative

sydnofen

WADA group
S1. STIMULANTS

CAS Registry number
3441-64-3

Short synonyms
sidnophen
sydnophen

Long synonyms
3 (beta phenylisopropyl)sydnonimine hydrochloride
3 (2 phenylisopropyl)sydnone imine

synthetic insulin

WADA group
S5. PEPTIDE HORMONES

Short synonyms
insulin,chemically synthesized

tabimorelin

WADA group
S5. PEPTIDE HORMONES

CAS Registry number
193079-69-5

Trade names and research codes
nn 703
nn703

Long synonyms
n (5 amino 5 methyl 1 oxo 2 hexenyl) n methyl 3 (2 naphthyl) dextro alanyl n,nalpha dimethyl dextro phenylalaninamide

talinolol

WADA group
P2. BETA-BLOCKERS

CAS Registry number
57460-41-0

Trade names and research codes
cordanum

Long synonyms
1 [4 (3 tert butylamino 2 hydroxypropoxy)phenyl] 3 cyclohexylurea
1 tert butylamino 3 [4 (3 cyclohexylureido)phenoxy] 2 propanol

tamoxifen

WADA group
S7. AGENTS WITH ANTI-OESTROGENIC ACTIVITY

MeSH descriptor
tamoxifen

CAS Registry number
10540-29-1

Trade names and research codes
kessar
tamoplac

tamoxasta

Short synonyms
nsc 180973
tamoxifene
trans tamoxifen

Long synonyms
1 [4 (2 diethylaminoethoxy)phenyl] 1,2 diphenylbut 1 ene
1 [4 (2 dimethylaminoethoxy)phenyl] 1,2 diphenyl 1 butene
1 [4 (2 dimethylaminoethoxy)phenyl] 1,2 diphenylbut 1 ene
1 [4 (2 dimethylaminoethoxy)phenyl] 1,2 diphenylbut 1 ene hydrobromide
2 [4 (1,2 diphenyl 1 buten 1 yl)phenoxy] n,n dimethylethylamine
1 para (2 dimethylaminoethoxyphenyl) 1,2 cis diphenylbut 1 ene hydrobromide
1 (para beta dimethylaminoethoxyphenyl) 1,2 diphenyl 1 butene
1 (para beta dimethylaminoethoxy phenyl) 1,2 diphenylbut 1 ene
1 (para beta dimethylaminoethoxyphenyl) 1,2 diphenylbut 1 ene
1 [para (beta dimethylaminoethoxy)phenyl] 1,2 diphenylbut 1 ene
trans 1 (para alpha dimethylaminoethoxyphenyl) 1,2 diphenylbut 1 ene
trans 1 (para beta dimethylaminoethoxyphenyl) 1,2 diphenyl 1 butene
trans 1 (para beta dimethylaminoethoxyphenyl) 1,2 diphenylbut 1 ene
trans 1 [para (beta dimethylaminoethoxy)phenyl] 1,2 diphenylbut 1 ene

tamoxifen aziridine

WADA group
S7. AGENTS WITH ANTI-OESTROGENIC ACTIVITY

CAS Registry number
79642-44-7

Long synonyms
1 [4 [2 (aziridin 1 yl)ethoxy]phenyl] 1,2 diphenyl 1 butene
1 [4 (2 aziridinoethoxy)phenyl] 1,2 diphenyl 1 butene
1 [4 [2 (1 aziridinyl)ethoxy]phenyl] 1,2 diphenyl 1 butene

tamoxifen citrate

WADA group
S7. AGENTS WITH ANTI-OESTROGENIC ACTIVITY

CAS Registry number
54965-24-1

Trade names and research codes
ici 46 474
ici 46,474
ici 46474
nolvadex
novadex
novaldex
tamofen
tamokadin
tamoplex
valodex
zemide
zemide 20
zitazonium

tamoxifen derivative

WADA group
S7. AGENTS WITH ANTI-OESTROGENIC ACTIVITY

Short synonyms
tamoxiphen derivative

tazolol

WADA group
S6. BETA-2 AGONISTS

CAS Registry number
39832-48-9

Short synonyms
rs 6245

Long synonyms
2 [2 hydroxy 3 (isopropylamino)propoxy]thiazole
1 isopropylamino 3 (2 thiazolyloxy) 2 propanol
1 isopropylamino 3 (thiazol 2 yloxy) 2 propanol

tensigradyl

WADA group
S8. MASKING AGENTS
P3. DIURETICS

Trade names and research codes
tensigradyl

Short synonyms
bemetizide plus guabenxan
guabenxan plus bemetizide

terbutaline

WADA group
S6. BETA-2 AGONISTS

MeSH descriptor
terbutaline

CAS Registry number
23031-25-6

Trade names and research codes
aerodur
brethine
bricanyl
bricanyl durules
bricanyl respules

Short synonyms
bricanyl durettes
bricanyl retard
terbutalin

Long synonyms
1 (3,5 dihydroxyphenyl) 2 (tert butylamino)ethanol
1 (3,5 dihydroxyphenyl) 2 tert butylaminoethanol
1 (3,5 dihydroxyphenyl) 2 tert butyliminoethanol
2 tert butylamino 1 (3,5 dihydroxyphenyl)ethanol

Terms and Synonyms

terbutaline sulfate

WADA group
S6. BETA-2 AGONISTS

CAS Registry number
23031-32-5

Trade names and research codes
arubendol
brethair
brethaire
kwd 2019
kwd2019
terbasmin

Short synonyms
spiranyl durules
terbutalin sulfate

Long synonyms
1 (3,5 dihydroxyphenyl) 2 (tert butylamino)ethanol sulfate

terracortril

WADA group
S9. GLUCOCORTICOSTEROIDS

CAS Registry number
62213-88-1

Trade names and research codes
terra cortril
terracortril
terracortril gel

Long synonyms
hydrocortisone plus oxytetracycline
oxytetracycline plus hydrocortisone

tertatolol

WADA group
P2. BETA-BLOCKERS

CAS Registry number
33580-30-2
34784-64-0

Trade names and research codes
artex
prenalex
s 2395
se 2395

Short synonyms
tertatolol hydrochloride

Long synonyms
8 [3 (tert butylamino) 2 hydroxypropoxy]thiochroman
1 (tert butylamino) 3 (thiochroman 8 yloxy) 2 propanol

tesmilifene

WADA group
S7. AGENTS WITH ANTI-OESTROGENIC ACTIVITY

CAS Registry number
92981-78-7
98774-23-3

Trade names and research codes
bms 217380
bms217380
bmy 33419
bmy33419

Short synonyms
tesmilifene hydrochloride

Long synonyms
2 (4 benzylphenoxy) n,n diethylethylamine
n,n diethyl 2 (4 benzylphenoxy)ethylamine
n,n diethyl 2 [4 (phenylmethyl)phenoxy]ethanamine
n,n diethyl 2 [4 (phenylmethyl)phenoxy]ethylamine

testolactone

WADA group
S7. AGENTS WITH ANTI-OESTROGENIC ACTIVITY

MeSH descriptor
testolactone

CAS Registry number
968-93-4

Trade names and research codes
fludestrin

Short synonyms
delta 1 testolactone
delta1 testolactone
delta 1 testololactone
delta1 testololactone
delta testolactone
nsc 12173
sq 9538
tes
teslac
testolactone propionate

Long synonyms
17a oxa d homoandrosta 1,4 diene 3,17 dione
d homo 17a oxaandrosta 1,4 diene 3,17 dione

testololactone

WADA group
S4. ANABOLIC AGENTS

CAS Registry number
4416-57-3

Long synonyms
d homo 17a oxaandrost 4 ene 3,17 dione

testosterone

WADA group
S4. ANABOLIC AGENTS

MeSH descriptor
testosterone

CAS Registry number
58-22-0

Trade names and research codes
adrotest
androderm
androgel
andronaq
andronaq 50
andropatch
fortigel
histerone
percutacrine androgine

Terms and Synonyms

sustanon
testamone
testaqua
testim
testoderm
testoderm ciii
testogel
testoject 50
tostrelle
tostrex
virilon
virormone

Short synonyms
andro 100
androfort
androlin
androst 4 en 17beta ol 3 one
4 androsten 17beta ol 3 one
androstenolone
androtest
andrusol
aquaviron
aquaviron b12
beta testosterone
free testosterone
geno cristaux
homosteron
hydroxyandrostenone
mertestate
neotestis
nsc 9700
oreton f
orquisteron
percutacrine androgenique
primotest
primoteston
primoteston depot
synandrol
teslen
testandrone
testerone
testoluton
testoluton forte
testosteron
testosterone chloride
testosterone conjugate
testrone
testryl
trans testosterone
virosterone

Long synonyms
17beta hydroxy 4 androsten 3 one
17beta hydroxyandrost 4 en 3 one
delta 4 androsten 17beta ol 3 one
percutacrine androgenique forte

1 testosterone

WADA group
S4. ANABOLIC AGENTS

Short synonyms
1 androsten 17beta ol 3 one
androst 1 en 17beta ol 3 one
delta1 dihydrotestosterone

Long synonyms
17beta hydroxy 5alpha androst 1 en 3 one

testosterone 4 butylcyclohexanecarboxylate

WADA group
S4. ANABOLIC AGENTS

CAS Registry number
105165-22-8

Trade names and research codes
20 aet 1

Short synonyms
testosterone buciclate

Long synonyms
4 butylcyclohexanecarboxylic acid testosterone ester
testosterone trans 4 butylcyclohexylcarboxylate

testosterone cipionate

WADA group
S4. ANABOLIC AGENTS

CAS Registry number
58-20-8

Trade names and research codes
andro cyp
andronaq la
ciclosterone
depandro
depotest
depo testosterone
duratest
testa c
testred cypionate

Short synonyms
depandro 100
depandro 200
depovirin
depoviron
malogen cyp 200
pertestis
testodrin prolongatum
testosterone 17beta cypionate
testosterone cypionate

Long synonyms
testosterone 17beta cyclopentanepropionate
testosterone beta cyclopentylpropionate
testosterone cyclopentylpropionate

testosterone derivative

WADA group
S4. ANABOLIC AGENTS

MeSH descriptor
hydroxytestosterones

Short synonyms
androstenolone derivative
hydroxytestosterones
testosterone congeners

Long synonyms
5alpha androsten 17beta ol 3 one derivative

testosterone enantate

WADA group
S4. ANABOLIC AGENTS

CAS Registry number
315-37-7

Trade names and research codes
androtardyl
delatestryl
durathate
everone
malogex
testosviron depot
testoviron depot

Short synonyms
androgyn la
andro la 200
androstenolone enanthate
malogen la 200
testosterone enanthane
testosterone enanthate
testosterone heptanoate
testosterone heptonate
testosterone heptylate
testosterone oenanthate
virormone depot

Long synonyms
testosterone 1 hexanecarboxylate
testosterone oenanthic acid derivative

testosterone enantate benziloylhydrazone

WADA group
S4. ANABOLIC AGENTS

Trade names and research codes
climacterion
climacteron

Long synonyms
17 enanthoyltestosterone 3 benziloylhydrazone
17 heptanoyltestosterone 3 benziloylhydrazone
17 heptanoyltestosterone benzilhydrazone
testosterone 17 enanthate 3 benzilic acid hydrazone
testosterone enantate benzilic acid hydrazone
testosterone enanthate benzilic acid hydrazone

testosterone ester

WADA group
S4. ANABOLIC AGENTS

Short synonyms
testosterone ester mixture

testosterone ether

WADA group
S4. ANABOLIC AGENTS

Trade names and research codes
triolandren

testosterone phenylpropionate

WADA group
S4. ANABOLIC AGENTS

CAS Registry number
1255-49-8

Trade names and research codes
androject
retandrol

testosterone propionate

WADA group
S4. ANABOLIC AGENTS

CAS Registry number
57-85-2

Trade names and research codes
enarmon
neo hombreol
neo-hombreol
neohombreol
nsc 9166
nsc9166
penandren
perandren
sterandryl

Short synonyms
akroteston
anderone
andronate
andronex amp
androsan amp
androteston
androtest p
androxid
androxil
andrusol p
anertar
bio testiculina
bio teston
cosex tp 50
entestil
gonadrone
homandren amp
hormandren
hormoteston
masenate
napionate
nasdol
okasa mascul
orchiol
orchiormon
orchisterone
orchisterone p
orchistin
oreton
oretone
oreton propionate
orquisterone p
orquisteron p
pantestin
perandren amp
perandrone
perandrone amp
primoniat
propiokan
recthormone
recthormone testosterone
sterandryl amp
sterandryl retard
sterotest
suprasteron amp
suprasterone
synerone
testaform
testex
testodet
testodrin
testogen
testonique
testormol

testormon
testosid
testosteronepropionate
testosteron propionate
testoviron amp
testoxyl
testrex
tostrin
uniteston
virormone x

Long synonyms
delta4 androstene 17beta propionate 3 one
3 (3 oxo 17beta hydroxy 4 androsten 17alpha yl)propanoate
propionic acid testosterone ester

testosterone undecanoate

WADA group
S4. ANABOLIC AGENTS

CAS Registry number
5949-44-0

Trade names and research codes
andriol
pantestone
restandol

Short synonyms
testosterone 17 undecylate
testosterone undecylate

tetrabenazine

WADA group
S1. STIMULANTS

MeSH descriptor
tetrabenazine

CAS Registry number
58-46-8

Trade names and research codes
nitoman

Short synonyms
ro 1 9569

Long synonyms
1,3,4,6,7,11b hexahydro 3 isobutyl 9,10 dimethoxy 2h benzo[a]quinolizin 2 one

☝ tetracosactide

WADA group
S5. PEPTIDE HORMONES

MeSH descriptor
cosyntropin

CAS Registry number
16960-16-0

Trade names and research codes
ba 30920
ba30920
cortrosyn
nuvacthen
nuvacthen depot
synacten
synacthen
synacthene
synacthen immediat
tetracosactrin

Short synonyms
acth 1 24
acth 1-24
acth [1 24]
acth [1-24]
acth(1 24)
acth[1-24]
adrenocorticotropin 1-24
alpha acth 1-24
beta 1 24 acth
beta 1,24 acth
beta 1 24 corticotrophin
beta 1,24 corticotrophin
beta 1 24 corticotropin
beta 1,24 corticotropin
beta 1,24 tetracosactide
1 24 corticotropin
corticotropin 1 24
corticotropin [1-24]
corticotropin b 1 24
cortrosyn retard
cosyntropin
depot tetracosactrin
synacthine
synathen
synthetic acth
tetracosactid
1 24 tetracosactide
tetracosactide retard
tetracosactin

Long synonyms
h ser tyr ser met glu his phe arg try gly lys pro val gly lys lys arg arg pro val lys val tyr pro oh

☝ tetracosactide zinc phosphate

WADA group
S5. PEPTIDE HORMONES

CAS Registry number
53468-06-7
66198-67-2

Trade names and research codes
cortrosyn depot
synacthen depot

Short synonyms
acth z[1-24]
corticotropin[1-24] zinc
corticotropin zinc[1-24]
cortrosin z
cortrosyn z
tetracosactide zinc
tetracosactrin zinc phosphate

Long synonyms
tetracosactide zinc phosphate complex
tetracosactrin zinc phosphate complex
zinc phosphate tetracosactide complex

3 [4 (1,2,3,4 tetrahydro 6 methoxy 2 phenyl 1 naphthyl)phenoxy] 1,2 propanediol

WADA group
S7. AGENTS WITH ANTI-OESTROGENIC ACTIVITY

CAS Registry number
22845-61-0

☝ probably not prohibited

Trade names and research codes
u 23469

n (1,2,3,4 tetrahydro 7 hydroxy 2 naphthyl)phenylethanolamine

WADA group
S6. BETA-2 AGONISTS

CAS Registry number
107758-36-1

Trade names and research codes
sr 58375a

tetrahydrocannabinol

WADA group
S3. CANNABINOIDS

MeSH descriptor
tetrahydrocannabinol

CAS Registry number
3-8-1972

Short synonyms
delta 2 tetrahydrocannabinol
delta 3 tetrahydrocannabinol
delta3 tetrahydrocannabinol
delta3 thc
delta 5 tetrahydrocannabinol
delta tetrahydrocannabinol
sp 104
tetrahydrocannabinal
tetrahydro cannabinol
7,8,9,10 tetrahydrocannabinol
tetrahydrocannabinol isomer
tetrahydrocannabiol
trans tetrahydrocannabinol

Long synonyms
delta 6a,10a tetrahydrocannabinol
1 trans delta 8 tetrahydrocannabinol

delta8 tetrahydrocannabinol

WADA group
S3. CANNABINOIDS

CAS Registry number
5957-75-5

Short synonyms
delta 1,6 tetrahydrocannabinol
delta1(6) tetrahydrocannabinol
delta1,6 tetrahydrocannabinol
delta 6 tetrahydrocannabinol
delta6 tetrahydrocannabinol
delta 8 tetrahydro cannabinol
delta 8 tetrahydrocannabinol

Long synonyms
delta 1 (6) tetrahydrocannabinol
delta 1(6) tetrahydrocannabinol
delta 6 3,4 trans tetrahydrocannabinol
delta6 3,4 trans tetrahydrocannabinol
delta 6alpha tetrahydrocannabinol
delta6 trans tetrahydrocannabinol
delta 8 trans tetrahydrocannabinol
delta8 trans tetrahydrocannabinol
l delta 8 trans tetrahydrocannabinol
trans delta8 tetrahydrocannabinol

delta9(11) tetrahydrocannabinol

WADA group
S3. CANNABINOIDS

Short synonyms
delta1(7) tetrahydrocannabinol

Long synonyms
delta 1(7) tetrahydrocannabinol
delta 9(11) tetrahydrocannabinol

tetrahydrocannabinol derivative

WADA group
S3. CANNABINOIDS

delta8 tetrahydrocannabinol derivative

WADA group
S3. CANNABINOIDS

Long synonyms
delta6 tetrahydrocannabinol derivative

tetrahydrocannabinolic acid

WADA group
S3. CANNABINOIDS

CAS Registry number
23978-85-0
37347-91-4

Short synonyms
11 carboxytetrahydrocannabinol
tetrahydrocannabinoic acid
tetrahydrocannabinolic acid a
tetrahydrocannabinolic acid b

Long synonyms
9 carboxy 11 nor delta 9 tetrahydrocannabinol
9 carboxy 11 nor delta9 tetrahydrocannabinol
9 carboxy delta9 tetrahydrocannabinol
delta1 tetrahydrocannabinol 7 oic acid
delta 1 tetrahydrocannabinolic acid
delta1 tetrahydrocannabinolic acid
delta 9 tetrahydrocannabinol 11 carboxylic acid
delta9 tetrahydrocannabinol 11 carboxylic acid
delta 9 tetrahydrocannabinol 11 oic acid
delta9 tetrahydrocannabinol 11 oic acid
delta 9 tetrahydrocannabinol 9 carboxylic acid
delta9 tetrahydrocannabinol 9 carboxylic acid
delta 9 tetrahydrocannabinolic acid
delta9 tetrahydrocannabinolic acid
11 nor 9 carboxy delta 9 tetrahydrocannabinol
11 nor 9 carboxy delta9 tetrahydrocannabinol
11 nor delta9 tetrahydrocannabinol 9 carboxylic acid
tetrahydrocannabinol 11 oic acid
tetrahydrocannabinol carboxylic acid

tetrahydrocortisol

WADA group
S9. GLUCOCORTICOSTEROIDS

MeSH descriptor
tetrahydrocortisol

CAS Registry number
53-02-1

Terms and Synonyms

Short synonyms
tetrahydro hydrocortisone
tetrahydrohydrocortisone

tetrahydrocortisone

WADA group
S9. GLUCOCORTICOSTEROIDS

MeSH descriptor
tetrahydrocortisone

CAS Registry number
53-05-4

Short synonyms
trihydroxypregnanedione

Long synonyms
3alpha,17alpha,21 trihydroxy 5beta pregnane 11,20 dione
5alpha pregnane 3alpha,17alpha,21 triol 11,20 dione
5beta pregnane 3alpha,17alpha,21 triol 11,20 dione
pregnane 3 alpha,17 alpha,21 triol 11,20 dione
pregnane 3alpha,17alpha,21 triol 11,20 dione

tetrahydrogestrinone

WADA group
S2. ANABOLIC AGENTS

Long synonyms
13beta,17alpha diethyl 17 hydroxygona 4,9,11 trien 3 one
13 ethyl 17 hydroxy 18,19 dinor 17alpha pregna 4,9,11 trien 3 one

tetramethylsuccinimide

WADA group
S1. STIMULANTS

CAS Registry number
3566-61-8

theodrenaline

WADA group
S1. STIMULANTS

CAS Registry number
13460-98-5

Short synonyms
l theodrenaline hydrochloride
noradrenalin ethyltheophylline
noradrenalin theophylline
theoadrenalin

Long synonyms
7 [2 [2 (3,4 dihydroxyphenyl) 2 hydroxyethylamino]ethyl]theophylline

thiazide diuretic agent

WADA group
S8. MASKING AGENTS
P3. DIURETICS

MeSH descriptor
diuretics, thiazide

Short synonyms
diuretics, thiazide
thiazide
thiazide derivative
thiazide diuretic

thrombocyte concentrate

WADA group
S8. MASKING AGENTS
M1. ENHANCEMENT OF OXYGEN TRANSFER

Short synonyms
platelet concentrate

tiamizide

WADA group
S8. MASKING AGENTS
P3. DIURETICS

CAS Registry number
3184-60-9
3688-85-5

Trade names and research codes
ci 456
ci456
cn 36,337
cn 36337
cn36,337
cn36337
d 1593
d-1593
d1593

Short synonyms
diapamide
thiamizide

Long synonyms
4 chloro n methyl 3 (methylsulfamoyl)benzamide
4 chloro n methyl 3 methylsulfamoylbenzamide

tibolone

WADA group
S4. ANABOLIC AGENTS

CAS Registry number
5630-53-5

Trade names and research codes
boltin
livial
liviella
org od 14
org od14
tibofem
xyvion

Long synonyms
17alpha ethynyl 17 hydroxy 7alpha methyl 5(10) estren 3 one
17beta hydroxy 7alpha methyl 19 norpregn 5(10) en 20 yn 3 one
17 hydroxy 7alpha methyl 19 nor 17alpha pregn 5(10) en 20 yn 3 one
17 hydroxy 7alpha methyl 19 norpregn 5(10) en 20 yn 3 one

ticabesone

WADA group
S9. GLUCOCORTICOSTEROIDS

CAS Registry number
74131-77-4

ticabesone propionate

WADA group
S9. GLUCOCORTICOSTEROIDS

CAS Registry number
73205-13-7

Trade names and research codes
rs 35909
rs 35909 00 00 0

Long synonyms
6alpha,9alpha difluoro 11beta,17alpha dihydroxy 16alpha methyl 17beta methylthiocarbonylandrosta 1,4 dien 3 one 17 propionate

tienilic acid

WADA group
S8. MASKING AGENTS
P3. DIURETICS

MeSH descriptor
ticrynafen

CAS Registry number
40180-04-9

Trade names and research codes
ticrynafen

Short synonyms
anp 3624
diflurex
selacryn
skf 62698
thienilic acid
thienylic acid
tricrynafen

Long synonyms
2 [2,3 dichloro 4 (2 thenoyl)phenoxy]acetic acid
2,3 dichloro 4 (2 thienyl carbonyl)phenoxyacetic acid
[2,3 dichloro 4 (2 thienylcarbonyl)phenoxy]acetic acid
2,3 dichloro 4 (2 thiophenoxy)phenoxyacetic acid
phenoxyacetic acid,2,3 dichloro 4 (2 thienylcarbonyl)

tienoxolol

WADA group
S8. MASKING AGENTS
P2. BETA-BLOCKERS
P3. DIURETICS

CAS Registry number
90055-97-3

Short synonyms
up 78842

Long synonyms
2 [3 [(1,1 dimethylethyl)amino] 2 hydroxypropoxy] 5 (2 thienylcarboxamido)benzoic acid ethyl ester

tilisolol

WADA group
P2. BETA-BLOCKERS

CAS Registry number
62774-96-3

Trade names and research codes
daim
n 696
selecal

Short synonyms
tilisolol hydrochloride

Long synonyms
4 (3 tert butylamino 2 hydroxypropoxy) 2 methyl 1(2h) isoquinolinone
4 [3 (tert butylamino) 2 hydroxypropoxy] 2 methylisocarbostyril
4 [3 (tert butylamino) 2 hydroxypropoxy] n methylisocarbostyril

timobesone

WADA group
S9. GLUCOCORTICOSTEROIDS

CAS Registry number
87116-72-1

Long synonyms
9 fluoro 11beta,17 dihydroxy 16beta methyl 3 oxoandrosta 1,4 diene 17beta carbothioic acid s methyl ester
s methyl 9 fluoro 11beta,17 dihydroxy 16beta methyl 3 oxoandrosta 1,4 diene 17beta carbothioate

timobesone acetate

WADA group
S9. GLUCOCORTICOSTEROIDS

CAS Registry number
79578-14-6

Short synonyms
rs 85446 007
rs 85446-007
rs 85446007

Long synonyms
17beta (methylthio)carbonyl 9 fluoro 11beta,17 dihydroxy 16beta methylandrosta 1,4 diene 3 one 17 acetate
9 fluoro 11beta,17alpha dihydroxy 16beta methyl 3 oxoandrosta 1,4 diene 17beta carbothioic acid 17alpha acetate 17beta s methyl ester
s methyl 17alpha acetyloxy 9alpha fluoro 11beta hydroxy 16beta methyl 3 oxoandrosta 1,4 diene 17beta carbothioate

timolol

WADA group
P2. BETA-BLOCKERS

MeSH descriptor
timolol

CAS Registry number
26839-75-8

Terms and Synonyms

Trade names and research codes
betimol
chibro timoptol
istalol
l 714465
l714465
moducren

Short synonyms
timolol hemihydrate

Long synonyms
3 (3 tert butylamino 2 hydroxypropoxy) 4 morpholino 1,2,5 thiadiazole
1 (tert butylamino) 3 (4 morpholino 1,2,5 thiadiazol 3 yloxy) 2 propanol
1 tert butylamino 3 (4 morpholino 1,2,5 thiadiazol 3 yloxy) 2 propanol
1 tert butylamino 3 (4 morpholino 1,2,5 thiadiazol 3 yloxy)propan 2 ol

timolol maleate

WADA group
P2. BETA-BLOCKERS

CAS Registry number
26921-17-5

Trade names and research codes
aquanil
arutimol
betim
blocadren
blocadrene
droptimol
mk 950
mk950
oftan timolol
temserin
timabak
timacor
timoptic
timoptic xe
timoptol
timpilo

Short synonyms
blocanol
timolate
timolol hydrogen maleate

Long synonyms
1 tert butylamino 3 (4 morpholino 1,2,5 thiadiazol 3 yloxy) 2 propanol hydrogen maleate

tipredane

WADA group
S9. GLUCOCORTICOSTEROIDS

CAS Registry number
85197-77-9

Trade names and research codes
sq 27239

Long synonyms
17alpha ethylthio 9 fluoro 11beta hydroxy 17beta (methylthio)androsta 1,4 dien 3 one
17alpha ethylthio 9 fluoro 11beta hydroxy 17 (methylthio)androsta 1,4 dien 3 one

tixocortol

WADA group
S9. GLUCOCORTICOSTEROIDS

CAS Registry number
61951-99-3

Short synonyms
cortisol 21 thiol
hydrocortisone 21 thiol
thixocortol

Long synonyms
11beta,17 dihydroxy 21 mercaptopregn 4 ene 3,20 dione
11beta,17 dihydroxy 21 mercaptoprogesterone
progesterone,11beta,17 dihydroxy 21 mercapto

tixocortol pivalate

WADA group
S9. GLUCOCORTICOSTEROIDS

CAS Registry number
55560-96-8

Trade names and research codes
pivalone
rectovalone
thiovalone
tiovalon

Short synonyms
jo 1016
thixocortol pivalate
tixocortol 21 pivalate
tixocortone 21 pivalate
tixocortone trimethylacetate

Long synonyms
11beta,17 dihydroxy 21 mercaptopregn 4 ene 3,20 dione pivalate
progesterone,11beta,17 dihydroxy 21 mercapto pivalate

tolamolol

WADA group
P2. BETA-BLOCKERS

CAS Registry number
38103-61-6

Short synonyms
tolamidol
tolamolol hydrochloride
uk 6558 01

Long synonyms
1 [2 (4 carbamoylphenoxy)ethylamino] 3 (2 methylphenoxy) 2 propanol
4 [2 [[2 hydroxy 3 (2 methylphenoxy)propyl]amino]ethoxy]benzamide
4 [2 (2 hydroxy 3 ortho tolyloxypropylamino)ethoxy]benzamide

toliprolol

WADA group
P2. BETA-BLOCKERS

CAS Registry number
2933-94-0

306-11-6
5711-18-2

Trade names and research codes
ko 592

Short synonyms
doberol
ici 45673
ici 45,763
ici 45763

Long synonyms
1 (beta methylphenoxy) 3 isopropylaminopropanol
3 hydroxy 1 isopropylamino 3 (4 tolyl)propane
3 isopropylamino 1 (3 methyl phenoxy) 2 propanol
3 isopropylamino 1 (3 methylphenoxy) 2 propanol
1 isopropylamino 3 (3 methylphenoxy) 2 propanol
1 isopropylamino 3 (3 tolyloxy) 2 propanol
1 isopropylamino 3 (3 tolyloxy)propan 2 ol
1 isopropylamino 3 (3 tolyloxy)propanol 2
1 isopropylamino 3 hydroxy 3 (4 tolyl)propane
1 (isopropylamino) 3 (meta toloxy) 2 propanol hydrochloride
1 (isopropylamino) 3 (metatoloxy) 2 propanol hydrochloride
1 (isopropylamino) 3 (meta tolyloxy) 2 propanol
1 isopropylamino 3 (meta tolyloxy) 2 propanol
1 isopropylamino 3 meta tolyloxy 2 propanol
1 isopropylamino 3 (meta tolyloxy) 2 propanol hydrochloride
1 (isopropylamino) 3 (meta tolyloxy) 2 propranol hydrochloride
1 isopropylamino 3 (m toloxy)2 propanol
1 isopropylamino 3 m toloxy 2 propanol
1 isopropylamino 3 (m toloxy) 2 propanolol
1 (3 methylphenoxy) 2 hydroxy 3 isopropylaminopropane hydrochloride
1 (meta methylphenoxy) 2 hydroxy 3 isopropylaminopropane
1 (3 methylphenoxy) 2 hydroxy 3 isopropylamine propane
1 (3 methylphenoxy) 2 hydroxy 3 isopropylamino 2 propanol hydrochloride
1 (3 methyl phenoxy) 2 hydroxy 3 isopropylaminopropane
1 (3 methylphenoxy) 2 hydroxy 3 isopropylamino propane
1 (3 methylphenoxy) 2 hydroxy 3 isopropylaminopropane
1 (3' methyl)phenoxy 2 hydroxy 3 isopropylaminopropane
1,3 methylphenoxy 2 hydroxy 3 isopropylamino propane
1 (3 methylphenoxy) 2 hydroxy 3 isopropylaminopropane hydrochloride
1 (3 methylphenoxy) 2 hydroxy 3 isopropylaminopropanol hydrochloride
1 (3 methylphenoxy) 2 hydroxy 3 isopropylo aminopropane
1 (3 methylphenoxy) 3 isopropylamino 2 propanol
1 (3' methylphenoxy) 3 isopropylamino 2 propanol
1 (3 methylphenoxy) 3 isopropylaminopropanol hydrochloride
1 (3 methylphenoxyl) 2 hydroxy 3 isopropylamine propane
1 (3 methylphenoxyl) 2 hydroxy 3 isopropylaminepropane

torasemide

WADA group
S8. MASKING AGENTS
P3. DIURETICS

CAS Registry number
56211-40-6

Trade names and research codes
bm 02015
bm02015
bm 2015
bm2015
demadex
jdl 464
jdl464
presaril
toradiur
torem
torrem
unat

Short synonyms
torsemide

Long synonyms
1 isopropyl 3 [(4 meta toluidino 3 pyridyl)sulfonyl]urea

toremifene

WADA group
S7. AGENTS WITH ANTI-OESTROGENIC ACTIVITY

MeSH descriptor
toremifene

CAS Registry number
89778-26-7

Trade names and research codes
estrimex
fareston
fc 1157 a
fc 1157a
fc1157a

Long synonyms
4 chloro 1,2 diphenyl 1 [4 [2 (n,n dimethylamino)ethoxy]phenyl] 1 butene
4 chloro 1 [4 (2 dimethylaminoethoxy)phenyl] 1,2 diphenyl 1 butene

torrat

WADA group
S8. MASKING AGENTS
P3. DIURETICS

CAS Registry number
72416-03-6

Trade names and research codes
torrat

Short synonyms
butizide plus metipranolol
butizide with metipranolol
metipranolol plus butizide

trasitensin

WADA group
S8. MASKING AGENTS
P2. BETA-BLOCKERS
P3. DIURETICS

Trade names and research codes
slow trasitensin

slow-trasitensin
sustained release trasitensin
trasitencin
trasitensin
trasitensin retard
trasitensin sr

Short synonyms
chlortalidone plus oxprenolol
oxprenolol plus chlortalidone

traxanox

WADA group
S8. MASKING AGENTS
P3. DIURETICS

CAS Registry number
58712-69-9
70502-82-8

Short synonyms
y 12141

Long synonyms
9 chloro 5 oxo 7 (1h tetrazol 5 yl) 5h 1 benzopyrano[2,3 b]pyridine
9 chloro 5 oxo 7 (1h tetrazol 5 yl) 5h 1 benzopyrano[2,3 b]pyridine sodium salt pentahydrate
9 chloro 7 (1h tetrazol 5 yl) 5h [1]benzopyrano[2,3 b]pyridin 5 one

trecadrine

WADA group
S6. BETA-2 AGONISTS

CAS Registry number
108767-50-6

Long synonyms
alpha [1 [[2 (10,11 dihydro 5h dibenzo[a,d]cyclohepten 5 ylidene)ethyl]methylamino]ethyl]benzenemethanol

trenbolone

WADA group
S4. ANABOLIC AGENTS

MeSH descriptor
trenbolone

CAS Registry number
10161-33-8

Trade names and research codes
parabolan
r 2580
r2580

Short synonyms
beta trenbolone
17beta trenbolone
trienbolone
trienolone

Long synonyms
17beta hydroxy 19 norandrosta 4,9,11 trien 3 one
17beta hydroxyestra 4,9,11 trien 3 one
3 oxo 17beta hydroxy 4,9,11 estratriene
3 oxo 17beta hydroxyestra 4,9,11 triene

17alpha trenbolone

WADA group
S4. ANABOLIC AGENTS

CAS Registry number
80657-17-6

Short synonyms
alpha trenbolone
epitrenbolone

trenbolone acetate

WADA group
S4. ANABOLIC AGENTS

CAS Registry number
10161-34-9

Trade names and research codes
finajet
finaplix
r 1697
r1697
ru 1697
ru1697

Short synonyms
trenbalone acetate
trienbolone acetate
trienolone acetate

Long synonyms
17beta hydroxy 19 norandrosta 4,9,11 trien 3 one acetate
17beta hydroxyestra 4,9,11 trien 3 one acetate
3 oxo 17beta hydroxy 4,9,11 estratriene acetate
3 oxo 17beta hydroxyestra 4,9,11 triene acetate

trepress

WADA group
S8. MASKING AGENTS
P2. BETA-BLOCKERS
P3. DIURETICS

Trade names and research codes
trepress

Long synonyms
chlortalidone plus hydralazine and oxprenolol
oxprenolol plus chlortalidone and hydralazine

trestolone

WADA group
S4. ANABOLIC AGENTS

CAS Registry number
3764-87-2

Trade names and research codes
ru 27333
ru27333

Short synonyms
7alpha methylnandrolone
MENT

Long synonyms
7alpha methyl 19 nortestosterone
7alpha methyl 3 oxo 4 estren 17beta ol
17beta hydroxy 7alpha methylestr 4 en 3 one

estr 4 en 17beta ol 3 one,7alpha methyl
19 nor 7alpha methyltestosterone

tretoquinol

WADA group
S6. BETA-2 AGONISTS

MeSH descriptor
tretoquinol

CAS Registry number
18559-59-6
18559-63-2
30418-38-3

Trade names and research codes
aq 110
aq110
aql 208
aql208
bentomex
vems

Short synonyms
expansolin
inolin
levo tretoquinol
levo trimetoquinol
tetroquinol
tretoguinol
tretoquinol hydrochloride
trimethochinol
trimethokinol
trimethoquinol
trimethoquinol hydrochloride
trimetoquinol
triquinol

Long synonyms
1,2,3,4 tetrahydro 1 (3,4,5 trimethoxybenzyl) 6,7
isoquinolinediol

tretoquinol derivative

WADA group
S6. BETA-2 AGONISTS

Short synonyms
trimethoquinol derivative
trimetoquinol derivative

triamcinolone

WADA group
S9. GLUCOCORTICOSTEROIDS

MeSH descriptor
triamcinolone

CAS Registry number
124-94-7

Trade names and research codes
adcortyl
aristocort
cl 19823
cl19823
delphicort
kenacort
kenacort retard
ledercort
omcilon
polcortolon
rp 8357
rp8357
triamcort
volon

Short synonyms
aristodan
celeste
fluoxiprednisolone
fluoxyprednisolone
tramcinolone
triacortyl
triamcinolon
triancinolon

Long synonyms
9alpha fluoro 11beta,16alpha,17alpha,21
tetrahydroxypregna 1,4 diene 3,20 dione
9alpha fluoro 1,4 pregnadiene 3,20 dione
11beta,16alpha,17alpha,21 tetrol
9alpha fluoro 16alpha hydroxyhydrocortisone
9alpha fluoro 16alpha hydroxyprednisolone

triamcinolone acetate

WADA group
S9. GLUCOCORTICOSTEROIDS

triamcinolone acetonide

WADA group
S9. GLUCOCORTICOSTEROIDS

MeSH descriptor
triamcinolone acetonide

CAS Registry number
76-25-5

Trade names and research codes
aristogel
azmacort
flutone
fougera
ftorocort
kenacort a
kena log
kenalog
kenalog 10
kenalog 40
kenalog a 40
kenalone
kenlog
kortikoid ratiopharm
nasacort
panalog
pokkortolon
solodelf
tibicorten
tramacin
triacet
triam
triamalone
tri anemul
trianide
trigon depot
trikort
vetalog
volon a
volonimat
yn 102

Short synonyms
aquatain
aristocort acetonide
aristoderm

fluoxiprednisolone acetonide
kenac
kenacort e
kenalog suspensoid
ledercort d
tibiocorten
triamcinolide acetonide
triamcinolon acetonide
triamcinolone 16,17 acetonide
triamcinolone acetamide
triamcinolone acetonamide
triamcinolone acetonid
triamcinolone benetonide
trymex
volon a 40
volon a 80
volon a tincture

Long synonyms
triamcinolone acetonide potassium phosphate
triamcinolone acetonide tincture
triamcinolone cyclic 16,17 acetal with acetone

triamcinolone diacetate

WADA group
S9. GLUCOCORTICOSTEROIDS

CAS Registry number
67-78-7

Trade names and research codes
aristocort intralesional
cenocort forte

Short synonyms
aristocort forte parenteral
kenocort diacetate syrup
tedarol

Long synonyms
triamcinolone 16alpha,21 diacetate

triamcinolone hexacetonide

WADA group
S9. GLUCOCORTICOSTEROIDS

CAS Registry number
5611-51-8

Trade names and research codes
aristospan
cl 34433
cl34433
hexatrione
lederlon
lederspan

Long synonyms
triamcinolone acetonide 21 (3,3 dimethylbutyrate)

triamterene

WADA group
S8. MASKING AGENTS
P3. DIURETICS

MeSH descriptor
triamterene

CAS Registry number
396-01-0

Trade names and research codes
dyrenium
dytac
jatropur
nsc 77625
nsc77625
sk and f 8542
skf 8542
skf8542
triamteril

Short synonyms
ademin
ademine
dyren
iatropur
noridyl
pterofen
pterophene
teriam
triampterene
triamterence
triamterens
triamterine
triteren
uretren
urocaudal

Long synonyms
6 phenyl 2,4,6 triaminopteridine
6 phenyl 2,4,7 triaminopteridine
2,4,7 triamino 6 phenylpteridine

triamterene plus xipamide

WADA group
S8. MASKING AGENTS
P3. DIURETICS

CAS Registry number
84272-17-3

Trade names and research codes
epitens
neotri
trirexan

Short synonyms
neotril
triamterene with xipamide
xipamide plus triamterene

tribendilol

WADA group
P2. BETA-BLOCKERS

CAS Registry number
96258-13-8

Trade names and research codes
bm 11604
bm11604

Long synonyms
1 (benzotriazol 4 yloxy) 3 [2 (2 methoxyphenoxy)ethylamino] 2 propanol
4 [2 hydroxy 3 [2 (2 methoxyphenoxy)ethylamino]propoxy]benzotriazol e

trichlormethiazide

WADA group
S8. MASKING AGENTS
P3. DIURETICS

MeSH descriptor
trichlormethiazide

CAS Registry number
133-67-5

Trade names and research codes
aquazide
diurese
esmarin
fluitran
flutra
methahydrin
naqua
triazide

Short synonyms
eurinol
gangesol
hydrotrichlorothiazide
metahydrin
naquasone
salurin (wadel)
trichlordiuride
trichlormethazide
trichloromethiazide
triflumen

Long synonyms
6 chloro 3 (dichloromethyl) 3,4 dihydro 1,2,4 benzothiadiazine 7 sulfonamide 1,1 dioxide
6 chloro 3 dichloromethyl 3,4 dihydro 7 sulfamoyl 1,2,4 benzothiadiazine 1,1 dioxide
6 chloro 3 dichloromethyl 7 sulfamoyl 3,4 dihydro 1,2,4 benzothiadiazine 1,1 dioxide
3 dichloromethylhydrochlorothiazide
trichloromethylhydrochlorothiazide

1,3,8 trichloro 6 methyldibenzofuran

WADA group
S7. AGENTS WITH ANTI-OESTROGENIC ACTIVITY

CAS Registry number
115039-00-4
118174-38-2

Short synonyms
MCDF

Long synonyms
6 methyl 1,3,8 trichlorodibenzofuran

11beta,17alpha,21 trihydroxy 3,20 dioxopregna 1,4 diene 16alpha carboxylic acid methyl ester

WADA group
S9. GLUCOCORTICOSTEROIDS

CAS Registry number
111802-47-2

Trade names and research codes
p16cm

Long synonyms
prednisolone 16alpha carboxylic acid methyl ester

n (3,4,5 trimethoxyphenethyl)noradrenalin

WADA group
S6. BETA-2 AGONISTS

CAS Registry number
108930-00-3

Trade names and research codes
t 1583

Long synonyms
3,4 dihydroxy alpha [[[2 (3,4,5 trimethoxyphenyl)ethyl]amino]methyl]benzenemethanol
n [2 (3,4,5 trimethoxyphenyl)ethyl]epinephrine
n [2 (3,4,5 trimethoxyphenyl)ethyl]noradrenalin
n (3,4,5 trimethoxyphenethyl)norepinephrine
noradrenalin,n (3,4,5 trimethoxyphenethyl)

triniton

WADA group
S8. MASKING AGENTS
P3. DIURETICS

CAS Registry number
81569-86-0

Trade names and research codes
triniton

trioxifene

WADA group
S7. AGENTS WITH ANTI-OESTROGENIC ACTIVITY

CAS Registry number
63619-84-1

Long synonyms
[3,4 dihydro 2 (4 methoxyphenyl) 1 naphthalenyl] [4 [2 (1 pyrrolidinyl)ethoxy]phenyl]methanone
3,4 dihydro 2 (4 methoxyphenyl) 1 naphthyl 4 [2 (1 pyrrolidinyl)ethoxy]phenyl ketone
[3,4 dihydro 2 (4 methoxyphenyl) 1 naphthyl] [4 (2 pyrrolidinoethoxy)phenyl] ketone
[3,4 dihydro 2 (4 methoxyphenyl)naphth 1 yl] [4 (2 pyrrolidinoethoxy)phenyl] ketone

trioxifene mesilate

WADA group
S7. AGENTS WITH ANTI-OESTROGENIC ACTIVITY

CAS Registry number
68307-81-3

Trade names and research codes
compound 133314

Short synonyms
trioxifene mesylate
trioxifene methanesulfonate

Long synonyms
[3,4 dihydro 2 (4 methoxyphenyl) 1 naphthyl] [4 [2 (1 pyrrolidinyl)ethoxy]phenyl] ketone mesilate
[3,4 dihydro 2 (4 methoxyphenyl) 1 naphthyl] [4 [2 (1 pyrrolidinyl)ethoxy]phenyl]methanone methylsulfonate

Terms and Synonyms

[3,4 dihydro 2 (4 methoxyphenyl)naphth 1 yl] [4 (2 pyrrolidinoethoxy)phenyl] ketone mesilate

tripamide

WADA group
S8. MASKING AGENTS
P3. DIURETICS

CAS Registry number
73803-48-2

Trade names and research codes
adr 033
adr033
e 614
e614

Long synonyms
4 chloro n (endo hexahydro 4,7 methanoisoindolin 2 yl) 3 sulfamoylbenzamide
n (4 aza endo tricyclodecan 4 yl) 4 chloro 3 sulfamoylbenzamide

1,1,2 triphenylethylene derivative

WADA group
S7. AGENTS WITH ANTI-OESTROGENIC ACTIVITY

Short synonyms
triphenylethylene derivative

triptorelin

WADA group
S5. PEPTIDE HORMONES

MeSH descriptor
triptorelin

CAS Registry number
57773-63-4

Trade names and research codes
arvekap
ay 25650
ay25650
decapeptyl
decapeptyl cr
trelstar

Short synonyms
detryptorelin
[d trp 6]lhrh
d trp 6 lhrh
lhrh[6 dextro tryptophan]
lhrh (d trp 6)
tryptorelin

Long synonyms
[6 dextro tryptophan]gonadorelin
6 dextro tryptophanylgonadorelin
d trp 6 luteinizing hormone releasing hormone
gonadorelin[6 dextro tryptophan]
gonadotropin releasing hormone[6 dextro tryptophan]
luteinizing hormone releasing hormone[6 dextro tryptophan]

trometamol

WADA group
S8. MASKING AGENTS
P3. DIURETICS

MeSH descriptor
tromethamine

CAS Registry number
1185-53-1
77-86-1

Trade names and research codes
trizma

Short synonyms
nsc 6365
peha norm
pehanorm
talatrol
tham
tham solution
thrometamol
tri(hydroxymethyl)aminomethane
trihydroxy methylaminomethane
trihydroxymethyl amino methane
trihydroxymethylaminomethane
trimethylol
trimethylolaminomethane
tris
trisamine
tris amino
trisaminol
tris buffer
tris chloride
tris cl
tris concentrate
tris hydrochloride
tris hydroxymethylaminomethan
trishydroxymethylamino methane
trishydroxymethylaminomethane
tris(hydroxymethyl)methylamine
tris steril
tris trometamol
trometamine
tromethamine
tromethamol
tromethane
tromethanine

Long synonyms
2 amino 2 (hydroxymethyl) 1,3 propanediol
2 amino 2 hydroxymethyl 1,3 propanediol
2 amino hydroxymethyl 1,3 propanediol
tris (hydroxymethyl) aminomethane
tris(hydroxymethyl)aminomethane
trishydroxy methylamino methane
1,1,1 tris(hydroxymethyl) methylamine

trometamol edetate

WADA group
S8. MASKING AGENTS
P3. DIURETICS

Short synonyms
tromethamine e

tulobuterol

WADA group
S6. BETA-2 AGONISTS

Terms and Synonyms

CAS Registry number
- 41570-61-0
- 56776-01-3

Trade names and research codes
- atenos
- brelomax
- bremax
- c 78
- c78

Short synonyms
- berachin
- hokumalin
- tolubuterol
- tuloboterol
- tulobuterol hydrochloride
- turobuterol

Long synonyms
- alpha (tert butylaminomethyl) 2 chlorobenzenemethanol
- alpha (tert butylaminomethyl) 2 chlorobenzyl alcohol
- ortho chloro alpha [(tert butylamino)methyl]benzylalcohol
- tert butyl beta (2 chlorophenyl) beta hydroxyethylamine

ulobetasol propionate

WADA group
- **S9. GLUCOCORTICOSTEROIDS**

CAS Registry number
- 66852-54-8

Trade names and research codes
- bmy 30056
- bmy30056
- cgp 14458
- cgp14458
- miracorten
- ultravate

Short synonyms
- halobetasol propionate

ultroser g

WADA group
- **S8. MASKING AGENTS**

Trade names and research codes
- ultroser g

uniderm

WADA group
- **S9. GLUCOCORTICOSTEROIDS**

Trade names and research codes
- uniderm

urofollitropin

WADA group
- **S5. PEPTIDE HORMONES**

CAS Registry number
- 97048-13-0

Trade names and research codes
- fertinex
- fertinorm
- follegon
- fostimon
- metrodin
- metrodine
- metrodin high purity
- metrodin hp

Short synonyms
- urofollitrophin

veratide

WADA group
- **S8. MASKING AGENTS**
- **P3. DIURETICS**

Trade names and research codes
- veratide

Long synonyms
- hydrochlorothiazide plus triamterene plus verapamil

viskaldix

WADA group
- **S8. MASKING AGENTS**
- **P2. BETA-BLOCKERS**
- **P3. DIURETICS**

CAS Registry number
- 71789-16-7

Trade names and research codes
- viskaldix

Short synonyms
- clopamide plus pindolol
- pindolol plus clopamide

vorozole

WADA group
- **S7. AGENTS WITH ANTI-OESTROGENIC ACTIVITY**

CAS Registry number
- 118949-22-7
- 129731-10-8

Trade names and research codes
- r 76713
- r 83839
- r 83842
- rivizor

Long synonyms
- 6 [(4 chlorophenyl)(1h 1,2,4 triazol 1 yl)methyl] 1 methyl 1h benzotriazole

xamoterol

WADA group
- **S1. STIMULANTS**
- **S6. BETA-2 AGONISTS**

MeSH descriptor
- xamoterol

CAS Registry number
- 81801-12-9

Terms and Synonyms

Long synonyms
1 (4 hydroxyphenoxy) 3 [2 (morpholinocarboxamido)ethyl]amino 2 propanol
1 (4 hydroxyphenoxy) 3 [2 (morpholinocarboxamido)ethyl]aminoisopropyl alcohol
1 (4 hydroxyphenoxy) 3 beta (morpholinocarboxamido)ethylamino 2 propanol
1 (para hydroxyphenoxy) 3 [beta (morpholinocarboxamido)ethylamino] 2 propanol

xamoterol hydrogen fumarate

WADA group
S1. STIMULANTS
S6. BETA-2 AGONISTS

CAS Registry number
73210-73-8

Trade names and research codes
carwin
corwil
corwin
ici 118587
xamtol

Short synonyms
xamoterol fumarate
xamoterol hemifumarate

Long synonyms
1 (4 hydroxyphenoxy) 3 [2 (morpholinocarboxamido)ethyl]amino 2 propanol hydrogen fumarate
1 (para hydroxyphenoxy) 3 [beta (morpholinocarboxamido)ethylamino] 2 propanol hemifumarate

xibenolol

WADA group
P2. BETA-BLOCKERS

CAS Registry number
15263-30-6
81584-06-7

Trade names and research codes
d 32
d32

Long synonyms
1 tert butylamino 3 (2,3 dimethylphenoxy) 2 propanol
1 tert butylamino 3 (2,3 xylyloxy) 2 propanol

xipamide

WADA group
S8. MASKING AGENTS
P3. DIURETICS

MeSH descriptor
xipamide

CAS Registry number
14293-44-8

Trade names and research codes
aquaphor
lumitens
zipix

Short synonyms
aquaforil
aquaphoril
aquavor
bei 1293
diurexan
mjf 10,938
mjf 10938
xypamide

Long synonyms
4 chloro 5 sulfamoyl 2',6' salicyloxylidide

zearalanone

WADA group
S4. ANABOLIC AGENTS

CAS Registry number
5975-78-0

zearalenone

WADA group
S4. ANABOLIC AGENTS

MeSH descriptor
zearalenone

CAS Registry number
17924-92-4

Short synonyms
toxin f2
zearalenon
zearalenone mycotoxin

Long synonyms
6 (10 hydroxy 6 oxo 1 undecenyl) beta resorcylic acid lactone
6 (10 hydroxy 6 oxo trans 1 undecenyl) beta resorcylic acid lactone

zeranol

WADA group
S4. ANABOLIC AGENTS

MeSH descriptor
zeranol

CAS Registry number
26538-44-3

Trade names and research codes
frideron
mk 188
mk188
p 1496
p1496
ralgro

Short synonyms
ralabol
zearalanol

Long synonyms
3,4,5,6,7,8,9,10,11,12 decahydro 7,14,16 trihydroxy 3 methyl 1h 2 benzoxacyclotetradecin 1 one
6 (6,10 dihydroxyundecyl) beta resorcylic acid lactone

zilpaterol

WADA group
S4. ANABOLIC AGENTS
S6. BETA-2 AGONISTS

Trade names and research codes
zilmax

Short synonyms
zilpaterol hydrochloride

Long synonyms
4,5,6,7 tetrahydro 7 hydroxy 6 (isopropylamino)imidazo[4,5,1 jk][1]benzazepin 2(1h) one

zindoxifene

WADA group
S7. AGENTS WITH ANTI-OESTROGENIC ACTIVITY

CAS Registry number
86111-26-4

Trade names and research codes
d 16726
d16726

Long synonyms
5 acetoxy 2 (4 acetoxyphenyl) 1 ethyl 3 methylindole
1 ethyl 5 hydroxy 2 (4 hydroxyphenyl) 3 methylindole diacetate

zinterol

WADA group
S6. BETA-2 AGONISTS

CAS Registry number
37000-20-7
38241-28-0

Short synonyms
mj 9184 1
mj 91841

Long synonyms
5 [2 (alpha,alpha dimethylphenethylamino) 1 hydroxyethyl] 2 hydroxymethanesulfonanilide
5 [1 hydroxy 2 (alpha,alpha dimethylphenethylamino)ethyl] 2 hydroxymethanesulfonanilide
2 hydroxy 5 [1 hydroxy 2 (2 methyl 1 phenyl 2 propylamino)ethyl]methanesulfonanilide

zuclomifene

WADA group
S7. AGENTS WITH ANTI-OESTROGENIC ACTIVITY

CAS Registry number
15690-55-8

Short synonyms
cis clomiphene
cisclomiphene
isomer a
rmi 16,312
rmi 16312
zu clomiphene
zuclomiphene

Long synonyms
2 [4 (2 chloro cis 1,2 diphenylvinyl)phenoxy]triethylamine
(z) 2 [4 (2 chloro 1,2 diphenylvinyl)phenoxy]triethylamine

zuclomifene citrate

WADA group
S7. AGENTS WITH ANTI-OESTROGENIC ACTIVITY

CAS Registry number
55491-35-5
7619-53-6

Short synonyms
cis clomifene citrate
cis clomiphene citrate

18-502
see: 1 tert butylamino 3 (2 methyl 4 indolyloxy) 2 propanol
a 21
see: isoprenaline
a 21 hf
see: isoprenaline
a2 hemoglobin
see: hemoglobin A2
a 4020 linz
see: midodrine
a4020 linz
see: midodrine
a 41 304
see: desoximetasone
a 41304
see: desoximetasone
a41304
see: desoximetasone
a 43818
see: leuprorelin
a43818
see: leuprorelin
a 46 745
see: gestrinone
a 46745
see: gestrinone
a46745
see: gestrinone
a 49816
see: 2 [4 (3 aminomethyl 4 hydroxybenzoyl) 2,3 dichlorophenoxy]acetic acid ethyl ester
a49816
see: 2 [4 (3 aminomethyl 4 hydroxybenzoyl) 2,3 dichlorophenoxy]acetic acid ethyl ester
a 56234
see: 8 chloro 3 (2 fluorophenyl) 5,6 dihydrofuro[3,2 f][1,2]benzisoxazole 6 carboxylate potassium
a56234
see: 8 chloro 3 (2 fluorophenyl) 5,6 dihydrofuro[3,2 f][1,2]benzisoxazole 6 carboxylate potassium
a575c
see: n [1 carboxy 5 [4 (2 hydroxy 3 isopropylaminopropoxy)indole 2 carboxamido]pentyl]alanylproline
a 66
see: phenmetrazine
a66
see: phenmetrazine
aarane
see: cromoglycate disodium plus reproterol
ab 01
see: bemegride
ab a 663
see: cimaterol
aba 663
see: cimaterol
aba663
see: cimaterol
abbolactone
see: spironolactone
abbott 30400
see: pemoline magnesium
abbott 31528
see: pemoline
abbott 41070
see: gonadorelin acetate
abbott 43326
see: carteolol
abbott 43818
see: leuprorelin
abbott 56234
see: 8 chloro 3 (2 fluorophenyl) 5,6 dihydrofuro[3,2 f][1,2]benzisoxazole 6 carboxylate potassium
abecor
see: celiprolol
abirol
see: metandienone
abnormal hemoglobin
see: hemoglobin variant
ac 263780
see: cimaterol
ac263780
see: cimaterol
acc 9089
see: flestolol
acc9089
see: flestolol
accuretic
see: hydrochlorothiazide plus quinapril
accuzide
see: hydrochlorothiazide plus quinapril

acebutolol

acebutolol hydrochloride
see: acebutolol

acebutolol plus nifedipine

acediur
see: captopril plus hydrochlorothiazide

acefluranol

acelat
see: spironolactone
aceplus
see: captopril plus hydrochlorothiazide
acepreval
see: prednival acetate
acetamox
see: acetazolamide
acetate,ammonium
see: ammonium acetate
acetazolam
see: acetazolamide
acetazolamid
see: acetazolamide

acetazolamide

acetazol amide
see: acetazolamide
acetazolamide sodium
see: acetazolamide
acetazolamine
see: acetazolamide
acetazoleamide
see: acetazolamide
acethropan
see: corticotropin
acetomorphine
see: diamorphine
acetophran
see: corticotropin
acetozolamide
see: acetazolamide
acetozolamine
see: acetazolamide
acetylated corticotropin
see: corticotropin
6 acetylmorphine
see: morphine 6 acetate
aclosone
see: alclometasone
aclovate
see: alclometasone dipropionate
acortan
see: corticotropin
acortan prolongatum
see: corticotropin
acorto
see: corticotropin
acrinor
see: cafedrine plus theodrenaline
actedron
see: amphetamine
actemin
see: amphetamine
ACTH
see: corticotropin
acth 1 10
see: corticotropin[1-10]
acth[1-10]
see: corticotropin[1-10]
acth [11-24]
see: corticotropin[11-24]
acth(11 24)
see: corticotropin[11-24]
acth[11 24]
see: corticotropin[11-24]
acth[11-24]
see: corticotropin[11-24]
acth 1-17
see: corticotropin[1-17]
ACTH[1-17]
see: corticotropin[1-17]
acth 1 24
see: tetracosactide
acth 1-24
see: tetracosactide
acth [1 24]
see: tetracosactide
acth [1-24]
see: tetracosactide
acth(1 24)
see: tetracosactide
acth[1-24]
see: tetracosactide
acth 1 39
see: corticotropin[1-39]
acth 1-39
see: corticotropin[1-39]
acth [1-39]
see: corticotropin[1-39]
acth[1-39]
see: corticotropin[1-39]
acth 18 39
see: corticotropin[18-39]
acth 18-39
see: corticotropin[18-39]

Index

acth [18-39]
see: corticotropin[18-39]
acth[18-39]
see: corticotropin[18-39]
acth 40
see: corticotropin
acth (4-10)
see: corticotropin[4-10]
ACTH 4-10
see: corticotropin[4-10]
acth(4 10)
see: corticotropin[4-10]
acth[4-10]
see: corticotropin[4-10]
acth [7-10]
see: corticotropin[7-10]
acth[7-10]
see: corticotropin[7-10]
acth[7-16]
see: corticotropin[7-16]
acth 80
see: corticotropin
acth,acetylated
see: corticotropin
acth albumin polymer
see: corticotropin derivative
ACTH analog
see: corticotropin derivative
acth analogue
see: corticotropin derivative
acthar
see: corticotropin
acth depot
see: corticotropin
ACTH derivative
see: corticotropin derivative
acthon
see: corticotropin
acth peptide
see: corticotropin derivative
ACTH releasing factor
see: corticotropin releasing factor
acth releasing hormone
see: corticotropin releasing factor
acth synthetic analog
see: corticotropin derivative
acth synthetic analogue
see: corticotropin derivative
acth z[1-24]
see: tetracosactide zinc phosphate
actocortin
see: hydrocortisone sodium phosphate
acton
see: corticotropin
actonar
see: corticotropin
acton prolongatum
see: corticotropin

actovegin

actovegin forte
see: actovegin
actraphane
see: isophane insulin
actrapid
see: neutral insulin
actrapid hm
see: monocomponent insulin
actrapid insulin
see: insulin
actrapid mc
see: insulin
actrope
see: corticotropin
acutrim
see: phenylpropanolamine
adactan
see: corticotropin
adanon
see: methadone
adanon hydrochloride
see: methadone
adato deca
see: perfluorodecalin
adbiol
see: bufetolol
adcortyl
see: triamcinolone
adderall
see: amphetamine
adderall xr
see: amphetamine
adelfan esidrex
see: dihydralazine plus hydrochlorothiazide plus reserpine
adelphane esidrex
see: dihydralazine plus hydrochlorothiazide plus reserpine
adelphan esidrex
see: dihydralazine plus hydrochlorothiazide plus reserpine
ademin
see: triamterene

ademine
see: triamterene

adenohypophysis hormone

adepresol
see: dihydralazine plus hydrochlorothiazide plus reserpine
adifax
see: dexfenfluramine

adimolol

adimolol hydrochloride hydrate
see: adimolol
adiol
see: androstanediol
adipan
see: amphetamine
adiparthrol
see: n ethylamphetamine
adipex
see: methamphetamine
adipex neu
see: phentermine resin
adipex p
see: phentermine
adiposetten
see: norpseudoephedrine
adiposettin
see: norpseudoephedrine
adiposon
see: amfepramone
adipost
see: phendimetrazine tartrate
adnephrin
see: adrenalin
adnephrine
see: adrenalin
adr 033
see: tripamide
adr033
see: tripamide

adrafinil

adrenal cortex trophic hormone
see: corticotropin
adrenal cortex tropic hormone
see: corticotropin
adrenalex
see: cortisone

adrenalin

adrenalin chloride
see: adrenalin
adrenalin dipivalate
see: dipivefrine
adrenaline
see: adrenalin
adrenaline chloride
see: adrenalin
adrenaline dipivalate
see: dipivefrine
adrenaline hydrochloride
see: adrenalin
adrenalin hydrochloride
see: adrenalin
adrenalon
see: adrenalone

adrenalone

adrenamine
see: adrenalin
adrenapax
see: adrenalin
adrenazin
see: adrenalin
adrenergic beta-agonists
see: beta adrenergic receptor stimulating agent
adrenergic beta-antagonists
see: beta adrenergic receptor blocking agent
adrenine
see: adrenalin
adrenocorticaltrophormon
see: corticotropin
adrenocorticotrope hormone
see: corticotropin
adrenocorticotrophic hormone
see: corticotropin
adrenocorticotrophin
see: corticotropin
adrenocorticotropic hormone
see: corticotropin
adrenocorticotropin
see: corticotropin
adrenocorticotropin[1-10]
see: corticotropin[1-10]
adrenocorticotropin[11-24]
see: corticotropin[11-24]
adrenocorticotropin 1-17
see: corticotropin[1-17]
adrenocorticotropin 1-24
see: tetracosactide

adrenocorticotropin derivative
see: corticotropin derivative
adrenocorticotropin hormone
see: corticotropin
adrenomone
see: corticotropin
adrenone
see: adrenalone
adrenor
see: noradrenalin

adrenosterone

adrenotropin
see: corticotropin
adreson
see: cortisone acetate
adrin
see: adrenalin
adrine
see: adrenalin
adrotest
see: testosterone
adroyd
see: oxymetholone
adult Hb
see: hemoglobin A
adurix
see: clopamide
advair
see: fluticasone propionate plus salmeterol
advantan
see: methylprednisolone aceponate
advaradin
see: adrenalin
adventan
see: methylprednisolone aceponate
adyston
see: pholedrine
aerobid
see: flunisolide
aero clenil
see: salbutamol
aeroclenil
see: salbutamol
aerodur
see: terbutaline
aerolin
see: salbutamol
aerolone
see: isoprenaline
aeromax
see: salmeterol xinafoate
aeroseb dex
see: dexamethasone
aeroseb hc
see: hydrocortisone
aerotrol
see: isoprenaline
20 aet 1
see: testosterone 4 butylcyclohexanecarboxylate
aethimizol
see: ethimizole
aethimizole
see: ethimizole
af 0104
see: perfluorooctyl bromide
af0104
see: perfluorooctyl bromide
af 45
see: anordiol
af45
see: anordiol
afagil
see: phenmetrazine
afatin
see: dexamphetamine
afema
see: fadrozole
afettine
see: dexamphetamine
aflucoson
see: dexamethasone
aflucosone
see: dexamethasone

afurolol

agent,anorexiant
see: anorexigenic agent
agn 190342
see: brimonidine
agn190342
see: brimonidine
agovirin
see: methyltestosterone
agovirin depot
see: methyltestosterone
agyrase
see: buphenine
ah 19501
see: dilevalol
ah 3365
see: salbutamol
ah3365
see: salbutamol

ah 5158
see: labetalol
ah5158
see: labetalol
ah 5158a
see: labetalol
ah5158a
see: labetalol
ahr 619
see: doxapram
ahr619
see: doxapram
ahr 965
see: fenfluramine
ahr965
see: fenfluramine
a hydrocort
see: hydrocortisone sodium succinate
ahydrocort
see: hydrocortisone sodium succinate
ai 27,303
see: cetamolol
ai 27303
see: cetamolol
aimax
see: methallibure
airomir
see: salbutamol sulfate

ajulemic acid

ak beta
see: levobunolol
akrinor
see: cafedrine plus theodrenaline
akroteston
see: testosterone propionate
aktamin
see: noradrenalin bitartrate
aktedrin
see: amphetamine
aktedron
see: amphetamine
alanase
see: beclometasone dipropionate
alaton
see: spironolactone
alatone
see: spironolactone
albemap
see: dexamphetamine
albetol
see: labetalol
albuterol
see: salbutamol
albuterol sulfate
see: salbutamol sulfate
alcinonide
see: halcinonide
alcinonidel
see: halcinonide

alclometasone

alclometasone dipropionate

alclomethasone
see: alclometasone
alclomethasone dipropionate
see: alclometasone dipropionate

alcohol

alcohol, ethyl
see: alcohol
alcohol vapor
see: alcohol
aldace
see: spironolactone
aldactazide
see: aldactazine

aldactazine

aldactone
see: spironolactone
aldactone 50
see: spironolactone
aldactone a
see: spironolactone
aldactone diurapid
see: spironolactone
aldactone saltucin
see: butizide plus spironolactone
aldadiene
see: canrenone
aldadiene k
see: canrenoate potassium
aldadiene kalium
see: canrenoate potassium
aldadiene potassium
see: canrenoate potassium
aldecin
see: beclometasone dipropionate

Index

aldecina
see: beclometasone dipropionate
aldecine
see: beclometasone dipropionate
alderlin
see: pronetalol
aldocorten
see: aldosterone
aldopur
see: spironolactone
aldosteron
see: aldosterone

aldosterone

aldozone
see: butizide plus spironolactone
aldozone forte
see: butizide plus spironolactone
alentol
see: amphetamine
alertec
see: modafinil
alertol
see: pipradol
alertonic
see: pipradol
aleudrin
see: isoprenaline
aleudrine
see: isoprenaline
aleudrin ingelheim
see: isoprenaline
alfa 6
see: paramethasone
alfa6
see: paramethasone
alfafluorone
see: fludrocortisone acetate
alfanonidrone
see: fludrocortisone acetate
alfason
see: hydrocortisone butyrate
alflorone
see: fludrocortisone
algidon
see: methadone
algil
see: pethidine
alginodia
see: noradrenalin
algolysin
see: methadone
algoxale
see: methadone
alidril
see: isoprenaline

alifedrine

alifedrine hydrochloride
see: alifedrine
alipid
see: amfepramone
alisactide
see: alsactide
allergospasmin
see: cromoglycate disodium plus reproterol
allodene
see: amphetamine
allodihydrocortisol
see: hydrallostane
allodihydro f
see: hydrallostane
allodihydrohydrocortisone
see: hydrallostane
alloprenalol
see: alprenolol
allylglycin
see: allylglycine

allylglycine

almarl
see: arotinolol
almeta
see: alclometasone dipropionate

almitrine

almitrine dimesilate

almitrine bismesilate
see: almitrine dimesilate
almitrine bismesylate
see: almitrine dimesilate
almitrine dimesylate
see: almitrine dimesilate
almitrine dimethanesulfonate
see: almitrine dimesilate
alo 1401 02
see: betaxolol
alo 2145
see: apraclonidine

Index

alo2145
see: apraclonidine
alodan
see: pethidine
alometasone
see: halometasone
alondra
see: paramethasone acetate
alotec
see: orciprenaline
alotex
see: isoprenaline
aloxicort
see: paramethasone
alpha 1-19 acth
see: corticotropin derivative
9alpha,11alpha epoxymexrenone
see: eplerenone
alpha 1 23 nh2 acth
see: corticotropin derivative
alpha 1,6 glucan
see: dextran
3alpha,17beta androstanediol
see: androstanediol
7alpha,17 dimethylnandrolone
see: mibolerone
7alpha,17 dimethyltestosterone
see: bolasterone
17alpha 19 nortestosterone
see: nandrolone
5alpha,3beta androstanediol
see: 3beta androstanediol
alpha 4 23 acth
see: corticotropin derivative
alpha 4 23 adrenocorticotropin
see: corticotropin derivative
alpha 4 23 corticotropin
see: corticotropin derivative
alpha 5 23 acth
see: corticotropin derivative
alpha 5 23 adrenocorticotropin
see: corticotropin derivative
alpha 5 23 corticotropin
see: corticotropin derivative
alpha 6 24 acth
see: corticotropin derivative
alpha 6 24 adrenocorticotropin
see: corticotropin derivative
alpha 6 24 corticotropin
see: corticotropin derivative
alpha 7 23 acth
see: corticotropin derivative
alpha 7 23 adrenocorticotropin
see: corticotropin derivative
alpha 7 23 corticotropin
see: corticotropin derivative
alpha acth 1-24
see: tetracosactide
alpha amphetamine
see: amphetamine
3alpha androstanediol
see: androstanediol
5 alpha androstanediol
see: androstanediol
5alpha androstanediol
see: androstanediol
5 alpha androstanedione
see: androstanedione
5alpha androstanedione
see: androstanedione
5alpha androstanolone
see: androstanolone
5alpha androstenedione
see: androstenedione
5alpha androsterone
see: androsterone
alpha chain,hemoglobin
see: hemoglobin alpha chain
11alpha cortisol
see: epihydrocortisone
7alpha dehydro epiandrosterone
see: prasterone
7alpha dehydroepiandrosterone
see: prasterone
alphaderm
see: hydrocortisone
alpha desoxyadrenalin
see: epinine
4,5alpha dihydrocortisol
see: hydrallostane
5alpha dihydrocortisol
see: hydrallostane
5alpha dihydrohydrocortisone
see: hydrallostane
5alpha dihydrotestosterone
see: androstanolone
alphadrol
see: fluprednisolone
9,11alpha epoxymexrenone
see: eplerenone
17alpha ethylnortestosterone
see: norethandrolone
9alpha fludrocortisone
see: fludrocortisone

6alpha fluorobetamethasone
see: diflorasone
9alpha fluorocortisal
see: fludrocortisone
9 alpha fluorocortisol
see: fludrocortisone
9alpha fluorocortisol
see: fludrocortisone
9alpha fluorocortisol acetate
see: fludrocortisone acetate
6alpha fluorodexamethasone
see: flumetasone
alpha fluorohydrocortisone
see: fludrocortisone
9alpha fluorohydro cortisone
see: fludrocortisone
9alpha fluorohydrocortisone
see: fludrocortisone
6 alpha fluoroprednisolone
see: fluprednisolone
6alpha fluoroprednisolone
see: fluprednisolone
9 alpha fluoroprednisolone
see: isoflupredone
9alpha fluoroprednisolone
see: isoflupredone
9alpha fluprednisolone
see: isoflupredone
alphagen
see: brimonidine
alpha hcg
see: chorionic gonadotropin alpha subunit
11alpha hydrocortisone
see: epihydrocortisone
3alpha hydroxy 17 androstanone
see: androsterone
11alpha hydroxycortexolone
see: epihydrocortisone
11alpha hydroxycortodoxone
see: epihydrocortisone
alpha lobeline
see: lobeline
17 alpha methylandrostenediol
see: methandriol
17alpha methylandrostenediol
see: methandriol
alpha methyl meta tyramine
see: gepefrine
alpha methyl m tyramine
see: gepefrine
7alpha methylnandrolone
see: trestolone
alpha methyl para tyramine
see: hydroxyamphetamine
alpha methylphenethylamine
see: amphetamine
alpha methylphenylethylamine
see: amphetamine
6 alpha methylprednisolone
see: methylprednisolone
6alpha methylprednisolone
see: methylprednisolone
17 alpha methyltestosterone
see: methyltestosterone
17alpha methyltestosterone
see: methyltestosterone
alpha methyl tyramine
see: hydroxyamphetamine
alpha methyltyramine
see: hydroxyamphetamine
alphamine
see: midodrine
alpha piperid 2 ylbenzhydrol
see: pipradol
7alpha propylspirolactone
see: 7alpha propylspironolactone
alpha testosterone
see: epitestosterone
17alpha testosterone
see: epitestosterone
alpha trenbolone
see: 17alpha trenbolone
alphatrex
see: betamethasone dipropionate
alpheprol
see: alprenolol
alprendol
see: alprenolol
alprenol
see: alprenolol

alprenolol

alprenolol derivative

alprenolol,dihydro
see: dihydroalprenolol
alprenolol hydrochloride
see: alprenolol
alprenolol isomer
see: alprenolol
alrex
see: loteprednol etabonate

Index

alsactide

althiazide
see: altizide
althiazide with spironolactone
see: aldactazine
althose
see: methadone
althose hydrochloride
see: methadone
altim
see: cortivazol

altizide

altizide plus spironolactone
see: aldactazine
aludrin
see: isoprenaline
aludrine
see: isoprenaline
alupent
see: orciprenaline
aluzine
see: furosemide
am 356
see: methanandamide
am356
see: methanandamide

amafolone

ambar
see: methamphetamine
ambinon
see: gonadotropin

ambroxol plus clenbuterol

amciderm
see: amcinonide

amcinonide

a methopred
see: methylprednisolone sodium succinate
amethopred
see: methylprednisolone sodium succinate

amfepramone

amfetamine
see: amphetamine
amfetaminil
see: amphetaminil
amfetasul
see: dexamphetamine
amfetyline
see: fenetylline
amfolenic acid
see: amfonelic acid

amfonelic acid

amicla
see: amcinonide
amiclaran
see: amiloride
amidon
see: methadone
amidone
see: methadone
amidosan
see: methadone
amilorid
see: amiloride

amiloride

amiloride chloride
see: amiloride
amiloride hcl
see: amiloride
amiloride hydrochlorhydrate
see: amiloride
amiloridehydrochlorhydrate
see: amiloride
amiloride hydrochloride
see: amiloride
amiloride hydroxychloride
see: amiloride

amiloride plus cyclopenthiazide

amiloride plus furosemide
see: frumil

amiloride plus hydrochlorothiazide

amiloridine
see: amiloride

4 amino 1 (6 bromo 2 pyridyl)piperidine

4 amino 1 (6 chloro 2 pyridyl)piperidine

2 amino 1 phenyl 1 propanol
see: phenylpropanolamine

2 amino 1 phenylpropane
see: amphetamine

6 amino 2 methyl 2 heptanol
see: heptaminol

1 [2 (2 amino 2 methylpropionylamino) 3 (1h indol 3 yl)propionyl] 3 benzyl 3 piperidinecarboxylic acid ethyl ester

3 amino 3 methyl n [2,3,4,5 tetrahydro 2 oxo 1 [[2' (1h tetrazol 5 yl) 1,1' biphenyl 4 yl]methyl] 1h 1 benzazepin 3 yl]butanamide

2 amino 4 (bicyclo[2.2.1]hept 2 ylamino) n (n isopropylcarbamoyl) 5 pyrimidinesulfonamide

2 amino 4 (methylsulfonyl)butyrylglutamylhistidylphenylalanyl dextro lysylphenylalanine

2 amino 4 pentenoic acid
see: allylglycine

2 amino 5 phenyl 2 oxazoline
see: aminorex

2 amino 5 phenyloxazoline
see: aminorex

6 amino alpha [[(1 methyl 3 phenylpropyl)amino]methyl] 3 pyridinemethanol

4 aminoclonidine
see: apraclonidine

aminocordin
see: nikethamide

4 (2 aminoethylpyrocatechol
see: dopamine

amino glutethimide
see: aminoglutethimide

aminoglutethimide

aminoglutethimide derivative

amino glutethimide phosphate
see: aminoglutethimide phosphate

aminoglutethimide phosphate

aminogluthimide
see: aminoglutethimide

2 [4 (3 aminomethyl 4 hydroxybenzoyl) 2,3 dichlorophenoxy]acetic acid ethyl ester

2 aminomethyl 4 tert butyl 6 iodophenol

7alpha (4 aminophenylthio)androstenedione

3 (2 aminopropyl)phenol
see: gepefrine

4 (2 aminopropyl)phenol
see: hydroxyamphetamine

aminorex

aminorex,4 methyl
see: 4 methylaminorex

aminorex fumarate
see: aminorex

aminorexfumarate
see: aminorex

aminorexum
see: aminorex

aminoxafen
see: aminorex

aminoxaphen
see: aminorex

amiphenazol
see: amiphenazole

amiphenazole

amipramidine
see: amiloride

amitrene
see: dexamphetamine

Index

ammonium acetate

amorphan depot
see: norpseudoephedrine

amosulalol

amosulalol hydrochloride
see: amosulalol
amphamed
see: amphetamine
amphamine
see: amphetamine
amphedrine
see: dexamphetamine
amphedroxyn
see: methamphetamine
amphepramon
see: amfepramone
amphetaime
see: amphetamine
amphetamin
see: amphetamine

amphetamine

amphetamine,2 methoxy n methyl
see: 2 methoxymethamphetamine
amphetamine,3 methoxy n methyl
see: 3 methoxymethamphetamine
amphetamine,4 methoxy
see: 4 methoxyamphetamine
amphetamine,4 methoxy n methyl
see: 4 methoxymethamphetamine
amphetamine base phosphate
see: amphetamine
amphetamine base sulfate
see: amphetamine

amphetamine derivative

amphetamine,furfuryl
see: furfurylamphetamine
amphetamine hydrochloride
see: amphetamine
amphetamine,meta hydroxy
see: gepefrine
amphetamine,n (2 chlorobenzyl)
see: clobenzorex
amphetamine,n (3 chloropropyl)
see: mefenorex
amphetamine,n formyl
see: formetorex
amphetamine,n hydroxy
see: n hydroxyamphetamine
amphetamine phosphate
see: amphetamine
amphetamines
see: amphetamine derivative
amphetamine sulfate
see: amphetamine

amphetaminil

amphetaminyl
see: amphetamine
amphethamine
see: amphetamine
amphetyline
see: fenetylline
amphex
see: dexamphetamine
amphezamin
see: amphetamine
amphonelic acid
see: amfonelic acid
amsolulol
see: amosulalol
amsustain
see: dexamphetamine
amunine
see: corticotropin releasing factor
amylopectin,hydroxyethyl
see: hetastarch
amyloride
see: amiloride
an 1
see: amphetaminil
an 148
see: methadone
an148
see: methadone
an 152
see: gonadorelin[6 dextro lysine] doxorubicin
an-152
see: gonadorelin[6 dextro lysine] doxorubicin
an152
see: gonadorelin[6 dextro lysine] doxorubicin
an 207
see: gonadorelin[6 dextro lysine] 2 pyrrolinodoxo-rubicin
an-207
see: gonadorelin[6 dextro lysine] 2 pyrrolinodoxo-rubicin
an207
see: gonadorelin[6 dextro lysine] 2 pyrrolinodoxo-

Index

rubicin
an 448
see: mazindol
an-448
see: mazindol
an448
see: mazindol
anabol
see: stanozolol
anaboleen
see: androstanolone
anabolex
see: androstanolone

anabolic agent

anabolic agents
see: anabolic agent
anabolic drug
see: anabolic agent
anabolic hormone
see: anabolic agent
anabolic steroid
see: anabolic agent
anabolic steroid agent
see: anabolic agent
anabolic steroids
see: anabolic agent
anabolicum
see: quinbolone
anabolin la
see: nandrolone decanoate
anabolizing agent
see: anabolic agent
anabolizing cream
see: anabolic agent
anabolizing drug
see: anabolic agent
anabol tablinen
see: androstanolone
anacardone
see: nikethamide
anacordone
see: nikethamide
anadon
see: methadone
anadrol
see: oxymetholone
anadrol 50
see: oxymetholone
anadur
see: nandrolone 4 hexyloxyhydrocinnamate
anaflogistico
see: dexamethasone
anaflogistico 17 valerate
see: dexamethasone 17 valerate
anaflogistico novobios
see: dexamethasone
analeptic
see: central stimulant agent
analeptic agent
see: central stimulant agent
analeptic combination
see: central stimulant agent
analeptic drug
see: central stimulant agent
analepticon
see: etamivan
analeptics
see: central stimulant agent
analgesic anesthetic agent
see: narcotic analgesic agent
analgesics, opioid
see: narcotic analgesic agent
analog ii
see: 1,1 dichloro 2,3 diphenylcyclopropane
analone
see: nandrolone decanoate
anamidol
see: oxymesterone

anandamide

anapetol
see: phenmetrazine
anapolon
see: oxymetholone
anapolon 50
see: oxymetholone
anaprilin
see: propranolol
anapriline
see: propranolol
anaprilinium
see: propranolol
anaprotin
see: androstanolone
anapryline
see: propranolol
anara
see: amphetamine
anastar
see: prasterone
anasterone
see: oxymetholone

anastrazole
see: anastrozole

anastrozole

anatrofin
see: stenbolone acetate
anavar
see: oxandrolone
ancortone
see: prednisone
anderone
see: testosterone propionate
andol
see: nandrolone cyclohexylpropionate
andractim
see: androstanolone
andrhormone
see: methyltestosterone
andriol
see: testosterone undecanoate
andro 100
see: testosterone
andro cyp
see: testosterone cipionate
androderm
see: testosterone
androdiol
see: methandriol
androfluorene
see: fluoxymesterone
androfluorone
see: fluoxymesterone
androfort
see: testosterone
androfurazanol
see: furazabol
androgel
see: testosterone

androgen

androgenic agent
see: androgen
androgenic hormone
see: androgen
androgenic steroid
see: androgen
androgens
see: androgen
androgens, synthetic
see: androgen
androgen sulfate
see: androgen
androgyn la
see: testosterone enantate
'android'
see: methyltestosterone
android f
see: fluoxymesterone
androject
see: testosterone phenylpropionate
andro la 200
see: testosterone enantate
androlin
see: testosterone
androlone
see: androstanolone
andrometh
see: methyltestosterone
andronaq
see: testosterone
andronaq 50
see: testosterone
andronaq la
see: testosterone cipionate
andronate
see: testosterone propionate
andronex
see: methyltestosterone
andronex amp
see: testosterone propionate
andropatch
see: testosterone
androral
see: methyltestosterone
androsan
see: methyltestosterone
androsan amp
see: testosterone propionate
androst 1 en 17beta ol 3 one
see: 1 testosterone

androst 1 ene 3,17 dione

androst 4 en 17alpha ol 3 one
see: epitestosterone
androst 4 en 17beta ol 3 one
see: testosterone
androst 4 en 19 ol 3,17 dione
see: 19 hydroxyandrostenedione
androst 4 en 19 ole 3,17 dione
see: 19 hydroxyandrostenedione
androst 4 en 3,17 dione
see: androstenedione

Index

androst 4 en 4 ol 3,17 dione
see: formestane
androst 4 ene 3,11,17 trione
see: adrenosterone
androst 4 ene 3,17 dione
see: androstenedione
androst 4 ene 3beta,17beta diol
see: 4 androstenediol
androst 4 enediol
see: 4 androstenediol
androst 5 en 3beta,17beta diol
see: androstenediol
androst 5 en 3 beta ol 17 one
see: prasterone
androst 5 en 3beta ol 17 one
see: prasterone
androst 5 ene 3,17beta diol
see: androstenediol
androst 5 ene 3beta ol 17 one
see: prasterone

androsta 1,4,6 triene 3,17 dione

androsta 1,4 dien 3,17 dione
see: boldione
androsta 1,4 diene 3,17 dione
see: boldione

androsta 4,16 dien 3 one

androsta 4,6,8(9) triene 3,17 dione

androstadiendione
see: boldione
androstadienedione
see: boldione
androstadienone
see: androsta 4,16 dien 3 one
1,4 androstadien 3,17 dione
see: boldione
4,16 androstadien 3 one
see: androsta 4,16 dien 3 one
1,4 androstadiene 3,17 dione
see: boldione
androstalone
see: mestanolone
androstan 17beta ol 3 one
see: androstanolone
5 androstan 17 beta ol 3 one
see: androstanolone
5 androstan 17beta ol 3 one
see: androstanolone
androstan 3alpha ol 17 one
see: androsterone
androstan 3beta,17beta diol
see: 3beta androstanediol
androstan 3beta ol 17 one
see: epiandrosterone
5 androstan 3beta ol 17 one
see: epiandrosterone
5 androstan 3 one 17b ol
see: androstanolone

5alpha androstan 3 one

androstanasol
see: stanozolol
androstanazole
see: stanozolol
androstandiol
see: androstanediol
androstandione
see: androstanedione
androstane 17 one
see: prasterone
androstane-3,17-diol
see: androstanediol
androstane 3alpha,17beta diol
see: androstanediol
androstane 3beta,17beta diol
see: 3beta androstanediol

androstanediol

3beta androstanediol

androstanedione

androstanolone

androstanolone 17 bromoacetate
see: androstanolone bromoacetate
androstanolone,17 deoxy
see: 5alpha androstan 3 one

5beta androstanolone

androstanolone bromoacetate

Index

androstanolone derivative

androstanolone propionate

androstanopyrazole
see: stanozolol
1,4,6 androstatrien 3,17 dione
see: androsta 1,4,6 triene 3,17 dione
androsten
see: methyltestosterone
androsten 11beta ol dione
see: 11beta hydroxyandrostenedione
4 androsten 11 ol 3,17 dione
see: 11beta hydroxyandrostenedione
4 androsten 17alpha ol 3 one
see: epitestosterone
1 androsten 17beta ol 3 one
see: 1 testosterone
4 androsten 17beta ol 3 one
see: testosterone
4 androsten 3,17 dione
see: androstenedione
4 androsten 3beta,17beta diol
see: 4 androstenediol
5 androsten 3beta,17beta diol
see: androstenediol
5 androsten 3 beta 17 one
see: prasterone
5 androsten 3 beta ol 17 one
see: prasterone
5 androsten 3beta ol 17 one
see: prasterone
5 androsten 3 ol 17 one
see: prasterone
androstendione
see: androstenedione
4 androstene 19 ol 3,17 dione
see: 19 hydroxyandrostenedione
4 androstene 3,11,17 trione
see: adrenosterone
5 androstene 3,17beta diol
see: androstenediol
4 androstene 3,17 dion 19 al
see: 19 oxoandrostenedione
androstene 3,17 dione
see: androstenedione
1 androstene 3,17 dione
see: androst 1 ene 3,17 dione
4 androstene 3,17 dione
see: androstenedione
5 androstene 3beta,17beta diol
see: androstenediol
5 androstene 3 beta ol 17 one
see: prasterone
5 androstene 3beta ol 17 one
see: prasterone
androstene 5 3b ol 17 one
see: prasterone

androstenediol

androstene diol
see: androstenediol

4 androstenediol

5 androstenediol
see: androstenediol

androstenediol derivative

5 androstenediol derivative
see: androstenediol derivative
androstenediols
see: androstenediol derivative
androstenedion 19 al
see: 19 oxoandrostenedione

androstenedione

androstene dione
see: androstenedione
4 androstenedione
see: androstenedione
androstenedione,4 hydroxy
see: formestane

androstenedione derivative

androstenetrione
see: adrenosterone
androstenolone
see: testosterone
androstenolone derivative
see: testosterone derivative
androstenolone enanthate
see: testosterone enantate
androsteron
see: androsterone

androsterone

Index

androsterone derivative

androsterone plus clofibrate
see: atromid
androtardyl
see: testosterone enantate
androtest
see: testosterone
androteston
see: testosterone propionate
androteston m
see: methandriol
androtest p
see: testosterone propionate
androtex
see: androstenedione
androviron
see: mesterolone
androxid
see: testosterone propionate
androxil
see: testosterone propionate
androxil oral
see: methyltestosterone
androyd f
see: oxymetholone
andrusol
see: testosterone
andrusol p
see: testosterone propionate
anertan
see: methyltestosterone
anertan perlingual
see: methyltestosterone
anertar
see: testosterone propionate
angeliq
see: drospirenone plus estradiol
angiazol
see: pentetrazole
angioton
see: pentetrazole
angium
see: bufuralol
anhydron
see: cyclothiazide
anhydrous caffeine
see: caffeine

4 anilino 2 methylthiopyrido[2,3 d]pyrimidine

animine
see: caffeine
anipryl
see: selegiline

anordiol

anorectic agent
see: anorexigenic agent
anorectic drug
see: anorexigenic agent
anorex
see: amfepramone
anorexant agent
see: anorexigenic agent
anorexiant
see: anorexigenic agent
anorexiant agent
see: anorexigenic agent
anorexiant drug
see: anorexigenic agent
anorexic agent
see: anorexigenic agent
anorexic drug
see: anorexigenic agent
anorexigen
see: anorexigenic agent

anorexigenic agent

anorexigenic compound
see: anorexigenic agent
anorexigenic drug
see: anorexigenic agent
anorexil
see: amfepramone
anp 235
see: meclofenoxate
anp 297
see: mefexamide
anp 3624
see: tienilic acid
anpec
see: morphine
anteron
see: seric gonadotropin
antex
see: seric gonadotropin
antasthmin kwizda
see: isoprenaline

anthrogon
see: gonadotropin
antiappetite agent
see: anorexigenic agent
antiasmatico serpero
see: isoprenaline
anticatabolin
see: nandrolone phenpropionate

antiestrogen

anti estrogen
see: antiestrogen
antiestrogen agent
see: antiestrogen
antiestrogenic agent
see: antiestrogen
antiobes retard
see: fenproporex
antiparkin
see: selegiline
antisolon
see: prednisolone
antisolone
see: prednisolone
antostab
see: seric gonadotropin
antuitrin s
see: chorionic gonadotropin
antuitrin t
see: growth hormone
anusol hc
see: hydrocortisone acetate
apetinil
see: n ethylamphetamine
apidra
see: insulin glulisine
apiquel
see: aminorex
apisate
see: amfepramone
apl
see: chorionic gonadotropin
apliobal
see: alprenolol
aplonidine
see: apraclonidine
aplonidine hydrochloride
see: apraclonidine
apodrine
see: phenylpropanolamine
apoephedrine
see: phenylpropanolamine
apokinon
see: apomorphine
'apolar'
see: desonide
apomorfine
see: apomorphine

apomorphine

apomorphine hydrochloride
see: apomorphine
aponeuron
see: amphetaminil
apophedrine
see: phenylpropanolamine
apormorphine
see: apomorphine
appedrine
see: phenylpropanolamine
appetite depressant agent
see: anorexigenic agent
appetite depressants
see: anorexigenic agent
appetite inhibitor
see: anorexigenic agent
appetite reducer
see: anorexigenic agent
appetite reducing drug
see: anorexigenic agent
appetite restrainer
see: anorexigenic agent
appetite suppressant
see: anorexigenic agent
appetite suppressing agent
see: anorexigenic agent

apraclonidine

aprednislon
see: prednisolone
aprednislone
see: prednisolone
aprenolol
see: alprenolol
apresazide
see: hydralazine plus hydrochlorothiazide
apresoline esidrex
see: hydralazine plus hydrochlorothiazide
apresoline plus esidrex
see: hydralazine plus hydrochlorothiazide
aprinox
see: bendroflumethiazide

Index

aptia
see: alprenolol
aptin
see: alprenolol
aptin durules
see: alprenolol
aptine
see: alprenolol
aptol
see: alprenolol
aptol duriles
see: alprenolol
aptrol
see: 4 methylamphetamine
aq 110
see: tretoquinol
aq110
see: tretoquinol
aql 208
see: tretoquinol
aql208
see: tretoquinol
aquadon
see: chlortalidone
aquaforil
see: xipamide
aquamox
see: quinethazone
aquanil
see: timolol maleate
aquaphor
see: xipamide
aquaphoril
see: xipamide
aquareduct
see: spironolactone
aquaretic
see: amiloride plus hydrochlorothiazide
aquarius
see: hydrochlorothiazide
aquatag
see: benzthiazide
aquatain
see: triamcinolone acetonide
aquatensen
see: methyclothiazide
aquaviron
see: testosterone
aquaviron b12
see: testosterone
aquavor
see: xipamide
aquazide
see: trichlormethiazide
aquazide h
see: hydrochlorothiazide
aquex
see: clopamide
arachidonoylethanolamide
see: anandamide

2 arachidonoylglycerol

arachidonylethanolamide
see: anandamide
2 arachidonylglycerol
see: 2 arachidonoylglycerol
aramercur
see: chlormerodrin
aramine
see: metaraminol
araminum
see: metaraminol
aranesp
see: novel erythropoiesis stimulating protein
ar c68397aa
see: 4 hydroxy 7 [2 [2 [3 (2 phenylethoxy)propylsulfonyl]ethylamino]ethyl]benzothiazol 2(3h) one
arc 68397aa
see: 4 hydroxy 7 [2 [2 [3 (2 phenylethoxy)propylsulfonyl]ethylamino]ethyl]benzothiazol 2(3h) one
arc68397aa
see: 4 hydroxy 7 [2 [2 [3 (2 phenylethoxy)propylsulfonyl]ethylamino]ethyl]benzothiazol 2(3h) one
ar c68397xx
see: 4 hydroxy 7 [2 [2 [3 (2 phenylethoxy)propylsulfonyl]ethylamino]ethyl]benzothiazol 2(3h) one
arc68397xx
see: 4 hydroxy 7 [2 [2 [3 (2 phenylethoxy)propylsulfonyl]ethylamino]ethyl]benzothiazol 2(3h) one
arcablock
see: propranolol
arcablock retard
see: propranolol
arcodexan
see: dexamethasone
arcodexane
see: dexamethasone
arcort
see: deoxycorticosterone acetate

ardex
see: dexamphetamine
arelix
see: piretanide
arensin
see: fadrozole
arial
see: salmeterol xinafoate
arifon
see: indapamide
arimidex
see: anastrozole
aristocort
see: triamcinolone
aristocort acetonide
see: triamcinolone acetonide
aristocort forte parenteral
see: triamcinolone diacetate
aristocort intralesional
see: triamcinolone diacetate
aristodan
see: triamcinolone
aristoderm
see: triamcinolone acetonide
aristogel
see: triamcinolone acetonide
aristospan
see: triamcinolone hexacetonide
arlibide
see: buphenine
arlidin
see: buphenine
arlix
see: piretanide
arm a med
see: orciprenaline
aromasin
see: exemestane

aromatase inhibitor

arotinolol

arotinolol hydrochloride
see: arotinolol
arsiprenol
see: isoprenaline
arteolol
see: carteolol
arteoptic
see: carteolol
arteoptik
see: carteolol
arterenal
see: noradrenalin
arterenol
see: noradrenalin
artex
see: tertatolol

artificial blood

artoron
see: ethylestrenol
arubendol
see: terbutaline sulfate
arumil
see: amiloride
arutimol
see: timolol maleate
arvekap
see: triptorelin

arzoxifene

arzoxifene hydrochloride
see: arzoxifene
asahydrin
see: chlormerodrin
asellacrin
see: human growth hormone
asenlix
see: clobenzorex
asialo chorionic gonadotropin
see: asialochorionic gonadotropin

asialochorionic gonadotropin

asialochorionogonadotropin
see: asialochorionic gonadotropin
asialo hCG
see: asialochorionic gonadotropin
asiprenol
see: isoprenaline
asl 279
see: dopamine
asl279
see: dopamine
asl 607
see: hetastarch
asl-607
see: hetastarch
asl607
see: hetastarch

Index

asl 8052
see: esmolol
asl8052
see: esmolol
asl 8052 001
see: esmolol
asl 8052-001
see: esmolol
asl8052-001
see: esmolol
asl8052001
see: esmolol
asl 8123
see: 3 [4 (2 hydroxy 3 isopropylaminopropoxy)phenyl]propionic acid
asl8123
see: 3 [4 (2 hydroxy 3 isopropylaminopropoxy)phenyl]propionic acid
aslera
see: prasterone
asmadren
see: isoprenaline
asmalar
see: isoprenaline
asmalidrina
see: isoprenaline
asmalin
see: salbutamol
asmanex
see: mometasone furoate
asmanor
see: isoprenaline
asmaterolo
see: reproterol
asmaven
see: salbutamol
asmol
see: salbutamol
asmolidrina
see: isoprenaline
asmolon
see: isoprenaline
asmonor
see: isoprenaline
assiprenol
see: isoprenaline
astedin
see: amphetamine
astenile
see: prasterone
asthmahaler
see: adrenalin
asthmalitan
see: isoetarine
asthmatermine
see: isoprenaline
asthmolytan
see: isoetarine
asthmopent
see: orciprenaline
asthone
see: clorprenaline
astmo
see: isoprenaline
astmopent
see: orciprenaline
astonin h
see: fludrocortisone
astra
see: alprenolol
astramorph
see: morphine sulfate
astrocar
see: nikethamide
at 101
see: isosorbide
at101
see: isosorbide

atamestane

atapryl
see: selegiline
atemur
see: fluticasone propionate
atenigron
see: atenolol plus chlortalidone
atenol
see: atenolol

atenolol

atenolol plus chlortalidone

atenolol plus nifedipine

atenos
see: tulobuterol
atock
see: formoterol fumarate
atomide
see: beclometasone dipropionate

Index

atriona
see: cortisone acetate

atromid

aturgyl delta
see: pemoline
authus
see: propranolol
auxiloson
see: dexamethasone isonicotinate
auxison
see: dexamethasone isonicotinate
avicol
see: chlorphentermine
avinza
see: morphine sulfate
avipron
see: chlorphentermine
avlocardyl
see: propranolol
avlocardyl retard
see: propranolol
axotide
see: fluticasone propionate
ay 21,011
see: practolol
ay 21011
see: practolol
ay21011
see: practolol
ay 24,031
see: gonadorelin
ay 24031
see: gonadorelin
ay24,031
see: gonadorelin
ay24031
see: gonadorelin
ay 25650
see: triptorelin
ay25650
see: triptorelin
ay 31906
see: 2 amino 4 (bicyclo[2.2.1]hept 2 ylamino) n (n isopropylcarbamoyl) 5 pyrimidinesulfonamide
ay31906
see: 2 amino 4 (bicyclo[2.2.1]hept 2 ylamino) n (n isopropylcarbamoyl) 5 pyrimidinesulfonamide
ay 61122
see: methallibure
ay61122
see: methallibure
ay 6204
see: pronetalol
ay6204
see: pronetalol
ay 64043
see: propranolol
ay64043
see: propranolol
azacort
see: deflazacort
azetazolamide
see: acetazolamide
azium
see: dexamethasone
azmacort
see: triamcinolone acetonide

azosemide

azoxodone
see: pemoline
b 1312
see: bupranolol
b1312
see: bupranolol
b 1500
see: mefruside
b1500
see: mefruside
b 24 76
see: 1 (2,4 dichlorophenoxy) 3 [2 (3,4 dimethoxyphenyl)ethylamino] 2 propanol
b 2476
see: 1 (2,4 dichlorophenoxy) 3 [2 (3,4 dimethoxyphenyl)ethylamino] 2 propanol
b2476
see: 1 (2,4 dichlorophenoxy) 3 [2 (3,4 dimethoxyphenyl)ethylamino] 2 propanol
b 436
see: prenylamine
b436
see: prenylamine
b 673
see: fluprednisolone
b673
see: fluprednisolone
b 9207 015
see: ciclesonide
b 9207015
see: ciclesonide

b9207 015
see: ciclesonide
b9207015
see: ciclesonide
ba 16038
see: aminoglutethimide
ba16038
see: aminoglutethimide
ba 29038
see: boldenone undecenoate
ba29038
see: boldenone undecenoate
ba 30920
see: tetracosactide
ba30920
see: tetracosactide
39089 ba
see: oxprenolol
39089ba
see: oxprenolol
ba 39,089
see: oxprenolol
ba 39089
see: oxprenolol
ba39,089
see: oxprenolol
ba39089
see: oxprenolol
bacarate
see: phendimetrazine tartrate
bacitracin oropivalone
see: oropivalone
badrin
see: amphetamine
balmadren
see: adrenalin
balnimax
see: oxymesterone
bambec
see: bambuterol

bambuterol

bamethan

bamethane
see: bamethan
bamethane sulfate
see: bamethan
bamethan succinate
see: bamethan
bamethan sulfate
see: bamethan
bantron
see: lobeline
barseb
see: hydrocortisone acetate
barseb hc
see: hydrocortisone
bay 1500
see: mefruside
bay1500
see: mefruside
bay c 7705
see: acebutolol
bay c7705
see: acebutolol
baycain green
see: noradrenalin
bay caron
see: mefruside
baycaron
see: mefruside
baycarone
see: mefruside

baycuten

bayer g 2821
see: muzolimine
bayer g2821
see: muzolimine
bay f 4797
see: baycuten
bay f4797
see: baycuten
bay g 2821
see: muzolimine
bay g2821
see: muzolimine
bay l 5240
see: acebutolol plus nifedipine
bay l5240
see: acebutolol plus nifedipine
bay r 1999
see: atenolol plus nifedipine
bay r1999
see: atenolol plus nifedipine

bazedoxifene

bazedoxifene acetate
see: bazedoxifene

bd 40a
see: formoterol fumarate
bd40a
see: formoterol fumarate
bdf 8186
see: brefonalol
bdf8186
see: brefonalol
be 14348b
see: 3 methylnaringenin
be14348b
see: 3 methylnaringenin
be 14348c
see: 3 methylnaringenin
be14348c
see: 3 methylnaringenin
be 14348d
see: 8 chloro 3 methylnaringenin
be14348d
see: 8 chloro 3 methylnaringenin
be 14348e
see: 8 chloro 3 methylnaringenin
be14348e
see: 8 chloro 3 methylnaringenin
be 724 a
see: bendroflumethiazide
be 724a
see: bendroflumethiazide
be724a
see: bendroflumethiazide
beben
see: betamethasone benzoate
beclamet
see: beclometasone dipropionate
beclate
see: beclometasone dipropionate
beclazone
see: beclometasone dipropionate
becloasma
see: beclometasone dipropionate
becloforte
see: beclometasone dipropionate
beclojet
see: beclometasone dipropionate
beclomet
see: beclometasone dipropionate

beclometasone

beclometasone dipropionate

beclomethasone
see: beclometasone
beclomethasone dipropionate
see: beclometasone dipropionate
beclomethazone dipropionate
see: beclometasone dipropionate
beclorhinol
see: beclometasone dipropionate
beclosol
see: beclometasone dipropionate
beclotaide
see: beclometasone dipropionate
becloturmant
see: beclometasone dipropionate
becloturmat
see: beclometasone dipropionate
beclovent
see: beclometasone dipropionate
becodisk
see: beclometasone dipropionate
becodisks
see: beclometasone dipropionate
beconase
see: beclometasone dipropionate
beconase aq
see: beclometasone dipropionate
beconasol
see: beclometasone dipropionate
becotide
see: beclometasone dipropionate
bedranol
see: propranolol
beef insulin
see: bovine insulin
befnolol
see: befunolol

befunolol

beglan
see: salmeterol
behyd ra
see: hydrochlorothiazide
bei 1293
see: xipamide
belidrin
see: buphenine
bellasthma medihaler
see: isoprenaline
bellasthman
see: isoprenaline

beloc
see: metoprolol tartrate
beloc comp
see: hydrochlorothiazide plus metoprolol tartrate
beloc duriles
see: metoprolol
beloderm
see: betamethasone dipropionate
belok zok
see: metoprolol

bemegride

bemequide
see: bemegride

bemetizide

bemetizide plus guabenxan
see: tensigradyl
bemetizide plus triamterene
see: diucomb
bemetson
see: betamethasone valerate
bemigride
see: bemegride

bemitradine

benatol
see: bevantolol

benazepril plus hydrochlorothiazide

bendrofluazide
see: bendroflumethiazide
bendrofluazide k
see: bendroflumethiazide

bendroflumethiazide

bendroflumethiazide plus nadolol

benemid
see: probenecid
benemide
see: probenecid
benemin
see: probenecid
benfuran
see: befunolol
benisolon
see: prednisolone
benisolone
see: prednisolone
benisone
see: betamethasone benzoate

benorterone

bentelan
see: betamethasone sodium phosphate
bentomex
see: tretoquinol
bentos
see: befunolol
bentos ophtadose
see: befunolol
bentox
see: befunolol
benzafinyl
see: amphetamine
benzebar
see: amphetamine
benzedrex
see: propylhexedrine
benzedrine
see: amphetamine
benzfetamine
see: benzphetamine
benzhydroflumethiazide
see: bendroflumethiazide
benzhydrylsulfinylacetamide
see: modafinil

alpha [[[3 (1 benzimidazolyl) 1,1 dimethylpropyl]amino]methyl] 2 fluoro 4 hydroxybenzyl alcohol

1 (1,3 benzodioxol 5 yl) n methyl 2 butanamine

benzolone
see: amphetamine
benzothiazide
see: benzthiazide
benzoylmethyl ecgonine
see: cocaine
1 benzoyltriethylamine
see: amfepramone

Index

benzphetamine

benzphetamine hydrochloride
see: benzphetamine
benzpropamin
see: amphetamine
benzpropamine
see: amphetamine

benzthiazide

benzthiazide plus triamterene

benzydroflumethiazide
see: bendroflumethiazide
2 benzyl 2 propylamine
see: phentermine
benzyl hydroflumethiazide
see: bendroflumethiazide
benzylhydroflumethiazide
see: bendroflumethiazide
benzylmetamphetamine
see: benzphetamine
benzylthiomethylchlorothiazide
see: benzthiazide
beprane
see: propranolol
berachin
see: tulobuterol
bercolol
see: propranolol
berisolon
see: prednisolone
berisolone
see: prednisolone
berkamil
see: amiloride
berkozide
see: bendroflumethiazide
berlinsulin
see: neutral insulin
berodual
see: fenoterol plus ipratropium bromide
berotec
see: fenoterol

besulpamide

beta 1 24 acth
see: tetracosactide
beta 1,24 acth
see: tetracosactide
beta 1 24 corticotrophin
see: tetracosactide
beta 1,24 corticotrophin
see: tetracosactide
beta 1 24 corticotropin
see: tetracosactide
beta 1,24 corticotropin
see: tetracosactide
beta 1,24 tetracosactide
see: tetracosactide
beta 19 nortestosterone
see: nandrolone
beta 1 adrenergic agonist
see: beta 1 adrenergic receptor stimulating agent
beta 1 adrenergic antagonist
see: beta 1 adrenergic receptor blocking agent
beta 1 adrenergic blocker
see: beta 1 adrenergic receptor blocking agent

beta 1 adrenergic receptor blocking agent

beta 1 adrenergic receptor stimulating agent

beta 1 adrenergic stimulant
see: beta 1 adrenergic receptor stimulating agent
beta 1 adrenoceptor blocker
see: beta 1 adrenergic receptor blocking agent
beta 2 adrenergic agent
see: beta 2 adrenergic receptor stimulating agent
beta 2 adrenergic agonist
see: beta 2 adrenergic receptor stimulating agent
beta 2 adrenergic antagonist
see: beta 2 adrenergic receptor blocking agent
beta 2 adrenergic blocker
see: beta 2 adrenergic receptor blocking agent

beta 2 adrenergic receptor blocking agent

beta 2 adrenergic receptor stimulating agent

beta 2 adrenergic stimulant
see: beta 2 adrenergic receptor stimulating agent
beta 3 adrenergic agonist
see: beta 3 adrenergic receptor stimulating agent
beta 3 adrenergic antagonist
see: beta 3 adrenergic receptor blocking agent

beta 3 adrenergic blocker
see: beta 3 adrenergic receptor blocking agent

beta 3 adrenergic receptor blocking agent

beta 3 adrenergic receptor stimulating agent

beta 3 adrenoceptor agonist
see: beta 3 adrenergic receptor stimulating agent
beta 3 adrenoceptor antagonist
see: beta 3 adrenergic receptor blocking agent
3beta,5alpha androstanediol
see: 3beta androstanediol
beta adalat
see: atenolol plus nifedipine
beta adalate
see: atenolol plus nifedipine
beta adrenergic agent
see: beta adrenergic receptor stimulating agent
beta adrenergic agonist
see: beta adrenergic receptor stimulating agent
beta adrenergic antagonist
see: beta adrenergic receptor blocking agent
beta adrenergic blocker
see: beta adrenergic receptor blocking agent
beta adrenergic blockers
see: beta adrenergic receptor blocking agent
beta adrenergic blocking agent
see: beta adrenergic receptor blocking agent
beta adrenergic blocking drug
see: beta adrenergic receptor blocking agent
beta adrenergic drug
see: beta adrenergic receptor stimulating agent
beta adrenergic receptor agent
see: beta adrenergic receptor stimulating agent

beta adrenergic receptor blocking agent

beta adrenergic receptor stimulating agent

beta adrenergic stimulant
see: beta adrenergic receptor stimulating agent
beta adrenergic stimulator
see: beta adrenergic receptor stimulating agent
beta adrenoceptor agonist
see: beta adrenergic receptor stimulating agent
beta adrenoceptor antagonist
see: beta adrenergic receptor blocking agent
beta adrenolytic
see: beta adrenergic receptor blocking agent
beta adrenolytic agent
see: beta adrenergic receptor blocking agent
beta agonist
see: beta adrenergic receptor stimulating agent
beta air
see: procaterol
beta aldopur
see: spironolactone
beta aminoisopropylbenzene
see: phentermine
beta aminopropylbenzene
see: amphetamine
5beta androstan 17 one
see: etiocholanone
5beta androstanone
see: etiocholanone
17 beta androstenediol
see: androstenediol
beta antagonist
see: beta adrenergic receptor blocking agent
beta antiadrenergic agent
see: beta adrenergic receptor blocking agent
beta blocker
see: beta adrenergic receptor blocking agent
beta blocking adrenergic agent
see: beta adrenergic receptor blocking agent
beta blocking agent
see: beta adrenergic receptor blocking agent
beta blocking drug
see: beta adrenergic receptor blocking agent
betacard
see: alprenolol
betacardone
see: sotalol
beta chain,hemoglobin
see: hemoglobin beta chain
beta chorionic gonadotropin
see: chorionic gonadotropin
beta cocaine
see: cocaine
betacor
see: cetamolol
beta corlan
see: betamethasone sodium phosphate
betacort
see: betamethasone valerate
beta corticotropin
see: corticotropin
betacortril
see: betamethasone

Index

betaderm
see: betamethasone valerate
betades
see: sotalol
betadexamethasone
see: betamethasone
5 beta dihydrotestosterone
see: 5beta androstanolone
5beta dihydrotestosterone
see: 5beta androstanolone
beta (dimethylamino)ethanol
see: deanol
beta dimethylaminoethanol
see: deanol
3beta diol
see: 3beta androstanediol
betadipresan
see: propranolol
betadol
see: nadolol
betadrenol
see: bupranolol
betafedrina
see: dexamphetamine
betafen
see: amphetamine
6beta flunisolide
see: flunisolide
betagan
see: levobunolol
betagon
see: mepindolol
beta hcg
see: chorionic gonadotropin beta subunit
3beta hydroxy 17 androstanone
see: prasterone
17beta hydroxy 4 estren 3 one
see: nandrolone
3beta hydroxy 5 pregnen 20 one
see: pregnenolone
3beta hydroxyandrostan 17 one
see: epiandrosterone
17beta hydroxyandrostan 3 one
see: androstanolone
11 beta hydroxyandrostenedione
see: 11beta hydroxyandrostenedione
11beta hydroxy androstenedione
see: 11beta hydroxyandrostenedione
6 beta hydroxycortisol
see: 6beta hydroxyhydrocortisone
6beta hydroxycortisol
see: 6beta hydroxyhydrocortisone
17beta hydroxyestr 4 en 3 one
see: nandrolone
3beta hydroxypregn 5 en 20 one
see: pregnenolone
beta isoket
see: isosorbide
betaloc
see: metoprolol
betalone
see: meprednisone
betamann
see: metipranolol
betamet
see: metipranolol
betametasone
see: betamethasone
beta metasone 17 valerate
see: betamethasone valerate
betametasone 17 valerate
see: betamethasone valerate
betametasone dipropionate
see: betamethasone dipropionate
betamethasolone
see: betamethasone
beta methason
see: betamethasone
betamethason
see: betamethasone
betamethason 17 valerate
see: betamethasone valerate

betamethasone

beta methasone
see: betamethasone
betamethasone 17 benzoate
see: betamethasone benzoate
beta methasone 17 valerate
see: betamethasone valerate
betamethasone 17 valerate
see: betamethasone valerate
betamethasone 17-valerate
see: betamethasone valerate
betamethasone 21 acetate
see: betamethasone acetate
betamethasone 21 phosphate
see: betamethasone sodium phosphate

betamethasone acetate

Index

betamethasone acetate plus betamethasone sodium phosphate

betamethasone alcohol
see: betamethasone

betamethasone benzoate

betamethasone derivative

betamethasone dipropionate

beta methasone phosphate
see: betamethasone sodium phosphate
betamethasone phosphate
see: betamethasone sodium phosphate

betamethasone sodium phosphate

betamethasone sodium phosphate plus neomycin

betamethasone valerate

beta methasone valerate
see: betamethasone valerate
betamethasone valerianate
see: betamethasone valerate
betamethasonium
see: betamethasone
betamethasonum
see: betamethasone
betamethazone
see: betamethasone
beta methazone 17 benzoate
see: betamethasone benzoate
betamethazone 17 valerate
see: betamethasone valerate
betamethazone valerate
see: betamethasone valerate
16beta methylprednisolene
see: 16beta methylprednisolone
beta methylprednisolone
see: methylprednisolone
16 beta methylprednisone
see: meprednisone
16beta methylprednisone
see: meprednisone
beta mimetic agent
see: beta adrenergic receptor stimulating agent
betanamin
see: pemoline
beta neg
see: propranolol
betaneg
see: propranolol
betanison
see: 16beta methylprednisolone
betanisone
see: 16beta methylprednisolone
betanol
see: metipranolol
betanolol
see: metipranolol
beta nortestosterone
see: nandrolone
17beta nortestosterone
see: nandrolone
11 beta oh androstenedione
see: 11beta hydroxyandrostenedione
beta ophtiole
see: metipranolol
betapace
see: sotalol
betapar
see: meprednisone
betaphedrine d
see: dexamphetamine
beta phenyl isopropylamine
see: amphetamine
beta phenylisopropylamine
see: amphetamine
beta phenyltert.butylamine
see: phentermine
betapin
see: alprenolol
betapindol
see: pindolol
betapred
see: meprednisone
betapressin
see: penbutolol
betaprol
see: propranolol
betapyrimidum
see: nikethamide
beta receptor blocker
see: beta adrenergic receptor blocking agent
beta receptor blocking agent
see: beta adrenergic receptor blocking agent

Index

betares
see: propranolol
betaryl
see: propranolol
betasite
see: levobunolol
beta stimulating drug
see: beta adrenergic receptor stimulating agent
beta subunit hcg
see: chorionic gonadotropin beta subunit
beta sympathetic agent
see: beta adrenergic receptor stimulating agent
beta sympathicolytic agent
see: beta adrenergic receptor blocking agent
beta sympathicolytics
see: beta adrenergic receptor blocking agent
beta sympathicomimetic
see: beta adrenergic receptor stimulating agent
beta sympathicomimetic agent
see: beta adrenergic receptor stimulating agent
beta sympatholytic agent
see: beta adrenergic receptor blocking agent
betasympatholytic agent
see: beta adrenergic receptor blocking agent
beta sympathomimetic agent
see: beta adrenergic receptor stimulating agent
beta sympathomimetic drug
see: beta adrenergic receptor stimulating agent
beta tablinen
see: propranolol
beta tablinen retard
see: propranolol
beta testosterone
see: testosterone
beta timelets
see: propranolol
beta trenbolone
see: trenbolone
17beta trenbolone
see: trenbolone
betatrex
see: betamethasone valerate
beta val
see: betamethasone valerate
betaval
see: betamethasone valerate

betaxolol

betaxolol hydrochloride
see: betaxolol
betaxon
see: betaxolol
betim
see: timolol maleate
betimol
see: timolol
betnasol
see: betamethasone
betnelan
see: betamethasone
betnelan v
see: betamethasone valerate
betnesol
see: betamethasone sodium phosphate
betnesol h
see: betamethasone
betnesol inj
see: betamethasone sodium phosphate
betnesol n
see: betamethasone sodium phosphate plus neomycin
betnesol v
see: betamethasone
betneval
see: betamethasone valerate
betnovat
see: betamethasone valerate
betnovate
see: betamethasone valerate
betnovate a
see: betamethasone
betnovate c
see: betamethasone valerate
betoptic
see: betaxolol
betoptima
see: betaxolol
betrilol
see: bunitrolol
betsolan
see: betamethasone
betsolon
see: betamethasone
betsopart
see: betamethasone

bevantolol

bevantolol hydrochloride
see: bevantolol
bextasol
see: betamethasone valerate

Index

bfe 55

bfe55
see: bfe 55

bfe 60
see: befunolol

bfe60
see: befunolol

bhang
see: cannabis

big insulin
see: proinsulin

bigonist
see: buserelin

binodrenal
see: noradrenalin bitartrate

biocapton
see: fenetylline

biocortone
see: prednisone

bioflutin
see: etilefrine

biomorphyl
see: hydromorphone

bionine
see: oxycodone

bionone
see: oxycodone

biophedrin
see: ephedrine

biorenine
see: adrenalin

biosynthetic erythropoietin
see: recombinant erythropoietin

biosynthetic growth hormone
see: recombinant growth hormone

biosynthetic human insulin
see: recombinant human insulin

biosynthetic human proinsulin

bio testiculina
see: testosterone propionate

bio teston
see: testosterone propionate

biotropin
see: human growth hormone

biphasic insulin

biphasic insulin injection
see: biphasic insulin

biphetamine
see: dexamphetamine

bird acth
see: corticotropin

bird corticotropin
see: corticotropin

1 [4 [n,n bis(2 chloroethyl)carbamoyloxy]phenyl] 1 (4 hydroxyphenyl) 2 phenyl 1 butene

2,3 bis(2 fluoro 4 hydroxyphenyl) 2,3 dimethylbutane

2,3 bis(2 fluoro 4 hydroxyphenyl) 2,3 dimethylbutane derivative

2,3 bis(4 hydroxyphenyl) 2,3 dimethylbutane

bis(4 hydroxyphenyl)cyclohexylidenemethane

bisalunil
see: hydrochlorothiazide

4 [3 [bis(beta hydroxyphenethyl)amino]butyl]benzamide

bisobloc
see: bisoprolol fumarate

bisocor
see: bisoprolol fumarate

bisoprolol

bisoprolol fumarate

bisoprolol fumarate plus hydrochlorothiazide

bis(perfluorohexyl)ethylene

bis(trifluoroethyl) ether
see: flurothyl

Index

biterol
see: bitolterol mesilate

bitolterol

bitolterol mesilate

bitolterol mesylate
see: bitolterol mesilate
bitolterol methanesulfonate
see: bitolterol mesilate
bl 343
see: 4 (2 hydroxy 3 isopropylaminopropoxy)carbanilic acid propyl ester
bl343
see: 4 (2 hydroxy 3 isopropylaminopropoxy)carbanilic acid propyl ester
bl 343 ac
see: 4 (2 hydroxy 3 isopropylaminopropoxy)carbanilic acid propyl ester
bl 343ac
see: 4 (2 hydroxy 3 isopropylaminopropoxy)carbanilic acid propyl ester
bl343 ac
see: 4 (2 hydroxy 3 isopropylaminopropoxy)carbanilic acid propyl ester
blocadren
see: timolol maleate
blocadrene
see: timolol maleate
blocanol
see: timolol maleate
blocotin
see: penbutolol
blokium
see: atenolol
blokium diu
see: atenolol plus chlortalidone
blood,artificial
see: artificial blood

blood derivative

blood extract

blood plasma substitute
see: plasma substitute

blood substitute

blood substitutes
see: blood substitute
blood volume expander
see: plasma substitute
bloxan
see: metoprolol tartrate
bluzedrin
see: amphetamine
bm 02015
see: torasemide
bm02015
see: torasemide
bm 10188
see: doxaminol
bm10188
see: doxaminol
bm 11604
see: tribendilol
bm11604
see: tribendilol
bm 14190
see: carvedilol
bm14190
see: carvedilol
bm 2015
see: torasemide
bm2015
see: torasemide
bm 51052
see: carazolol
bm51052
see: carazolol
bms 217380
see: tesmilifene
bms217380
see: tesmilifene
bmy 30056
see: ulobetasol propionate
bmy30056
see: ulobetasol propionate
bmy 33419
see: tesmilifene
bmy33419
see: tesmilifene
bmy 5763 1
see: sotalol
bmy 57631
see: sotalol
bmy5763 1
see: sotalol

Index

bmy57631
see: sotalol
bogadin tm
see: ibogaine

bolandiol

bolasterone

boldane
see: boldenone

boldenone

boldenone 10 undecenoate
see: boldenone undecenoate

boldenone undecenoate

boldenone undecylenate
see: boldenone undecenoate

boldione

bolodorm
see: oxycodone
boltin
see: tibolone
bolusacplus
see: hydrochlorothiazide plus telmisartan
bonpro
see: sotalol
bontril
see: phendimetrazine tartrate

bopindolol

bornaprolol

bosmin
see: adrenalin
bovine growth hormone
see: growth hormone
bovine icsh
see: luteinizing hormone

bovine insulin

bovine proinsulin
see: proinsulin

brain stimulant
see: central stimulant agent
brassel 1000
see: citicoline
brefanolol
see: brefonalol

brefonalol

brelomax
see: tulobuterol
bremax
see: tulobuterol
bremil
see: hydrochlorothiazide
brethair
see: terbutaline sulfate
brethaire
see: terbutaline sulfate
brethine
see: terbutaline
brevibloc
see: esmolol
bricanyl
see: terbutaline
bricanyl durettes
see: terbutaline
bricanyl durules
see: terbutaline
bricanyl respules
see: terbutaline
bricanyl retard
see: terbutaline

brimonidine

brimonidine tartrate
see: brimonidine
brinaldix
see: clopamide
brinedine
see: briserin
brinerdin
see: briserin
brinerdine
see: briserin
briserim
see: briserin

briserin

briserine
see: briserin

bristab
see: hydroflumethiazide
bristuron
see: bendroflumethiazide
brl 26830
see: 4 [2 [(2 hydroxy 2 phenylethyl)amino]propyl]benzoic acid methyl ester
brl26830
see: 4 [2 [(2 hydroxy 2 phenylethyl)amino]propyl]benzoic acid methyl ester
brl 26830a
see: 4 [2 [(2 hydroxy 2 phenylethyl)amino]propyl]benzoic acid methyl ester hydrogen maleate
brl26830a
see: 4 [2 [(2 hydroxy 2 phenylethyl)amino]propyl]benzoic acid methyl ester hydrogen maleate
brl 28410
see: 4 [2 [(2 hydroxy 2 phenylethyl)amino]propyl]benzoic acid
brl28410
see: 4 [2 [(2 hydroxy 2 phenylethyl)amino]propyl]benzoic acid
brl 35135
see: 4 [2 [[2 (3 chlorophenyl) 2 hydroxyethyl]amino]propyl]phenoxyacetic acid methyl ester
brl35135
see: 4 [2 [[2 (3 chlorophenyl) 2 hydroxyethyl]amino]propyl]phenoxyacetic acid methyl ester
brl 35135a
see: 4 [2 [[2 (3 chlorophenyl) 2 hydroxyethyl]amino]propyl]phenoxyacetic acid methyl ester
brl35135a
see: 4 [2 [[2 (3 chlorophenyl) 2 hydroxyethyl]amino]propyl]phenoxyacetic acid methyl ester
brl 37344
see: 4 [2 [[2 (3 chlorophenyl) 2 hydroxyethyl]amino]propyl]phenoxyacetic acid
brl37344
see: 4 [2 [[2 (3 chlorophenyl) 2 hydroxyethyl]amino]propyl]phenoxyacetic acid

brocrinat

brolamfetamine

bromantan

8 bromoacetamido 1 [2 hydroxy 3 (4 indolyloxy)propylamino] para menthane

bromoacetylalprenololmenthane

2 (4 bromoanilino)adamantane
see: bromantan

4 [n (4 bromobenzyl) n (1,2,4 triazol 4 yl)amino]benzonitrile

bromoheptadecafluorooctane
see: perfluorooctyl bromide
bronalide
see: flunisolide
bronchodil
see: reproterol
bronchodilatin
see: isoprenaline
bronchodual
see: fenoterol plus ipratropium bromide
broncholysin
see: hexoprenaline
bronchomister
see: isoprenaline
bronchosol
see: isoetarine
bronchospasmin
see: reproterol
broncho spray
see: salbutamol
broncodal
see: oxycodone
broncosol
see: isoetarine
bronilide
see: flunisolide
bronitin mist
see: adrenalin
bronkaid
see: adrenalin
bronkometer
see: isoetarine
bronkosol
see: isoetarine
bronsecur
see: carbuterol

Index

broxaterol

broxaterol hydrochloride
see: broxaterol

brucine

bta 243
see: 5 [2 [[2 (3 chlorophenyl) 2 hydroxyethyl]amino]propyl] 1,3 benzodioxole 2,2 dicarboxylic acid
bta243
see: 5 [2 [[2 (3 chlorophenyl) 2 hydroxyethyl]amino]propyl] 1,3 benzodioxole 2,2 dicarboxylic acid
buccalsone
see: hydrocortisone sodium succinate

bucindolol

bucindolol hydrochloride
see: bucindolol
bucodal
see: oxycodone
bucumarol
see: bucumolol

bucumolol

budecol
see: budesonide
budecort
see: budesonide
budefat
see: budesonide
budenoside
see: budesonide
budes
see: budesonide
budeson
see: budesonide

budesonide

budesonide plus formoterol

budiair
see: budesonide
budon
see: budesonide
bufarolol
see: bufuralol
bufedon
see: buphenine
bufenine
see: buphenine

bufetolol

bufuralol

bukorti
see: hydrocortisone butyrate
bukumolol
see: bucumolol
bumetamide
see: bumetanide

bumetanide

bumetidine
see: bumetanide
bumex
see: bumetanide

bunitrolol

bunitrolol hydrochloride
see: bunitrolol

bunolol

bunolol hydrochloride
see: bunolol
bunulol
see: bunolol
bunulol hydrochloride
see: bunolol
bupatol
see: bamethan
buphedrin
see: buphenine
buphenin
see: buphenine

buphenine

buphenine hydrochloride
see: buphenine
buphenin hydrochloride
see: buphenine

bupranolol

bupranolol hydrochloride
see: bupranolol

buprenex
see: buprenorphine

buprenorphine

buprex
see: buprenorphine

burinex
see: bumetanide

buserelin

buserelin acetate

buserelin carbazamide
see: goserelin

buserelline
see: buserelin

buserelin monoacetate
see: buserelin acetate

butalgin
see: methadone

butaxamine
see: butoxamine

butedrin
see: bamethan

butedrine
see: bamethan

buthiazide
see: butizide

butizide

butizide plus metipranolol
see: torrat

butizide plus spironolactone

butizide with metipranolol
see: torrat

butizide with spironolactone
see: butizide plus spironolactone

butofilolol

butovent
see: salbutamol

butoxamide
see: butoxamine

butoxamine

butoxomine hydrochloride
see: butoxamine

n butyl 11 (16alpha chloro 3,17beta dihydroxyestra 1,3,5(10) trien 7alpha yl) n methylundecanamide

n butyl 11 (3,17beta dihydroxyestra 1,3,5(10) trien 7alpha yl) n methylundecanamide

4 (3 tert butylamino 2 hydroxypropoxy) 2 benzimidazolone

1 tert butylamino 3 (2 chlorophenoxy) 2 propanol

1 tert butylamino 3 (2 methyl 4 indolyloxy) 2 propanol

1 tert butylamino 3 (3 methyl 2 nitrophenoxy) 2 propanol

9 (1 tert butylamino 3 hydroxy 2 propyloxyimino)fluorene

tert butylbicycloorthobenzoate

tert butylbicyclophosphorothioate

butyl norsynephrine
see: bamethan

butyloctopamine
see: bamethan

butylsympathol
see: bamethan

butylsympatol
see: bamethan

buventol
see: salbutamol

Index

bw 64 9
see: butoxamine
bw 64-9
see: butoxamine
bw 649
see: butoxamine
bw64-9
see: butoxamine
bw649
see: butoxamine
bw a575c
see: n [1 carboxy 5 [4 (2 hydroxy 3 isopropylaminopropoxy)indole 2 carboxamido]pentyl]alanylproline
bwa575c
see: n [1 carboxy 5 [4 (2 hydroxy 3 isopropylaminopropoxy)indole 2 carboxamido]pentyl]alanylproline
bw b385c
see: n [1 carboxy 5 [4 (2 hydroxy 3 isopropylaminopropoxy)indole 2 carboxamido]pentyl]alanylproline
bwb385c
see: n [1 carboxy 5 [4 (2 hydroxy 3 isopropylaminopropoxy)indole 2 carboxamido]pentyl]alanylproline
bx 591
see: acefluranol
bx591
see: acefluranol
by 9010
see: ciclesonide
by9010
see: ciclesonide
byk 1512
see: hexoprenaline
byk1512
see: hexoprenaline
bymex
see: bumetanide
c 1628
see: nitromifene
c1628
see: nitromifene
c 17309
see: metandienone
c17309
see: metandienone
c 4311-b
see: methylphenidate
c4311-b
see: methylphenidate
c4311b
see: methylphenidate
c 78
see: tulobuterol
c78
see: tulobuterol
caa 40
see: isoxsuprine
caa40
see: isoxsuprine
caberdelta
see: prednisolone
cafacodal
see: oxycodone
cafcit
see: caffeine citrate
cafedrine and theodrenaline
see: cafedrine plus theodrenaline

cafedrine plus theodrenaline

cafeine
see: caffeine
caffein
see: caffeine
caffein benzoate
see: caffeine benzoate

caffeine

caffeine benzoate

caffeine benzoate sodium
see: caffeine benzoate
caffeine calcium complex
see: caffeine

caffeine citrate

caffeine sodium benzoate
see: caffeine benzoate
calcium caffeine
see: caffeine
calcort
see: deflazacort
caldecort
see: hydrocortisone acetate
calmurid hc
see: hydrocortisone plus urea
calonat
see: dexamethasone

calonat 17 valerate
see: dexamethasone 17 valerate

calusterone

calvan
see: bevantolol
calvisken
see: pindolol
camphozone
see: nikethamide

cannabichromene

cannabidiol

cannabidiol derivative

cannabidiol dimethyl ether

cannabidiol methyl ether

cannabidiol monomethyl ether
see: cannabidiol methyl ether

cannabielsoin

cannabigerol

cannabinoid

cannabinoid derivative

cannabinoids
see: cannabinoid

cannabinol

cannabinol derivative

cannabis

cannabis alkaloid
see: cannabis
cannabis component
see: cannabis derivative
cannabis constituent
see: cannabis

cannabis derivative

cannabis extract
see: cannabis
cannabis herba
see: cannabis
cannabis indica
see: cannabis
cannabis indicae
see: cannabis
cannabis leaf
see: cannabis
cannabis sativa
see: cannabis
cannabis sativa derivative
see: cannabis derivative
cannabis sativa extract
see: cannabis
cannabis sativa leaf
see: cannabis
cannabis sativa var. indica
see: cannabis
cannabis substitution
see: cannabis
canrenoate
see: canrenoic acid

canrenoate potassium

canrenoate sodium
see: canrenoic acid

canrenoic acid

canrenol
see: canrenoate potassium

canrenone

canrenone,6,7 dihydro
see: 6,7 dihydrocanrenone

canrenone derivative

capozide
see: captopril plus hydrochlorothiazide

captagon
see: fenetylline
captea
see: captopril plus hydrochlorothiazide

captopril plus hydrochlorothiazide

carazolol

carbamidal
see: nikethamide
carbamoylinsulin
see: insulin derivative
carbamylinsulin
see: insulin derivative
carbon monoxide hemoglobin
see: carboxyhemoglobin
carbon monoxyhemoglobin
see: carboxyhemoglobin
carbonmonoxyhemoglobin
see: carboxyhemoglobin
carbonolol
see: carteolol
carbonyl bis methionyl insulin
see: insulin derivative
carbonyl hemoglobin
see: carboxyhemoglobin
carbonylhemoglobin
see: carboxyhemoglobin

n [1 carboxy 5 [4 (2 hydroxy 3 isopropylaminopropoxy)indole 2 carboxamido]pentyl]alanylproline

carboxyhaemoglobin
see: carboxyhemoglobin

carboxyhemoglobin

carboxy hemoglobin
see: carboxyhemoglobin
carboxyphen
see: dexamphetamine
11 carboxytetrahydrocannabinol
see: tetrahydrocannabinolic acid

carbuterol

carcinil
see: leuprorelin
cardamin
see: nikethamide
cardanon
see: oxycodone
cardiagen
see: nikethamide
cardiamid
see: nikethamide
cardiamin
see: nikethamide
cardiamina
see: nikethamide
cardiamine
see: nikethamide
cardiazol
see: pentetrazole
cardiazole
see: pentetrazole
cardiazolum
see: pentetrazole
cardifortan
see: pentetrazole
cardimon
see: nikethamide
cardinol
see: propranolol
cardiopiridina
see: nikethamide
cardiovanil
see: etamivan
cardosal
see: pentetrazole
cardosan
see: pentetrazole
cardrase
see: ethoxzolamide
cardrax
see: ethoxzolamide
cardraze
see: ethoxzolamide
carfedon
see: carphedon
carfedone
see: carphedon
caridian
see: mepindolol
carnigen
see: oxilofrine
carnigen forte
see: oxilofrine

carphedon

carphedone
see: carphedon

carp pituitary gonadotropin
see: gonadotropin
carteol
see: carteolol

carteolol

carteolol,8 hydroxy
see: 8 hydroxycarteolol
carteolol hydrochloride
see: carteolol
cartrol
see: carteolol

carvedilol

carvisken
see: pindolol
carwin
see: xamoterol hydrogen fumarate
catabon
see: dopamine
cathin
see: norpseudoephedrine
cathine
see: norpseudoephedrine
catovit
see: prolintane
caurenoate
see: canrenoic acid
caurenoic acid
see: canrenoic acid
caurenone
see: canrenone
cb 311
see: human growth hormone
cb311
see: human growth hormone
cb 7432
see: idoxifene
cb7432
see: idoxifene
8109 cb
see: canrenoate potassium
8109cb
see: canrenoate potassium
cb 8109
see: canrenoate potassium
cb8109
see: canrenoate potassium
cci 18781
see: fluticasone propionate
cci18781
see: fluticasone propionate
cci 22277
see: 2beta ethoxy 3alpha hydroxy 11alpha isopentylamino 5alpha androstane 17beta carboxylic acid methyl ester
cci22277
see: 2beta ethoxy 3alpha hydroxy 11alpha isopentylamino 5alpha androstane 17beta carboxylic acid methyl ester
cci 4725
see: clobetasol propionate
cci4725
see: clobetasol propionate
cci 5537
see: clobetasone butyrate
cci5537
see: clobetasone butyrate
cddd 5604
see: loteprednol etabonate
cddd5604
see: loteprednol etabonate
CDP choline
see: citicoline
cdri 85 287
see: 2 [4 (2 piperidinoethoxy)phenyl] 3 phenyl 2h 1 benzopyran
cdri 85-287
see: 2 [4 (2 piperidinoethoxy)phenyl] 3 phenyl 2h 1 benzopyran
cdri 85287
see: 2 [4 (2 piperidinoethoxy)phenyl] 3 phenyl 2h 1 benzopyran
cdri85 287
see: 2 [4 (2 piperidinoethoxy)phenyl] 3 phenyl 2h 1 benzopyran
cdri85-287
see: 2 [4 (2 piperidinoethoxy)phenyl] 3 phenyl 2h 1 benzopyran
cdri85287
see: 2 [4 (2 piperidinoethoxy)phenyl] 3 phenyl 2h 1 benzopyran
cebedex
see: dexamethasone
cecostrate
see: deoxycorticosterone
celectol
see: celiprolol

celestamine

celestan
see: betamethasone

celestan depot
see: betamethasone
celestan v
see: betamethasone
celeste
see: triamcinolone
celestene
see: betamethasone
celestoderm
see: betamethasone valerate
celestoderm v
see: betamethasone valerate
celestona
see: betamethasone
celestona c
see: betamethasone valerate
celeston chronodose
see: betamethasone
celestone
see: betamethasone
celestone soluspan
see: betamethasone acetate plus betamethasone sodium phosphate
celestone valerate
see: betamethasone valerate

celiprolol

celiprolol hydrochloride
see: celiprolol
cenalene m
see: pentetrazole
cenazol
see: pentetrazole
cenocort forte
see: triamcinolone diacetate

centchroman

centedrin
see: methylphenidate
centonuron
see: bendroflumethiazide
centralgin
see: pethidine
centralgine
see: pethidine
central stimulant
see: central stimulant agent

central stimulant agent

central stimulating agent
see: central stimulant agent
centramine
see: amphetamine
centrazole
see: pentetrazole
centron
see: centchroman
centrophenoxin
see: meclofenoxate
centrophenoxine
see: meclofenoxate
centrophenoxine hydrochloride
see: meclofenoxate
centroton
see: pyrovalerone
centyl
see: bendroflumethiazide
CERA
see: continuous erythropoiesis receptor activator
ceraxon
see: citicoline
cerson
see: flumetasone pivalate
cersone
see: flumetasone pivalate
certadyn
see: buphenine
cerutil
see: meclofenoxate
cetacort
see: hydrocortisone

cetamolol

cgp 12177
see: 4 (3 tert butylamino 2 hydroxypropoxy) 2 benzimidazolone
cgp12177
see: 4 (3 tert butylamino 2 hydroxypropoxy) 2 benzimidazolone
cgp 12177a
see: 4 (3 tert butylamino 2 hydroxypropoxy) 2 benzimidazolone
cgp12177a
see: 4 (3 tert butylamino 2 hydroxypropoxy) 2 benzimidazolone
cgp 14458
see: ulobetasol propionate
cgp14458
see: ulobetasol propionate

Index

cgp 17582
see: salcardolol
cgp17582
see: salcardolol
cgp 17582 b
see: salcardolol
cgp 17582b
see: salcardolol
cgp17582b
see: salcardolol
cgp 20712
see: 5 [2 [[2 hydroxy 3 [4 (1 methyl 4 trifluoromethyl 2 imidazolyl)phenoxy]propyl]amino]ethoxy]salicylamide
cgp20712
see: 5 [2 [[2 hydroxy 3 [4 (1 methyl 4 trifluoromethyl 2 imidazolyl)phenoxy]propyl]amino]ethoxy]salicylamide
cgp 20712 a
see: 5 [2 [[2 hydroxy 3 [4 (1 methyl 4 trifluoromethyl 2 imidazolyl)phenoxy]propyl]amino]ethoxy]salicylamide
cgp 20712a
see: 5 [2 [[2 hydroxy 3 [4 (1 methyl 4 trifluoromethyl 2 imidazolyl)phenoxy]propyl]amino]ethoxy]salicylamide
cgp20712a
see: 5 [2 [[2 hydroxy 3 [4 (1 methyl 4 trifluoromethyl 2 imidazolyl)phenoxy]propyl]amino]ethoxy]salicylamide
cgp 2175e
see: metoprolol tartrate
cgp2175e
see: metoprolol tartrate
cgp 25827a
see: formoterol fumarate
cgp25827a
see: formoterol fumarate
cgp 25827 a-e
see: formoterol fumarate
cgp 25827a-e
see: formoterol fumarate
cgp25827a-e
see: formoterol fumarate
cgp 30 083
see: eplerenone
cgp 30083
see: eplerenone
cgp30083
see: eplerenone
cgp 32349
see: formestane
cgp32349
see: formestane
cgp 361 a
see: isamoltane
cgp 361a
see: isamoltane
cgp361a
see: isamoltane
cgp 7760b
see: prenalterol
cgp7760b
see: prenalterol
cgs 16949
see: fadrozole
cgs16949
see: fadrozole
cgs 16949 a
see: fadrozole
cgs 16949a
see: fadrozole
cgs16949a
see: fadrozole
cgs 18320b
see: 1 (4,4' dicyanobenzhydryl)imidazole
cgs18320b
see: 1 (4,4' dicyanobenzhydryl)imidazole
cgs 20267
see: letrozole
cgs20267
see: letrozole
ch 103
see: 4 cyclohexylamino 1 (1 naphthyloxy) 2 butanol
ch103
see: 4 cyclohexylamino 1 (1 naphthyloxy) 2 butanol
chara
see: cannabis
charas
see: cannabis
chelafrin
see: adrenalin
'cheque'
see: mibolerone
chetovis
see: prasterone
17 chetovis
see: prasterone
17 chetovis 3 sulfate
see: prasterone sulfate
chf 023
see: ambroxol plus clenbuterol

Index

chf023
see: ambroxol plus clenbuterol
chibro timoptol
see: timolol
chinethazon
see: quinethazone
chinethazone
see: quinethazone
chinoin 103
see: 4 cyclohexylamino 1 (1 naphthyloxy) 2 butanol
chinoin103
see: 4 cyclohexylamino 1 (1 naphthyloxy) 2 butanol
chlomerodrin
see: chlormerodrin

chloramphetamine

chlorfentermine
see: chlorphentermine

chlormerodrin

chlormerodrine
see: chlormerodrin
chlormeroprin
see: chlormerodrin
chlormethamphetamine
see: 4 chloromethamphetamine

4 chloro 17beta hydroxy 17 methylandrosta 1,4 dien 3 one

4 chloro 19 nortestosterone
see: norclostebol
4 chloro 19 nortestosterone acetate
see: norclostebol acetate

8 chloro 1 [alpha (2 dimethylaminoethyl)benzyl] 6 phenyl 4h 1,2,4 triazolo[4,3 a][1,4]benzodiazepine

8 chloro 3 (2 fluorophenyl) 5,6 dihydrofuro[3,2 f][1,2]benzisoxazole 6 carboxylate potassium

[[5 chloro 3 (2 methylphenyl) 4 oxo 4h benzopyran 7 yl]oxy]acetic acid

8 chloro 3 methylnaringenin

8 chloro 5 (4 chlorophenyl) 5h indeno[1,2 d]pyrimidine

chloroamphetamine
see: chloramphetamine
4 chloroamphetamine
see: chloramphetamine
4 chlorodeoxyephedrine
see: 4 chloromethamphetamine
4 chloro desoxyephedrine
see: 4 chloromethamphetamine
4 chlorodesoxyephedrine
see: 4 chloromethamphetamine
chloromerodrin
see: chlormerodrin
4 chlorometandienone
see: 4 chloro 17beta hydroxy 17 methylandrosta 1,4 dien 3 one
chloromethamphetamine
see: 4 chloromethamphetamine

4 chloromethamphetamine

4 chloromethandienone
see: 4 chloro 17beta hydroxy 17 methylandrosta 1,4 dien 3 one
4 chloromethylamphetamine
see: 4 chloromethamphetamine
chlorometrodrine
see: chlormerodrin

3 chloro n (1,2,3,4 tetrahydro 7 hydroxy 2 naphthyl)phenylethanolamine

3 chloro n (7 ethoxycarbonylmethoxy 1,2,3,4 tetrahydro 2 naphthyl)phenylethanolamine

4 chloronandrolone
see: norclostebol
4 chloronandrolone acetate
see: norclostebol acetate
4 chloronortestosterone
see: norclostebol
4 chloronortestosterone acetate
see: norclostebol acetate
chlorophentermine
see: chlorphentermine

[[7 [[2 (3 chlorophenyl) 2 hydroxyethyl]amino] 5,6,7,8 tetrahydro 2 naphthyl]oxy]acetic acid ethyl ester

5 [2 [[2 (3 chlorophenyl) 2 hydroxyethyl]amino]propyl] 1,3 benzodioxole 2,2 dicarboxylic acid

4 [2 [[2 (3 chlorophenyl) 2 hydroxyethyl]amino]propyl]phenoxyacetic acid

4 [2 [[2 (3 chlorophenyl) 2 hydroxyethyl]amino]propyl]phenoxyacetic acid methyl ester

chloroprednisone

chlorosal
see: chlorothiazide

chlorosulthiadil
see: hydrochlorothiazide

chlorotestosterone
see: clostebol

4 chlorotestosterone
see: clostebol

chlorotestosterone acetate
see: clostebol acetate

4 chlorotestosterone acetate
see: clostebol acetate

chlorothiazid
see: chlorothiazide

chlorothiazide

chlorothiazide derivative

chlorothiazide diuretic agent
see: chlorothiazide derivative

chlorothiazide sodium
see: chlorothiazide

chlorothiazide sodium salt
see: chlorothiazide

chlorothiazidum
see: chlorothiazide

chlorothiazine
see: chlorothiazide

chlorphentarmine hydrochloride
see: chlorphentermine

chlorphentermin
see: chlorphentermine

chlorphentermine

chlorphentermine hydrochloride
see: chlorphentermine

chlorphentermine sl
see: chlorphentermine

chlorphenterminumhydrochlorid
see: chlorphentermine

chlorphthalidolone
see: chlortalidone

chlorphthalidone
see: chlortalidone

chlorprednisone
see: chloroprednisone

chlorprenaline
see: clorprenaline

chlortalidon
see: chlortalidone

chlortalidone

chlortalidone plus atenolol
see: atenolol plus chlortalidone

chlortalidone plus metoprolol

chlortalidone plus oxprenolol
see: trasitensin

chlortalidone plus reserpine

chlortermine
see: clortermine

chlortestosterone
see: clostebol

4 chlortestosterone
see: clostebol

chlortestosterone acetate
see: clostebol acetate

4 chlortestosterone acetate
see: clostebol acetate

chlorthalidine
see: chlortalidone

chlorthalidon
see: chlortalidone

chlorthalidone
see: chlortalidone

chlorthialidone
see: chlortalidone
chlorthiazide
see: chlorothiazide
chlosudimeprimylum
see: clopamide
chlotride
see: chlorothiazide
choice 7
see: centchroman
choragon
see: chorionic gonadotropin
chorigon
see: chorionic gonadotropin
choriogonadotrophin
see: chorionic gonadotropin
choriogonadotropin
see: chorionic gonadotropin
choriogonin
see: chorionic gonadotropin
chorion gonadotrophic hormone
see: chorionic gonadotropin
chorion gonadotrophin
see: chorionic gonadotropin
chorion gonadotropin
see: chorionic gonadotropin
chorionic gonadotrophin
see: chorionic gonadotropin
chorionic gonadotropic hormone
see: chorionic gonadotropin

chorionic gonadotropin

chorionic gonadotropin alpha subunit

chorionic gonadotropin beta subunit

chorionic gonadropin
see: chorionic gonadotropin
choron
see: chorionic gonadotropin
chorulon
see: chorionic gonadotropin
chronogyn
see: danazol
ci 406
see: oxymetholone
ci406
see: oxymetholone
ci 456
see: tiamizide
ci456
see: tiamizide
ci 628
see: nitromifene
ci628
see: nitromifene
ci 755
see: bevantolol
ci755
see: bevantolol
ci 775
see: bevantolol
ci775
see: bevantolol
ci 888
see: procaterol
ci888
see: procaterol
ciba 29038
see: boldenone
ciba29038
see: boldenone
ciba 39089
see: oxprenolol
ciba39089
see: oxprenolol
ciba 39 089 b
see: oxprenolol
ciba 39089 b
see: oxprenolol
ciba 39089b
see: oxprenolol
ciba39089b
see: oxprenolol
ciba 39 089 ba
see: oxprenolol
ciba 39 089ba
see: oxprenolol
ciba 39,089 ba
see: oxprenolol
ciba 39,089ba
see: oxprenolol
ciba 39.089 ba
see: oxprenolol
ciba 39.089ba
see: oxprenolol
ciba 39089 ba
see: oxprenolol
ciba 39089ba
see: oxprenolol
ciba39,089 ba
see: oxprenolol

ciba39.089 ba
see: oxprenolol
ciba39089ba
see: oxprenolol
ciba 39.889 ba
see: alprenolol
ciba 42.244 ba
see: oxprenolol
ciba 42.244ba
see: oxprenolol
ciba42.244ba
see: oxprenolol
cibacthen
see: corticotropin
cibadrex
see: benazepril plus hydrochlorothiazide
cibutamol
see: salbutamol

ciclesonide

cicloprolol

ciclosterone
see: testosterone cipionate
cidamex
see: acetazolamide
cidifos
see: citicoline
cidiphos
see: citicoline
cidoten
see: betamethasone
cidrex
see: hydrochlorothiazide

cilazapril plus hydrochlorothiazide

cilder
see: clocortolone pivalate

cimaterol

cimatrol
see: cimaterol
c.indica
see: cannabis
ciplar
see: propranolol

ciprocinonide

circovenil
see: buphenine
circupon
see: etilefrine
cis clomifene citrate
see: zuclomifene citrate
cis clomiphene
see: zuclomifene
cisclomiphene
see: zuclomifene
cis clomiphene citrate
see: zuclomifene citrate
cis morphine
see: morphine
citicholine
see: citicoline
citicolin
see: citicoline
citicolina
see: citicoline

citicoline

citocor
see: nikethamide
cl 112,302
see: buprenorphine
cl 112302
see: buprenorphine
cl112,302
see: buprenorphine
cl112302
see: buprenorphine
cl 19823
see: triamcinolone
cl19823
see: triamcinolone
cl 263780
see: cimaterol
cl263780
see: cimaterol
cl 297939
see: bisoprolol fumarate
cl297939
see: bisoprolol fumarate
cl 314514
see: 5 [2 [[2 (3 chlorophenyl) 2 hydroxyethyl]amino]propyl] 1,3 benzodioxole 2,2 dicarboxylic acid
cl314514
see: 5 [2 [[2 (3 chlorophenyl) 2 hydroxyethyl]ami-

Index

no]propyl] 1,3 benzodioxole 2,2 dicarboxylic acid
cl 316243
see: 5 [2 [[2 (3 chlorophenyl) 2 hydroxyethyl]amino]propyl] 1,3 benzodioxole 2,2 dicarboxylic acid
cl316243
see: 5 [2 [[2 (3 chlorophenyl) 2 hydroxyethyl]amino]propyl] 1,3 benzodioxole 2,2 dicarboxylic acid
cl 34433
see: triamcinolone hexacetonide
cl34433
see: triamcinolone hexacetonide
cl 34699
see: amcinonide
cl34699
see: amcinonide
cl 628
see: nitromifene
cl628
see: nitromifene
cl 68
see: clocortolone pivalate
cl68
see: clocortolone pivalate
cl 68 creme
see: clocortolone pivalate
cl68 creme
see: clocortolone pivalate
cl 775
see: bevantolol
cl775
see: bevantolol
cl 8490
see: methazolamide
cl8490
see: methazolamide
cl 911 c
see: dexoxadrol
cl 911c
see: dexoxadrol
cl911c
see: dexoxadrol
clairvan
see: etamivan
clear aid
see: hydrocortisone acetate
clemodril
see: prenylamine
clenasma
see: clenbuterol

clenbuterol

clenbuterol hydrochloride
see: clenbuterol
clenbuterol pharmachim
see: clenbuterol
clenbuterol plus ambroxol
see: ambroxol plus clenbuterol
clenbutol
see: clenbuterol
clenil
see: beclometasone dipropionate
climacterion
see: testosterone enantate benziloylhydrazone
climacteron
see: testosterone enantate benziloylhydrazone

clioquinol plus dexamethasone

clioquinol plus flumetasone pivalate

c.l.i.p.
see: corticotropin[18-39]
clobederm
see: clobetasol propionate

clobenzorex

clobenzorex hydrochloride
see: clobenzorex
clobesol
see: clobetasol propionate

clobetasol

clobetasol 17 propionate
see: clobetasol propionate

clobetasol butyrate

clobetasol propionate

clobetasone

clobetasone 17 butyrate
see: clobetasone butyrate

Index

clobetasone butyrate

clocinnamox

clocortolon
see: clocortolone

clocortolone

clocortolone 21 pivalate
see: clocortolone pivalate

clocortolone pivalate

clocortolone trimethylacetate
see: clocortolone pivalate
cloderm
see: clocortolone pivalate
clofibrate plus androsterone
see: atromid
clomid
see: clomifene citrate
clomifen
see: clomifene

clomifene

clomifene acid
see: clomifene

clomifene citrate

clomifene citrate isomer
see: clomifene citrate
clomifene dihydrogen citrate
see: clomifene citrate
clomifene isomer
see: clomifene
clomiphen
see: clomifene
clomiphene
see: clomifene
clomiphene citrate
see: clomifene citrate
clomiphene citrate isomer
see: clomifene citrate
clomivid
see: clomifene citrate
clonidine,4 amino
see: apraclonidine
clopamid
see: clopamide

clopamide

clopamide plus pindolol
see: viskaldix
clopamidum
see: clopamide
clopamine
see: clopamide
clopane
see: cyclopentamine
clopane hydrochloride
see: cyclopentamine

cloprednol

cloranolol

clorfentermina
see: chlorphentermine

clorprenaline

clorprenaline hydrochloride
see: clorprenaline
clortalidone
see: chlortalidone

clortermine

clortermine hydrochloride
see: clortermine

clostebol

clostebol acetate

clostilbegyt
see: clomifene citrate
clovate
see: clobetasol propionate
cm 57227
see: 4 amino 1 (6 chloro 2 pyridyl)piperidine
cm57227
see: 4 amino 1 (6 chloro 2 pyridyl)piperidine
cm 57373
see: 4 amino 1 (6 bromo 2 pyridyl)piperidine
cm57373
see: 4 amino 1 (6 bromo 2 pyridyl)piperidine
cm 9155
see: difluprednate

Index

cm9155
see: difluprednate
cn 36,337
see: tiamizide
cn 36337
see: tiamizide
cn36,337
see: tiamizide
cn36337
see: tiamizide
cn 55,945
see: nitromifene
cn 55945
see: nitromifene
cn55,945
see: nitromifene
cn55945
see: nitromifene
cn 55 945 27
see: nitromifene
cn 55945 27
see: nitromifene
cn 5594527
see: nitromifene
cn55945 27
see: nitromifene
cn5594527
see: nitromifene
CNS stimulant
see: central stimulant agent
co amilofruse
see: frumil
co amilozide
see: amiloride plus hydrochlorothiazide
co aprovel
see: hydrochlorothiazide plus irbesartan
coaprovel
see: hydrochlorothiazide plus irbesartan
cobadex
see: hydrocortisone
cobeloc
see: hydrochlorothiazide plus metoprolol tartrate
co betaloc
see: hydrochlorothiazide plus metoprolol tartrate
cobetaloc
see: hydrochlorothiazide plus metoprolol tartrate
cobutolin
see: salbutamol sulfate
cocaethylene
see: homococaine
cocaethylin
see: homococaine
cocain
see: cocaine

cocaine

cocaine hydrochloride
see: cocaine
cocaine methiodide
see: cocaine
cocain hydrochloride
see: cocaine
cocculin
see: picrotoxin
cocethyline
see: homococaine
codelcortone
see: prednisolone
codelsol
see: prednisolone sodium phosphate
codenon
see: oxycodone
codidramol
see: codydramol
co diovan
see: hydrochlorothiazide plus valsartan
co-diovan
see: hydrochlorothiazide plus valsartan
codiovan
see: hydrochlorothiazide plus valsartan
codrenine
see: cocaine

codydramol

cofalaudid
see: hydromorphone
coffein
see: caffeine
coffeine
see: caffeine
coffeine sodium benzoate
see: caffeine benzoate
co hydeltra
see: prednisolone
colectril
see: amiloride
colifoam
see: hydrocortisone acetate
colisone
see: prednisone
colloidal plasma substitute
see: plasma substitute

colofoam
see: dexamethasone
colterol 3,4 di para toluate
see: bitolterol

combivent

compound 133314
see: trioxifene mesilate
compound 6063
see: acetazolamide
compound 81929
see: dobutamine
compound e (kendall)
see: cortisone
compound f
see: hydrocortisone
concerta
see: methylphenidate
concerta xl
see: methylphenidate
concor
see: bisoprolol fumarate
conducton
see: carazolol
confidol
see: etilefrine
conovliss
see: isosorbide
contaren
see: canrenone

continuous erythropoiesis receptor activator

contrasmina
see: clenbuterol
contraspasmin
see: clenbuterol
convulsant
see: convulsant agent

convulsant agent

convulsant compound
see: convulsant agent
convulsant drug
see: convulsant agent
convulsants
see: convulsant agent
convulsive agent
see: convulsant agent
cophedrine
see: racephedrine
co prenozide
see: cyclopenthiazide plus oxprenolol
co-prenozide
see: cyclopenthiazide plus oxprenolol
coprenozide
see: cyclopenthiazide plus oxprenolol
coracon
see: nikethamide
coraethamide
see: nikethamide
coraethamidum
see: nikethamide
coralept
see: nikethamide
coramine
see: nikethamide
coranormol
see: pentetrazole
corasole
see: pentetrazole
coravita
see: nikethamide
corazol
see: pentetrazole
corazole
see: pentetrazole
corazone
see: nikethamide
corbeta
see: propranolol
cordanum
see: talinolol
cordes h
see: hydrocortisone acetate
cordexol
see: oxprenolol
cordiamid
see: nikethamide
cordiamin
see: nikethamide
cordiamine
see: nikethamide
cordin
see: nikethamide
corditon
see: nikethamide
cordran
see: fludroxycortide
cordran n
see: fludroxycortide

cordynil
see: nikethamide
corediol
see: nikethamide
coreg
see: carvedilol
co renitec
see: enalapril plus hydrochlorothiazide
coreopsin
see: nikethamide
coreptil
see: heptaminol
corespin
see: nikethamide
coretal
see: oxprenolol
corethamide
see: nikethamide
corethamidum
see: nikethamide
co retinec
see: enalapril plus hydrochlorothiazide
coretone
see: nikethamide
corgard
see: nadolol
corgaretic
see: bendroflumethiazide plus nadolol
corgaretic n
see: bendroflumethiazide plus nadolol
corgaretic s
see: bendroflumethiazide plus nadolol
coriantin
see: chorionic gonadotropin
corindolan
see: mepindolol
corivanil
see: etamivan
corlan
see: hydrocortisone sodium succinate
corlin
see: cortisone
corlopam
see: fenoldopam mesilate
cormed
see: nikethamide
cormid
see: nikethamide
cormotyl
see: nikethamide
corotonin
see: nikethamide
corpormon
see: human growth hormone
corson 17 valerate
see: dexamethasone 17 valerate
corsotalol
see: sotalol
cortadeltona
see: prednisolone
cortadeltone
see: prednisolone
cortadren
see: cortisone
cortagen
see: cortisone
cortaid
see: hydrocortisone acetate
cortal
see: cortisone acetate
cortancyl
see: prednisone acetate
cortandren
see: cortisone
cortane
see: cortisone
cortarmour
see: deoxycorticosterone
cortate
see: deoxycorticosterone acetate
cort dome
see: hydrocortisone
cortef
see: hydrocortisone
cortef acetate
see: hydrocortisone acetate
cortelan
see: cortisone acetate
cortelinter
see: prednisolone
cortenema
see: hydrocortisone
cortenil
see: deoxycorticosterone acetate
cortensor
see: heptaminol
cortesan
see: deoxycorticosterone acetate
cortexilar
see: flumetasone
cortexon
see: deoxycorticosterone
cortexone
see: deoxycorticosterone

cortibel
see: hydrocortisone
corti clyss
see: prednisolone 3 sulfobenzoate
corticobiss
see: corticotropin releasing factor
corticoderm
see: fluprednidene acetate
corticoliberin
see: corticotropin releasing factor
corticorelin
see: corticotropin releasing factor
corticotrophin
see: corticotropin
1,39 corticotrophin
see: corticotropin
corticotrophin analog
see: corticotropin derivative
corticotrophine
see: corticotropin
corticotrophin gelatin
see: corticotropin
corticotropic hormone
see: corticotropin

corticotropin

corticotropin[1-10]

corticotropin 1 10
see: corticotropin[1-10]
corticotropin [1-10]
see: corticotropin[1-10]

corticotropin[11-24]

corticotropin [11-24]
see: corticotropin[11-24]

corticotropin[1-17]

corticotropin 1 17
see: corticotropin[1-17]
1 24 corticotropin
see: tetracosactide
corticotropin 1 24
see: tetracosactide
corticotropin [1-24]
see: tetracosactide
corticotropin[1-24] zinc
see: tetracosactide zinc phosphate

corticotropin[1-39]

corticotropin (1-39)
see: corticotropin[1-39]
corticotropin 1 39
see: corticotropin[1-39]
corticotropin 1-39
see: corticotropin[1-39]
corticotropin [1 39]
see: corticotropin[1-39]
corticotropin [1-39]
see: corticotropin[1-39]

corticotropin[18-39]

corticotropin [18 39]
see: corticotropin[18-39]

corticotropin[4-10]

corticotropin (4-10)
see: corticotropin[4-10]
corticotropin 4 10
see: corticotropin[4-10]
corticotropin 4-10
see: corticotropin[4-10]
corticotropin [4 10]
see: corticotropin[4-10]

corticotropin[7-10]

corticotropin[7-16]

corticotropin analog
see: corticotropin derivative
corticotropin analogue
see: corticotropin derivative
corticotropin b 1 24
see: tetracosactide

corticotropin derivative

corticotropine
see: corticotropin
corticotropin hormone
see: corticotropin
corticotropin peptide
see: corticotropin derivative
corticotropin release factor
see: corticotropin releasing factor

corticotropin releasing factor

corticotropin releasing factor[9-41]

corticotropin releasing factor derivative

corticotropin synthetic analog
see: corticotropin derivative
corticotropin zinc[1-24]
see: tetracosactide zinc phosphate
cortidelt
see: prednisone
cortiden
see: paramethasone
cortidene
see: paramethasone acetate
cortidrona
see: dexamethasone
cortidrone
see: dexamethasone
cortifan
see: hydrocortisone
cortifat
see: deoxycorticosterone
cortifoam
see: hydrocortisone
cortigel
see: corticotropin
cortigen
see: deoxycorticosterone acetate
cortilet
see: fluorometholone
cortilin
see: corticotropin
cortiment
see: hydrocortisone
cortinaq
see: deoxycorticosterone acetate
cortineff
see: fludrocortisone acetate
cortiphate
see: hydrocortisone
cortiphyson
see: corticotropin
cortiron
see: deoxycorticosterone acetate
cortisal
see: cortisone
cortisate
see: cortisone
cortisol
see: hydrocortisone
cortisol 17 butyrate
see: hydrocortisone butyrate
cortisol 21 acetate
see: hydrocortisone acetate
cortisol 21 hemisuccinate
see: hydrocortisone sodium succinate
cortisol 21 phosphate
see: hydrocortisone sodium phosphate
cortisol 21 succinate
see: hydrocortisone sodium succinate
cortisol 21 thiol
see: tixocortol
cortisol,5alpha dihydro
see: hydrallostane
cortisol acetate
see: hydrocortisone acetate
cortisol derivative
see: hydrocortisone derivative
cortisole
see: hydrocortisone
cortisol hemisuccinate
see: hydrocortisone sodium succinate
cortisolone
see: prednisolone
cortisol phosphate
see: hydrocortisone sodium phosphate
cortisol sodium succinate
see: hydrocortisone sodium succinate
cortisol succinate
see: hydrocortisone sodium succinate
cortison
see: cortisone

cortisone

cortisone 21 acetate
see: cortisone acetate
cortisone 2' acetate
see: cortisone acetate

cortisone acetate

cortisone derivative

cortisone derivatives
see: cortisone derivative
cortisone sodium
see: cortisone

cortisporin

cortisporin otic
see: cortisporin
cortispray
see: hydrocortisone
cortistab
see: cortisone acetate
cortistal
see: cortisone
cortisumman
see: dexamethasone
cortisyl
see: cortisone acetate

cortivazol

cortivazol acetate
see: cortivazol
cortivis
see: deoxycorticosterone acetate
cortivite
see: cortisone
cortixyl
see: deoxycorticosterone acetate
cortoderm
see: hydrocortisone
cortogen
see: cortisone
cortogen acetate
see: cortisone acetate
cortone
see: cortisone
cortone acetate
see: cortisone acetate
cortril
see: hydrocortisone
cortril acetate as
see: hydrocortisone acetate
cortrophin
see: corticotropin
cortrophin gel acth
see: corticotropin
cortropin
see: corticotropin
cortrosin z
see: tetracosactide zinc phosphate
cortrosyn
see: tetracosactide
cortrosyn depot
see: tetracosactide zinc phosphate
cortrosyn retard
see: tetracosactide
cortrosyn z
see: tetracosactide zinc phosphate
corty clyss
see: prednisolone 3 sulfobenzoate
corvasol
see: pentetrazole
corvin
see: nikethamide
corvis
see: pentetrazole
corvitan
see: nikethamide
corvitin
see: methamphetamine
corvotone
see: nikethamide
corwil
see: xamoterol hydrogen fumarate
corwin
see: xamoterol hydrogen fumarate
corywas
see: nikethamide
corzepin
see: perhexiline maleate
corzide
see: bendroflumethiazide plus nadolol
cosex tp 50
see: testosterone propionate
cosyntropin
see: tetracosactide
cotareg
see: hydrochlorothiazide plus valsartan
co tenidone
see: atenolol plus chlortalidone
co triamterzide
see: hydrochlorothiazide plus triamterene
cotriamterzide
see: hydrochlorothiazide plus triamterene
cotrophin
see: corticotropin
cozidocapt
see: captopril plus hydrochlorothiazide
cp 24314
see: pirbuterol
cp24314
see: pirbuterol
cp 24,314 1
see: pirbuterol
cp 24314 1
see: pirbuterol
cp 243141
see: pirbuterol

cp24,314 1
see: pirbuterol
cp24314 1
see: pirbuterol
cp243141
see: pirbuterol
cp 24,314 14
see: pirbuterol acetate
cp 24314 14
see: pirbuterol acetate
cp 24314-14
see: pirbuterol acetate
cp24,314 14
see: pirbuterol acetate
cp24314 14
see: pirbuterol acetate
cp24314-14
see: pirbuterol acetate
cp 336156
see: lasofoxifene
cp336156
see: lasofoxifene
cp 44001
see: nantradol
cp44001
see: nantradol
cp 44,001 1
see: nantradol
cp 44001 1
see: nantradol
cp 440011
see: nantradol
cp44,001 1
see: nantradol
cp44001 1
see: nantradol
cp440011
see: nantradol
cp 50556
see: levonantradol
cp50556
see: levonantradol
cp 50,556 1
see: levonantradol
cp 50556 1
see: levonantradol
cp 505561
see: levonantradol
cp50,556 1
see: levonantradol
cp50556 1
see: levonantradol
cp505561
see: levonantradol
cp 53870 1
see: dextronantradol
cp 538701
see: dextronantradol
cp53870 1
see: dextronantradol
cp538701
see: dextronantradol
cp 55243
see: 5 (1,1 dimethylheptyl) 2 (3 hydroxy 7 hydroxymethyldecahydro 1 naphthyl)phenol
cp55243
see: 5 (1,1 dimethylheptyl) 2 (3 hydroxy 7 hydroxymethyldecahydro 1 naphthyl)phenol
cp 55244
see: 5 (1,1 dimethylheptyl) 2 (3 hydroxy 7 hydroxymethyldecahydro 1 naphthyl)phenol
cp55244
see: 5 (1,1 dimethylheptyl) 2 (3 hydroxy 7 hydroxymethyldecahydro 1 naphthyl)phenol
cp 55940
see: 4 (1,1 dimethylheptyl) 1',2',3',4',5',6' hexahydro 2,3' dihydroxy 6' (3 hydroxypropyl)biphenyl
cp55940
see: 4 (1,1 dimethylheptyl) 1',2',3',4',5',6' hexahydro 2,3' dihydroxy 6' (3 hydroxypropyl)biphenyl
cp 56667
see: 4 (1,1 dimethylheptyl) 1',2',3',4',5',6' hexahydro 2,3' dihydroxy 6' (3 hydroxypropyl)biphenyl
cp56667
see: 4 (1,1 dimethylheptyl) 1',2',3',4',5',6' hexahydro 2,3' dihydroxy 6' (3 hydroxypropyl)biphenyl
cp 73
see: norclostebol acetate
cp 97587
see: 5 (1,1 dimethylheptyl) 2 (3 hydroxy 7 hydroxymethyldecahydro 1 naphthyl)phenol
cp97587
see: 5 (1,1 dimethylheptyl) 2 (3 hydroxy 7 hydroxymethyldecahydro 1 naphthyl)phenol
'crack'
see: cocaine
crack cocaine
see: cocaine
cre 10904
see: 2 [2 (4 fluorophenoxy)ethyl]phenol

cre10904
see: 2 [2 (4 fluorophenoxy)ethyl]phenol
cre 11296
see: [2 [2 (4 fluorophenoxy)ethyl]phenyl] sulfate
cre11296
see: [2 [2 (4 fluorophenoxy)ethyl]phenyl] sulfate
crescormon
see: human growth hormone
c rf
see: corticotropin releasing factor
CRF
see: corticotropin releasing factor
crf 41
see: corticotropin releasing factor
crf 9-41
see: corticotropin releasing factor[9-41]
crf analog
see: corticotropin releasing factor derivative
crf derivative
see: corticotropin releasing factor derivative
cristepin
see: briserin
cristerona
see: androstanolone
cristerone mb
see: androstanolone
crl 40028
see: adrafinil
crl40028
see: adrafinil
crl 40476
see: modafinil
crl40476
see: modafinil
crl 635
see: spironolactone
crl635
see: spironolactone

cromoglycate disodium plus reproterol

cropropamide

cropropamide plus crotetamide
see: prethcamide
cross linked insulin
see: insulin

crotamiton plus hydrocortisone

crotetamide

crotetamide plus cropropamide
see: prethcamide
crotethamide
see: crotetamide
crothetamide
see: crotetamide
cryptocur
see: gonadorelin
cryptolin
see: gonadorelin acetate
crystalline zinc insulin
see: insulin zinc suspension
crystepin
see: briserin
cs 359
see: bucumolol
cs359
see: bucumolol
ct 3
see: ajulemic acid
ct3
see: ajulemic acid
cutivate
see: fluticasone propionate

cyanoiodopindolol

1 (2 cyanophenoxy) 3 [2 (3 phenylureido)ethylamino] 2 propanol

cyanopindolol

cyclert
see: pemoline
cyclexedrine
see: propylhexedrine
cyclocort
see: amcinonide

cyclofenil

cyclofenil diphenol
see: bis(4 hydroxyphenyl)cyclohexylidenemethane
cyclofenyl
see: cyclofenil

Index

cyclohexyl[4 [2 [2 hydroxy 3 (4 hydroxyphenoxy)propylamino]ethyl]phenoxymethyl]phosphinic acid

4 cyclohexylamino 1 (1 naphthyloxy) 2 butanol

5 (2 cyclohexylideneethyl) 5 ethylbarbituric acid

cyclomen
see: danazol
cyclomethiazide
see: cyclopenthiazide
cyclonarol
see: cyclopentamine
cyclopentadrin
see: cyclopentamine

cyclopentamine

cyclopentamine hydrochloride
see: cyclopentamine

cyclopenthiazide

cyclopenthiazide plus guanethidine

cyclopenthiazide plus oxprenolol

cyclopenthiazine
see: cyclopenthiazide
cyclopentiazide
see: cyclopenthiazide
cyclophenil
see: cyclofenil
cyclophenthiazide
see: cyclopenthiazide
cyclophenyl
see: cyclofenil
cycloprolol
see: cicloprolol

n [2 [3 [4 [2 (2 cyclopropylmethoxyethoxy)ethyl]phenoxy] 2 hydroxypropylamino]ethyl] 4 hydroxy 1 piperidinecarboxamide

6 [4 [3 [[3 [4 [2 (cyclopropylmethoxy)ethyl]phenoxy] 2 hydroxypropyl]amino]propionamido] phenyl] 4,5 dihydro 5 methyl 3(2h) pyridazinone

cycloteriam

cyclothiazide

cyclothiazide plus triamterene
see: cycloteriam
cyklosan
see: cyclopentamine
cylert
see: pemoline magnesium
cyntaris
see: flunisolide
cystorelin
see: gonadorelin acetate
cytadren
see: aminoglutethimide
cytadren ag
see: aminoglutethimide
cyticholine
see: citicoline
cytidine diphosphate choline
see: citicoline
cytidine 5 diphosphocholine
see: citicoline
cytidine 5' diphosphocholoni
see: citicoline
cytidine diphosphocholine
see: citicoline
cytocholine
see: citicoline
d 13 625
see: alifedrine
d 13625
see: alifedrine
d13 625
see: alifedrine
d13625
see: alifedrine
d 1593
see: tiamizide
d-1593
see: tiamizide
d1593
see: tiamizide

Index

d 16726
see: zindoxifene
d16726
see: zindoxifene
d 18954
see: 2,3 bis(2 fluoro 4 hydroxyphenyl) 2,3 dimethylbutane
d18954
see: 2,3 bis(2 fluoro 4 hydroxyphenyl) 2,3 dimethylbutane
d 1959
see: reproterol
d1959
see: reproterol
d 1 phenyl 2 aminoproprane
see: dexamphetamine
d 2083
see: desonide
d2083
see: desonide
d 32
see: xibenolol
d32
see: xibenolol
d 4 androstenedione
see: androstenedione
d 563
see: oxyfedrine
d563
see: oxyfedrine
dacortin
see: prednisolone
dacortina fuerte
see: dexamethasone
dacortine fuerte
see: dexamethasone
dacortin h
see: prednisolone
dacrotin
see: prednisolone
dadex
see: dexamphetamine
daftazol
see: amiphenazole
daim
see: tilisolol

daktacort

dalalone
see: dexamethasone
d adrenalin
see: adrenalin
d aldosterone
see: aldosterone
d alpha methylphenethylamin
see: dexamphetamine
d amfetasul
see: dexamphetamine
d amphetamine
see: dexamphetamine
d amphetamine sulfate
see: dexamphetamine
d amphetamine sulphate
see: dexamphetamine
danabol
see: metandienone
danamine
see: nikethamide
danatrol
see: danazol

danazol

danocrine
see: danazol
danokrin
see: danazol
danol
see: danazol
daprisal
see: dexamphetamine
daptazile
see: amiphenazole
daptazole
see: amiphenazole
daranide
see: diclofenamide
darbepoetin alfa
see: novel erythropoiesis stimulating protein
darebon
see: chlortalidone plus reserpine
darob
see: sotalol
daropervamin
see: methamphetamine
dasten
see: mazindol
d ate
see: dexamphetamine
dazamide
see: acetazolamide
d beta phenylisopropylamine
see: dexamphetamine
d bunolol
see: bunolol

d bunolol hydrochloride
see: bunolol
dca
see: deoxycorticosterone acetate
dci
see: dichlorisoprenaline
d dioxadrol
see: dexoxadrol

deacetyllevonantradol

deacetylmetipranolol

deamin
see: methadone

deanol

deanol p chlorophenoxyacetate
see: meclofenoxate
deanol teststreifen g
see: deanol
decacortin
see: dexamethasone
decacortin 17 valerate
see: dexamethasone 17 valerate
decadeltosona
see: dexamethasone
decadeltosone
see: dexamethasone
decadion
see: dexamethasone
decadran
see: dexamethasone
decadron
see: dexamethasone
decadron 17 valerate
see: dexamethasone 17 valerate
decadronal
see: dexamethasone
decadrone
see: dexamethasone
decadron la
see: dexamethasone
deca durabolin
see: nandrolone decanoate
decadurabolin
see: nandrolone decanoate
decaesadril
see: dexamethasone
decamethasone
see: dexamethasone
decapeptide corticotropin 1-10
see: corticotropin derivative
decapeptyl
see: triptorelin
decapeptyl cr
see: triptorelin
decasone
see: dexamethasone
decasone 17 valerate
see: dexamethasone 17 valerate
decaspray
see: dexamethasone
decasterolone
see: dexamethasone
decilone
see: dexamethasone
decoderm
see: fluprednidene acetate
decoderm trivalent
see: fluprednidene acetate
decoderm trivalent cream
see: fluprednidene acetate
decofluor
see: dexamethasone
decortacete
see: deoxycorticosterone
decortancyl
see: prednisone
decortilen
see: prednylidene
decortin
see: prednisone
decortine
see: prednisone
decortin e merck
see: prednisone
decortin h
see: prednisolone
de cortisyl
see: prednisone
decorton
see: deoxycorticosterone
decortril
see: prednisolone
decosterone
see: deoxycorticosterone acetate
decreten
see: pindolol
dectancyl
see: dexamethasone
dectanyl 17 valerate
see: dexamethasone 17 valerate

Index

defencin
see: isoxsuprine
defencin cp
see: isoxsuprine
deflamene
see: formocortal
deflan
see: deflazacort

deflazacort

defluorofluazacort
see: deflazacort
9 defluorofluazacort
see: deflazacort

deglycochorionic gonadotropin

degonan
see: mazindol
dehydratin
see: acetazolamide
dehydratin neo
see: hydrochlorothiazide
dehydrochloromethyltestosterone
see: 4 chloro 17beta hydroxy 17 methylandrosta 1,4 dien 3 one
dehydro cortex
see: prednisolone
dehydrocortex
see: prednisolone
dehydrocortisol
see: prednisolone
dehydrocortisole
see: prednisolone
dehydrocortisone
see: prednisone
1,2 dehydrocortisone
see: prednisone
dehydroepiandrosteron
see: prasterone
dehydro epiandrosterone
see: prasterone
dehydroepiandrosterone
see: prasterone
dehydroepiandrosterone acetate
see: prasterone acetate
dehydroepiandrosterone sulfate
see: prasterone sulfate
dehydro hydrocortison
see: prednisolone
dehydrohydrocortison
see: prednisolone
1,2 dehydro hydrocortison
see: prednisolone
dehydro hydrocortisone
see: prednisolone
dehydrohydrocortisone
see: prednisolone
dehydroisoandrosterone
see: prasterone
dehydroisoandrosterone sulfate
see: prasterone sulfate
dehydrotestosterone
see: boldenone
1 dehydrotestosterone
see: boldenone
1,2 dehydrotestosterone
see: boldenone
dehyroepiandrosterone
see: prasterone
dekacort
see: dexamethasone
dekacort 17 valerate
see: dexamethasone 17 valerate
dekortin
see: prednisone
delaprem
see: hexoprenaline
delatestryl
see: testosterone enantate
delcortin
see: prednisone acetate
delcortol
see: prednisolone
delimon
see: morazone
delitisone
see: prednisone
delladec
see: dexamethasone
delmeson
see: fluorometholone
delmesone
see: fluorometholone
delmit
see: betamethasone valerate
delonal
see: alclometasone dipropionate
delphicort
see: triamcinolone
delta 1,2 tetrahydrocannabinol
see: dronabinol
delta 1,6 tetrahydrocannabinol
see: delta8 tetrahydrocannabinol

delta1(6) tetrahydrocannabinol
see: delta8 tetrahydrocannabinol
delta1,6 tetrahydrocannabinol
see: delta8 tetrahydrocannabinol
delta1(7) tetrahydrocannabinol
see: delta9(11) tetrahydrocannabinol
delta 1 androstene 3,17 dione
see: androst 1 ene 3,17 dione
delta1 androstene 3,17 dione
see: androst 1 ene 3,17 dione
delta1 dehydrocortisol
see: prednisolone
delta 1 dehydrocortisone
see: prednisone
delta1 dehydrohydrocortisone
see: prednisolone
delta1 dihydrotestosterone
see: 1 testosterone
delta 1 hydrocortisone
see: prednisolone
delta1 hydrocortisone
see: prednisolone
delta 1 testolactone
see: testolactone
delta1 testolactone
see: testolactone
delta 1 testololactone
see: testolactone
delta1 testololactone
see: testolactone
delta 1 tetrahydrocannabinol
see: dronabinol
delta1 tetrahydrocannabinol
see: dronabinol
delta1 thc
see: dronabinol
delta 2 tetrahydrocannabinol
see: tetrahydrocannabinol
delta 3 tetrahydrocannabinol
see: tetrahydrocannabinol
delta3 tetrahydrocannabinol
see: tetrahydrocannabinol
delta3 thc
see: tetrahydrocannabinol
delta4,16 androstadien 3 one
see: androsta 4,16 dien 3 one
delta 4 androsten 3,17 dione
see: androstenedione
delta 4 androstene 3,17 dione
see: androstenedione
delta 4 androstenediol
see: 4 androstenediol
delta4 androstenediol
see: 4 androstenediol
delta 4 androstenedione
see: androstenedione
delta4 androstenedione
see: androstenedione
delta5 androsten 3 beta 17 one
see: prasterone
delta5 androsten 3beta 17 one
see: prasterone
delta 5 androstenediol
see: androstenediol
delta5 androstenediol
see: androstenediol
delta5 pregnen 3beta ol 20 one
see: pregnenolone
delta 5 pregnenolone
see: pregnenolone
delta 5 tetrahydrocannabinol
see: tetrahydrocannabinol
delta 6 tetrahydrocannabinol
see: delta8 tetrahydrocannabinol
delta6 tetrahydrocannabinol
see: delta8 tetrahydrocannabinol
delta 8 tetrahydro cannabinol
see: delta8 tetrahydrocannabinol
delta 8 tetrahydrocannabinol
see: delta8 tetrahydrocannabinol
delta 9 tetrahydrocannabinol
see: dronabinol
delta9 tetrahydro cannabinol
see: dronabinol
delta9 tetrahydrocannabinol
see: dronabinol
delta amphetamine
see: amphetamine
delta cortef
see: prednisolone
deltacortef
see: prednisolone
delta cortelan
see: prednisone
deltacorten
see: prednisone
delta cortene beta
see: meprednisone
deltacortenolo
see: prednisolone
deltacortil
see: prednisolone
delta cortisone
see: prednisone

deltacortisone
see: prednisone
deltacortoil
see: prednisolone
deltacortone
see: prednisone
delta cortril
see: prednisolone
deltaderm
see: prednisolone
delta dome
see: prednisone
delta e
see: prednisone
delta ef cortelan
see: prednisolone
delta f
see: prednisolone
deltafluoren
see: dexamethasone
deltafluorene
see: dexamethasone
delta fluorene 17 valerate
see: dexamethasone 17 valerate
deltaglycortril
see: prednisolone
delta hycortol
see: prednisolone
deltahycortol
see: prednisolone
delta hydrocortison
see: prednisolone
deltahydrocortison
see: prednisolone
delta hydrocortisone
see: prednisolone
deltahydrocortisone
see: prednisolone
deltalone
see: prednisone acetate
deltamine
see: pemoline
delta ophticor
see: prednisolone
deltaophticor
see: prednisolone
deltaplasmat 40
see: dextran 40
deltaplasmat 70
see: dextran 70
delta prenovis
see: prednisone
deltasolone
see: prednisolone
deltasone
see: prednisone
delta stab
see: prednisolone
deltastab
see: prednisolone
delta testolactone
see: testolactone
delta tetrahydrocannabinol
see: tetrahydrocannabinol
deltelan
see: prednisolone sodium phosphate
deltidrosol
see: prednisolone
deltisilone
see: prednisolone
deltisolon
see: prednisolone
deltisolone
see: prednisolone
deltisone b
see: meprednisone
deltolasson
see: prednisolone
deltolassone
see: prednisolone
deltosona
see: prednisolone
deltosone
see: prednisolone
deltra
see: prednisone
demadex
see: torasemide
demanol
see: deanol
demelon
see: nandrolone furylpropionate
demerol
see: pethidine
demerol hydrochloride
see: pethidine
demethyltamoxifen
see: nortamoxifen
demi regroton
see: chlortalidone plus reserpine
demi-regroton
see: chlortalidone plus reserpine
demiregroton
see: chlortalidone plus reserpine

denmacard
see: pentetrazole

denopamine

denopamine, 3 hydroxy
see: 3 hydroxydenopamine
deofed
see: methamphetamine
deoxyadrenalin
see: epinine
deoxyadrenaline
see: epinine
17 deoxyandrostanolone
see: 5alpha androstan 3 one
deoxycortan
see: deoxycorticosterone
deoxycorten
see: deoxycorticosterone

deoxycorticosterone

11 deoxycorticosterone
see: deoxycorticosterone

deoxycorticosterone acetate

deoxycorticosterone phenpropionate plus nandrolone phenpropionate

deoxycorticosterone pivalate

deoxycortone
see: deoxycorticosterone
deoxycortone acetate
see: deoxycorticosterone acetate
deoxycortone pivalate
see: deoxycorticosterone pivalate
17 deoxydexamethasone
see: desoximetasone
17 deoxydihydrotestosterone
see: 5alpha androstan 3 one
deoxyephedrine
see: methamphetamine
deoxyepinephrine
see: epinine
deoxyhaemoglobin
see: deoxyhemoglobin

deoxyhemoglobin

deoxymethasone
see: desoximetasone
17 deoxymethasone
see: desoximetasone
deoxymethazone
see: desoximetasone
depandro
see: testosterone cipionate
depandro 100
see: testosterone cipionate
depandro 200
see: testosterone cipionate
depersolon
see: mazipredone
depersolone
see: mazipredone
dephadren
see: dexamphetamine
depmedalone 40
see: methylprednisolone acetate
depmedalone 80
see: methylprednisolone acetate
depo acth
see: corticotropin
depodillar
see: paramethasone acetate
depo lupron
see: leuprorelin
depo medrate
see: methylprednisolone acetate
depo medrol
see: methylprednisolone acetate
depomedrol
see: methylprednisolone acetate
depomedron
see: methylprednisolone acetate
depo medrone
see: methylprednisolone acetate
depomedrone
see: methylprednisolone acetate
depomorphine
see: morphine sulfate
depotest
see: testosterone cipionate
depo testosterone
see: testosterone cipionate
depot medrate
see: methylprednisolone acetate
depot tetracosactrin
see: tetracosactide

depovirin
see: testosterone cipionate
depoviron
see: testosterone cipionate
deppredalone
see: prednisolone acetate
deprenaline
see: selegiline
deprenil
see: selegiline
deprenyl
see: selegiline
depridol
see: methadone
deproteinized blood extract
see: blood extract
deralin
see: propranolol
derfon
see: amfepramone
dergramin
see: dexamethasone
dergramin 17 valerate
see: dexamethasone 17 valerate
dermacort
see: hydrocortisone acetate
dermatop
see: prednicarbate
dermolate
see: hydrocortisone
dermoval
see: clobetasol propionate
dermovate
see: clobetasol propionate
derolin 17 valerate
see: dexamethasone 17 valerate
deronil
see: dexamethasone
desacetyllevonantradol
see: deacetyllevonantradol
desacetylmetipranolol
see: deacetylmetipranolol
desacort
see: dexamethasone
desacortone
see: dexamethasone
desadrene
see: dexamethasone
desalark
see: dexamethasone
desameton
see: dexamethasone
desametone
see: dexamethasone
desamine
see: methamphetamine
descon
see: phenylpropanolamine
descorterone
see: deoxycorticosterone acetate
descotone
see: deoxycorticosterone acetate
deseronil 17 valerate
see: dexamethasone 17 valerate
desfedrin
see: methamphetamine
desialo hcg
see: asialochorionic gonadotropin

deslorelin

desmethyltamoxifen
see: nortamoxifen
desobesi
see: fenproporex
desoctapeptide insulin
see: insulin deoctapeptide
desoctapeptideinsulin
see: insulin deoctapeptide

desonide

desopimon
see: chlorphentermine
desowen
see: desonide
desoxicorticosterone acetate
see: deoxycorticosterone acetate

desoximetasone

desoximethasone
see: desoximetasone
desoxo 5
see: methamphetamine
desoxycortane
see: deoxycorticosterone
desoxycorticosteron
see: deoxycorticosterone
desoxycorticosterone
see: deoxycorticosterone
11 desoxycorticosterone
see: deoxycorticosterone
desoxycorticosterone acetate
see: deoxycorticosterone acetate

Index

desoxycortone
see: deoxycorticosterone
desoxycortone acetate
see: deoxycorticosterone acetate
desoxycortone pivalate
see: deoxycorticosterone pivalate
desoxycortone trimethylacetate
see: deoxycorticosterone pivalate
desoxydexamethasone
see: desoximetasone
17 desoxydexamethasone
see: desoximetasone
desoxyephedrine
see: methamphetamine
desoxyepinephrine
see: epinine
desoxyfed
see: methamphetamine
desoxymetasone
see: desoximetasone
desoxymethasone
see: desoximetasone
desoxyn
see: methamphetamine
desoxynorephedrin
see: amphetamine
destim
see: methamphetamine
destripeptide insulin
see: insulin
desyphed
see: methamphetamine
detensiel
see: bisoprolol
detrex
see: methamphetamine
detryptorelin
see: triptorelin
deumacard
see: pentetrazole
dexachel
see: dexamethasone
dexacort
see: dexamethasone
dexacortal
see: dexamethasone
dexacortal 17 valerate
see: dexamethasone 17 valerate
dexacorten
see: dexamethasone
dexacortin
see: dexamethasone
dexa cortisyl
see: dexamethasone
dexacortisyl
see: dexamethasone
dexa dabrosan
see: dexamethasone
dexadabroson
see: dexamethasone
dexadecadrol
see: dexamethasone
dexadreson
see: dexamethasone sodium phosphate
dexadrine
see: dexamphetamine
dexadrol
see: dexamethasone
dexagen
see: dexamethasone
dexahelvacort
see: dexamethasone
dexair
see: dexamethasone sodium phosphate
dexa korti
see: dexamethasone
dexakorti
see: dexamethasone
dexaline
see: dexamphetamine
dexalme
see: dexamphetamine
dexalocal
see: dexamethasone
dexalone
see: dexamphetamine
dexamecortin
see: dexamethasone
dexamed
see: dexamphetamine
dexameson
see: dexamethasone
dexameson 17 valerate
see: dexamethasone 17 valerate
dexamesone
see: dexamethasone
dexametason
see: dexamethasone
dexametasone
see: dexamethasone
dexameth
see: dexamethasone
dexameth 17 valerate
see: dexamethasone 17 valerate

dexamethason
see: dexamethasone
dexamethason 21 isonicotinate
see: dexamethasone isonicotinate

dexamethasone

dexamethasone 17,21 dipropionate

dexamethasone 17 valerate

dexamethasone 21 acetate
see: dexamethasone acetate
dexamethasone 21 isonicotinate
see: dexamethasone isonicotinate

dexamethasone 21 mesilate

dexamethasone 21 mesylate
see: dexamethasone 21 mesilate
dexamethasone 21 phosphate
see: dexamethasone sodium phosphate
dexamethasone 2 isonicotinate
see: dexamethasone isonicotinate
dexamethasone,6alpha fluoro
see: flumetasone

dexamethasone acetate

dexamethasone alcohol
see: dexamethasone

dexamethasone derivative

dexamethasone ester
see: dexamethasone derivative

dexamethasone isonicotinate

21 dexamethasone isonicotinate
see: dexamethasone isonicotinate
dexamethasone isonioatinate
see: dexamethasone isonicotinate
dexamethasone phosphate
see: dexamethasone sodium phosphate
dexamethasone phosphate sodium
see: dexamethasone sodium phosphate
dexamethasone plus clioquinol
see: clioquinol plus dexamethasone

dexamethasone plus tobramycin

dexamethasone sodium phosphate

dexamethasone valerate
see: dexamethasone 17 valerate
dexamethazon
see: dexamethasone
dexamethazone
see: dexamethasone
dexamethazone phosphate
see: dexamethasone sodium phosphate
dexamethonium
see: dexamethasone
dexamfetamine
see: dexamphetamine

dexamphetamine

dexamphetamine sulfate
see: dexamphetamine
dexamphetamin sulphate
see: dexamphetamine
dexamphethamine
see: dexamphetamine
dexamphoid
see: dexamphetamine
dexamyl
see: dexamphetamine
dexan
see: dexamethasone

dexanabinol

dexane
see: dexamethasone
dexapot
see: dexamethasone
dexa scherosan
see: dexamethasone
dexascherosan 17 valerate
see: dexamethasone 17 valerate
dexascheroson
see: dexamethasone
dexa scherozon
see: dexamethasone
dexascherozon
see: dexamethasone
dexa scherozone
see: dexamethasone
dexascherozone
see: dexamethasone

dexason
see: dexamethasone
dexason 17 valerate
see: dexamethasone 17 valerate
dexasone
see: dexamethasone
dexaspan b
see: dexamphetamine

dexatopic

dexatrim
see: phenylpropanolamine
dexavet
see: dexamethasone sodium phosphate
dexeamphetanine
see: dexamphetamine
dexedrine
see: dexamphetamine
dexedrine spansules
see: dexamphetamine
dexedrine sulfate
see: dexamphetamine

dexfenfluramine

dexfenfluramine hydrochloride
see: dexfenfluramine
dexfenmetrazin
see: phenmetrazine
dexinoral
see: dexamethasone
dexinoral 17 valerate
see: dexamethasone 17 valerate
dexionil
see: dexamethasone

dexmethylphenidate

dexnorfenfluramine

dexone
see: dexamethasone
dexoval
see: dexamphetamine

dexoxadrol

dexoxadrol hydrochloride
see: dexoxadrol
dexphenmetrazine
see: phenmetrazine
dexphenmetrazine hydrochloride
see: phenmetrazine
dexsotalol
see: sotalol
dexsotalol hydrochloride
see: sotalol
dextelan
see: dexamethasone
dextelan 17 valerate
see: dexamethasone 17 valerate

dextran

dextran 40

dextran 40,000
see: dextran 40
dextran 40000
see: dextran 40
dextran 45
see: dextran

dextran 60

dextran 70

dextrane
see: dextran
dextran ebewe
see: dextran 40
dextran k 300000
see: dextran
dextran k 40000
see: dextran
dextran k 500000
see: dextran
dextran k 70000
see: dextran
dextrans
see: dextran
dextraven
see: dextran
dextraven 150
see: dextran
dextrim
see: methamphetamine
dextro adrenalin
see: adrenalin
dextro aldosterone
see: aldosterone

dextro amphetamine
see: dexamphetamine
dextroamphetamine
see: dexamphetamine
dextro amphetamine sulfate
see: dexamphetamine
dextroamphetamine sulfate
see: dexamphetamine
dextro benzphetamine
see: benzphetamine
dextro bunolol
see: bunolol
dextro desoxyephedrine
see: methamphetamine
dextro fenfluramine
see: dexfenfluramine
dextro inpea
see: nifenalol
dextro isoprenaline
see: isoprenaline
dextro levo amphetamine
see: amphetamine
dextrolevo amphetamine
see: amphetamine
dextrolevo deoxyephedrine
see: methamphetamine
dextro levo fenfluramine
see: fenfluramine
dextro levo inpea
see: nifenalol
dextro,levo oxyfedrine
see: oxyfedrine
dextro levo phendimetrazine
see: phendimetrazine
dextro levo practolol
see: practolol
dextrolevo propranolol
see: propranolol
dextro mannitol
see: mannitol
dextro metaraminol
see: metaraminol
dextro metaraminol bitartrate
see: metaraminol

dextromethorphan plus morphine

dextro methylamphetamine
see: methamphetamine

dextromoramide

dextro moramide
see: dextromoramide
dextromoramide bitartras
see: dextromoramide
dextromoramide bitartrate
see: dextromoramide
dextromoramide tartrate
see: dextromoramide
dextromoramine
see: dextromoramide

dextronantradol

dextro noradrenalin
see: noradrenalin
dextro noradrenaline
see: noradrenalin
dextro norfenfluramine
see: norfenfluramine
dextro oxyprenolol
see: oxprenolol
dextro phenmetrazine
see: phenmetrazine
dextro pipradol
see: pipradol
dextro sorbitol
see: sorbitol
dextro sotalol
see: sotalol
dextrosotalol
see: sotalol
dextrostat
see: dexamphetamine
dexyfed
see: methamphetamine
dezone
see: dexamethasone
d fenfluramine
see: dexfenfluramine
d glucitol
see: sorbitol
d glucohexitol
see: sorbitol
dha 245
see: amiphenazole
dha245
see: amiphenazole
DHEA
see: prasterone
DHEA acetate
see: prasterone acetate

dheas
see: prasterone sulfate
DHEA sulfate
see: prasterone sulfate
diacarb
see: acetazolamide
diacephine
see: diamorphine
diacetoacetyl insulin
see: insulin derivative

diacetolol

diacetolol hydrochloride
see: diacetolol
diacetylinsulin
see: insulin derivative
diacetyl morphine
see: diamorphine
diacetylmorphine
see: diamorphine
3,6 diacetylmorphine
see: diamorphine
diacetylmorphine hydrochloride
see: diamorphine
diachlor
see: chlorothiazide
diacort
see: diflorasone diacetate
di ademil
see: hydroflumethiazide
di-ademil
see: hydroflumethiazide
diademil
see: hydroflumethiazide
di adreson
see: prednisone
di-adreson
see: prednisone
diadreson
see: prednisone
di adresone f
see: prednisolone
diadresone f
see: prednisolone
di adreson f
see: prednisolone
diadreson f
see: prednisolone
diakarmon
see: sorbitol
dialens
see: dextran
diamazon
see: furosemide
2,4 diamino 5 phenylthiazole
see: amiphenazole

3,5 diamino 6 chloro n [1 [n [2 [2 hydroxy 3 (1 naphthoxy)propylamino]ethyl]carbamoyl] 1 methylethyl]pyrazine 2 carboxamide

diaminon
see: methadone
diaminosuberoyl insulin
see: insulin derivative

diamorphine

diamorphine hydrochloride
see: diamorphine
diamox
see: acetazolamide
dianabol
see: metandienone
diandron
see: prasterone
diandron 3 sulfate
see: prasterone sulfate
diandrone
see: prasterone
1,4:3,6 dianhydro d glucitol
see: isosorbide
1,4:3,6 dianhydrosorbitol
see: isosorbide
dianone
see: methadone
diapamide
see: tiamizide
diaphorin
see: diamorphine
diaqua
see: hydrochlorothiazide

diaspirin crosslinked hemoglobin

diaster
see: cortivazol
diberal
see: 5 (1,3 dimethylbutyl) 5 ethylbarbituric acid
dicel
see: fenproporex

dichlorisoprenaline

dichlorisopropylnoradrenalin
see: dichlorisoprenaline
dichlorisoproterenol
see: dichlorisoprenaline

6,7 dichloro 2,3 dihydro 5 (n,n dimethylsulfamoyl)coumarilic acid

1,1 dichloro 2,3 diphenylcyclopropane

2,6 dichloro 4 dimethylaminoamphetamine

dichlorofenamide
see: diclofenamide
dichloroisoprenalin
see: dichlorisoprenaline
dichloro isoprenaline
see: dichlorisoprenaline
dichloroisoprenaline
see: dichlorisoprenaline
dichloro isoproterenol
see: dichlorisoprenaline
dichloroisoproterenol
see: dichlorisoprenaline
dichlorophenamide
see: diclofenamide

1 (2,4 dichlorophenoxy) 3 [2 (3,4 dimethoxyphenyl)ethylamino] 2 propanol

dichlorosal
see: hydrochlorothiazide
dichlorphenamide
see: diclofenamide
dichlotride
see: hydrochlorothiazide
dichlotride k
see: hydrochlorothiazide

diclofenamide

diclotride
see: hydrochlorothiazide
dicortol
see: prednisolone

1 (4,4' dicyanobenzhydryl)imidazole

dideral
see: propranolol
didrex
see: benzphetamine
diepropon
see: amfepramone
dietac premeal
see: phenylpropanolamine
diet gard
see: phenylpropanolamine
diethamine
see: amphetamine
diethanine
see: amphetamine

4 (2 diethylaminoethoxy) alpha' ethyl alpha (4 hydroxyphenyl) 4' methoxystilbene

diethylaminopropiophenone
see: amfepramone
2 diethylaminopropiophenone
see: amfepramone
diethylnicotinamide
see: nikethamide
diethyl propion
see: amfepramone
diethylpropion
see: amfepramone
diethylpropione
see: amfepramone
diethylpropione hydrochloride
see: amfepramone
diethylpropion hydrochloride
see: amfepramone
diflal
see: diflorasone diacetate

diflorasone

diflorasone 17,21 diacetate
see: diflorasone diacetate

diflorasone diacetate

diflucortolone

diflucortolone 21 valerate
see: diflucortolone valerate

Index

diflucortolone valerate

diflucortolone valerianate
see: diflucortolone valerate
difluocortolone
see: diflucortolone
difluocortolone valerate
see: diflucortolone valerate

6alpha,9alpha difluoro 11beta,17alpha dihydroxy 16beta methyl 17beta methylthiocarbonylandrosta 1,4 dien 3 one 17 acetate

6alpha,9alpha difluoro 11beta,17alpha dihydroxy 16beta methyl 17beta methylthiocarbonylandrosta 1,4 dien 3 one 17 propionate

difluorocortolone valerate
see: diflucortolone valerate
difluorocortolone valerianate
see: diflucortolone valerate

difluprednate

diflurex
see: tienilic acid

dihydralazine plus hydrochlorothiazide plus reserpine

dihydralazine plus oxprenolol

2,3 dihydro 5 methyl 3 (morpholinomethyl) 6 (1 naphthoyl)pyrrolo[1,2,3 de][1,4]benzoxazine

2,4 dihydro 6,8 dinitro 1,2,4 triazolo[3,4 c][1,4]benzoxazin 1 one

dihydroalprenolol

dihydroandrosteron
see: androstanediol

6,7 dihydrocanrenone

dihydrochlorothiazide
see: hydrochlorothiazide
dihydrocortisol
see: hydrallostane
dihydrodiuril
see: hydrochlorothiazide
dihydroepiandrosterone
see: prasterone
dihydroepiandrosterone sulfate
see: prasterone sulfate
dihydroflumethiazide
see: hydroflumethiazide
dihydroisoandrosterone
see: prasterone
dihydromorphinone
see: hydromorphone
7,8 dihydromorphinone hcl
see: hydromorphone
dihydromorphone
see: hydromorphone
dihydrone
see: oxycodone

20 dihydroprednisolonic acid methyl ester

1,2 dihydrospirorenone
see: drospirenone
dihydrotestosterone
see: androstanolone
5 dihydrotestosterone
see: androstanolone
dihydrotestosterone derivative
see: androstanolone derivative
dihydrotestosterone propionate
see: androstanolone propionate

11beta,17beta dihydroxy 17 (1 propynyl)androsta 1,4,6 trien 3 one

11beta,17beta dihydroxy 6 methyl 17alpha (1 propynyl)androsta 1,4,6 trien 3 one

3,4 dihydroxyphenethylamine
see: dopamine

1 (3,4 dihydroxyphenoxy) 3 (3,4 dimethoxyphenethylamino) 2 propanol

3 (3,4 dihydroxyphenyl) 2 [3 (4 fluorophenyl)propylamino] 3 hydroxypropionic acid pyrrolidine amide

6 [2 (3,4 dihydroxyphenyl) 2 hydroxyethylamino] n [4 (trifluoromethyl)phenyl]heptanamide

dihydroxyphenylethylamine
see: dopamine
3,4 dihydroxyphenylethylamine
see: dopamine
dilabron
see: isoetarine
dilanorm
see: celiprolol
dilar
see: paramethasone acetate
dilatal
see: buphenine
dilatol
see: buphenine
dilatrend
see: carvedilol
dilatropin
see: buphenine
dilatropon
see: buphenine
dilaudid
see: hydromorphone
dilavase
see: isoxsuprine
dilbloc
see: carvedilol

dilevalol

dilevalon
see: dilevalol
dillar
see: paramethasone acetate
dilovasan
see: isoxsuprine
diluran
see: acetazolamide
dilydrin
see: buphenine
dimafen
see: fenfluramine

dimefline

dimefline chloride
see: dimefline
dimefline hydrochloride
see: dimefline

dimetamfetamine

dimethofrine
see: dimetofrine
dimethophrine
see: dimetofrine
dimethoxy 4 methylamphetamine
see: 2,5 dimethoxy 4 methylamphetamine

2,5 dimethoxy 4 methylamphetamine

n (3,5 dimethoxyphenethyl) 5 methoxy 2 (phenylethynyl)amphetamine

dimethylaminoethanol
see: deanol
2 (dimethylamino)ethanol
see: deanol
2 dimethyl amino ethanol
see: deanol
2 dimethylaminoethanol
see: deanol
2(dimethylamino)ethanol
see: deanol

11 [4 (2 dimethylaminoethoxy)phenyl]estradio l

dimethylamphetamine
see: dimetamfetamine

5 (1,3 dimethylbutyl) 5 ethylbarbituric acid

dimethylcannabidiol
see: cannabidiol dimethyl ether
dimethylethanolamine
see: deanol

Index

4 (1,1 dimethylheptyl) 1',2',3',4',5',6' hexahydro 2,3' dihydroxy 6' (3 hydroxypropyl)biphenyl

5 (1,1 dimethylheptyl) 2 (3 hydroxy 7 hydroxymethyldecahydro 1 naphthyl)phenol

dimethylphenethylamine
see: phentermine
dimethylphenetylamine
see: phentermine

dimethylstilbestrol

dimetofrine

dimetophrine
see: dimetofrine
dimetriose
see: gestrinone
dimetrose
see: gestrinone
dimitone
see: carvedilol
dimorlin
see: dextromoramide
dimorphone
see: hydromorphone
dinacoryl
see: nikethamide
dinarkon
see: oxycodone
3,6 dinicotinoylmorphine
see: nicomorphine
dinintel
see: clobenzorex
d inpea
see: nifenalol
diocarb
see: dexamphetamine
diocurb
see: dexamphetamine
dioderm
see: hydrocortisone
diolandrone
see: methandriol
diolostene
see: methandriol
diomax
see: acetazolamide
diopine
see: dipivefrine
diovan comp
see: hydrochlorothiazide plus valsartan
diovan d
see: hydrochlorothiazide plus valsartan
diovan hct
see: hydrochlorothiazide plus valsartan
diovascole
see: pentetrazole
3,17 dioxoandrost 4 en 19 al
see: 19 oxoandrostenedione
dipan
see: amphetamine
diphenorciprenaline
see: fenoterol
dipivaloyl epinephrine
see: dipivefrine
dipivalyladrenalin
see: dipivefrine
dipivalylepinephrine
see: dipivefrine
dipivefrin
see: dipivefrine

dipivefrine

diprocel
see: betamethasone dipropionate
diproderm
see: betamethasone dipropionate
diprolene
see: betamethasone dipropionate
diprophos
see: betamethasone dipropionate
diprosalic
see: betamethasone dipropionate
diprosis
see: betamethasone dipropionate
diprosone
see: betamethasone dipropionate
diprospan
see: betamethasone sodium phosphate
diraudixin
see: hydroflumethiazide
direma
see: hydrochlorothiazide
disalunil
see: hydrochlorothiazide
disaluril
see: hydrochlorothiazide
'discoid'
see: furosemide

disodium isosorbide
see: isosorbide
d isoprenaline
see: isoprenaline
disorat
see: metipranolol
dispadol
see: pethidine
dispnoesan
see: isoprenaline
ditalyl
see: buphenine

ditec

diteriam
see: benzthiazide plus triamterene
diube
see: atenolol plus chlortalidone
diucardin
see: hydroflumethiazide

diucomb

diulo
see: metolazone
diu melusin
see: hydrochlorothiazide
diu-melusin
see: hydrochlorothiazide
diumelusin
see: hydrochlorothiazide
diumide
see: furosemide
diural
see: furosemide
diuramide
see: acetazolamide
diuregan
see: mersalyl
diuresal
see: furosemide
diurese
see: trichlormethiazide
diuretic
see: diuretic agent

diuretic agent

diuretic agent,loop
see: loop diuretic agent
diuretic drug
see: diuretic agent
diuretics
see: diuretic agent
diuretics, mercurial
see: diuretic agent
diuretics, osmotic
see: osmotic diuretic agent
diuretics, sulfamyl
see: diuretic agent
diuretics, thiazide
see: thiazide diuretic agent
diureticum
see: diuretic agent
diurexan
see: xipamide
diurgan
see: mersalyl
diuril
see: chlorothiazide
diurilix
see: chlorothiazide
diuril lyovac
see: chlorothiazide
diuriwas wassermann barcelona
see: acetazolamide
diuriwas wassermann milano
see: chlorothiazide
diurix
see: furosemide
diurone
see: chlormerodrin
diursal
see: mersalyl
diursan
see: amiloride plus hydrochlorothiazide
diutazol
see: acetazolamide
diutensat
see: hydrochlorothiazide plus triamterene
diu tonolytril
see: hydrochlorothiazide plus triamterene
diutonolytril
see: hydrochlorothiazide plus triamterene
diutrix
see: furosemide plus triamterene
divanal
see: etamivan
dizol
see: amiphenazole
dk line
see: perfluorodecalin
dl 458
see: deflazacort

dl458
see: deflazacort
dl 458 it
see: deflazacort
dl 458it
see: deflazacort
dl458it
see: deflazacort
dl 5458
see: deflazacort
dl5458
see: deflazacort
dl adrenalin
see: adrenalin
d,l alpha methyl meta tyramine
see: gepefrine
d l amphetamine
see: amphetamine
dl arterenol
see: noradrenalin
dl ephedrine
see: ephedrine
dl fenfluramine
see: fenfluramine
dl inpea
see: nifenalol
dl isoprenaline
see: isoprenaline
dl isoprenaline hydrochloride
see: isoprenaline
dl isoproterenol sulfate
see: isoprenaline
dl mefruside
see: mefruside
dl methamphetamine
see: methamphetamine
dl noradrenalin
see: noradrenalin
dl noradrenalin hydrochloride
see: noradrenalin
dl norephedrine
see: phenylpropanolamine
dl oxyfedrine
see: oxyfedrine
dl pentazocine
see: pentazocine
dl practolol
see: practolol
dl propanolol hydrochloride
see: propranolol
dl propranolol
see: propranolol
dl threo methylphenidate
see: methylphenidate
d mannitol
see: mannitol
DMCM
see: 4 ethyl 6,7 dimethoxy beta carboline 3 carboxylic acid methyl ester
d mefruside
see: mefruside
d methamphetamine
see: methamphetamine
d moramide
see: dextromoramide
d moramide bitartrate
see: dextromoramide
d noradrenalin
see: noradrenalin
d noradrenalin bitartrate
see: noradrenalin bitartrate
doberol
see: toliprolol
dobesin
see: amfepramone
dobuject
see: dobutamine
doburil
see: cyclothiazide
dobutamide
see: dobutamine

dobutamine

dobutamine hydrochloride
see: dobutamine
dobutrex
see: dobutamine
doc
see: deoxycorticosterone
doca
see: deoxycorticosterone acetate
doca acetate
see: deoxycorticosterone acetate
docabolin
see: deoxycorticosterone phenpropionate plus nandrolone phenpropionate
dociton
see: propranolol
docitone
see: propranolol
dociton retard
see: propranolol
doe
see: methamphetamine

dohycamon
see: deoxycorticosterone
DOI
see: 4 iodo 2,5 dimethoxyamphetamine
dolafin
see: methadone
dolamid
see: methadone
dolanquifa
see: pethidine
dolantal
see: pethidine
dolantin
see: pethidine
dolantine
see: pethidine
dolapent
see: pentazocine
dolargan
see: pethidine
dolcontin
see: morphine sulfate
dolcontral
see: pethidine
dolenal
see: pethidine
dolesone
see: methadone
dolestin
see: pethidine
dolin
see: pethidine
dolocontral
see: pethidine
dolomit
see: isoprenaline
doloneurin
see: pethidine
doloneurotrat
see: pethidine
dolophine
see: methadone
dolophine hydrochloride
see: methadone
dolor
see: pethidine
dolosa
see: pethidine
dolosal
see: pethidine
dolosan
see: pethidine
dolsin
see: pethidine
dolvanol
see: pethidine
DOM
see: 2,5 dimethoxy 4 methylamphetamine
domafate
see: dexamphetamine
domefate
see: dexamphetamine

domoprednate

domucortone
see: prednisolone
dopacard
see: dopexamine
dopachard
see: dopexamine
dopamin
see: dopamine

dopamine

dopamine hydrochloride
see: dopamine
dopastat
see: dopamine

dopexamine

dopexamine dihydrochloride
see: dopexamine
dopexamine hydrochloride
see: dopexamine
dopmin
see: dopamine
dopram
see: doxapram
dopram v
see: doxapram
doracil
see: mefenorex
dorcostrin
see: deoxycorticosterone acetate
dorex
see: methadone
dorexol
see: methadone
dosauxison
see: dexamethasone isonicotinate
dosberotec
see: fenoterol

dosberotec inhaletten
see: fenoterol
doxamethasone
see: dexamethasone

doxaminol

doxapram

doxapram chlorhydrate
see: doxapram
doxapram hydrochloride
see: doxapram
doxapram hydrochloride hydrate
see: doxapram
doxapril
see: doxapram
doxedrine
see: dexamphetamine
doxephrin
see: methamphetamine
doxo
see: deoxycorticosterone acetate
doxopram
see: doxapram
doxycamon
see: deoxycorticosterone acetate
doxyfed
see: methamphetamine
d oxyprenolol
see: oxprenolol
dpe
see: dipivefrine
d pentazocine
see: pentazocine
d phe 7 corticotropin 1-10
see: corticotropin derivative
d phenmetrazine
see: phenmetrazineS
dq 2466
see: carvedilol
dq2466
see: carvedilol
dr 3438
see: [[5 chloro 3 (2 methylphenyl) 4 oxo 4h benzopyran 7 yl]oxy]acetic acid
dr3438
see: [[5 chloro 3 (2 methylphenyl) 4 oxo 4h benzopyran 7 yl]oxy]acetic acid
drenamist
see: adrenalin
drenison
see: fludroxycortide
drenusil
see: polythiazide
drinalfa
see: methamphetamine
drinamyl
see: mazindol
dristan inhaler
see: propylhexedrine

drocinonide

drocort
see: fludroxycortide
drolban
see: drostanolone propionate

droloxifene

dromostanolone
see: drostanolone
dromostanolone propionate
see: drostanolone propionate
dromstanolone
see: drostanolone

dronabinol

dronabinol,11 hydroxy
see: 11 hydroxydronabinol
droptimol
see: timolol maleate

drospirenone

drospirenone plus estradiol

drospirenone plus ethinylestradiol

drostanediol
see: 3beta androstanediol

drostanolone

drostanolone propionate

d sotalol
see: sotalol

Index

dt 327
see: clopamide
dt327
see: clopamide
d threo methylphenidate
see: dexmethylphenidate
d trp 6 lhrh
see: triptorelin
[d trp 6]lhrh
see: triptorelin
d trp 6 pro 9 net lhrh
see: gonadorelin[1-9] ethylamide[6 dextro tryptophan]
du 21 220
see: ritodrine
du 21220
see: ritodrine
du21220
see: ritodrine
dualid
see: amfepramone
duomedihaler
see: hydrocortisone
duovent
see: fenoterol plus ipratropium bromide
durabetason
see: betamethasone sodium phosphate
durabeton
see: propranolol
durabolic
see: methandriol dipropionate
durabolin
see: nandrolone phenpropionate
duraboral
see: ethylestrenol
duradiuret
see: hydrochlorothiazide plus triamterene
durafurid
see: furosemide
duraludrin
see: isoprenaline
duramorph
see: morphine sulfate
duramorple
see: morphine sulfate
durapindol
see: pindolol
durarese
see: amiloride plus hydrochlorothiazide
duraspiron
see: spironolactone
duratest
see: testosterone cipionate
durathate
see: testosterone enantate
duromine
see: phentermine resin
duromorph
see: morphine

dutimelan

dutimelan 8 15
see: dutimelan
dutimelan 815
see: dutimelan
duvadilan
see: isoxsuprine
duvadilan retard
see: isoxsuprine
dw 62
see: dimefline
dw62
see: dimefline
dyazide
see: hydrochlorothiazide plus triamterene
dylephrin
see: adrenalin
dynabolon
see: nandrolone undecanoate
dynacoryl
see: nikethamide
dynalert
see: pemoline
dynamicarde
see: nikethamide
dynaphenyl
see: dexamphetamine
dynepo
see: recombinant erythropoietin
dyneric
see: clomifene citrate
dyren
see: triamterene
dyrenium
see: triamterene
dysemide
see: furosemide plus triamterene
dyspne inhal
see: adrenalin
dyspnoesan
see: isoprenaline
dytac
see: triamterene
dyta urese
see: spironolactone

dytaurese
see: spironolactone
dytenzide
see: hydrochlorothiazide plus triamterene
dytid
see: benzthiazide plus triamterene
dytide
see: benzthiazide plus triamterene
dytide h
see: hydrochlorothiazide plus triamterene
dytide n
see: benzthiazide
e 111
see: propylhexedrine
e111
see: propylhexedrine
e 241
see: clorprenaline
e241
see: clorprenaline
e 250
see: selegiline
e250
see: selegiline
e 614
see: tripamide
e614
see: tripamide
ea 1477
see: dronabinol
ea1477
see: dronabinol

ebiratide

ebiratide acetate

ecazide
see: captopril plus hydrochlorothiazide
ecgonine methyl ester benzoate
see: cocaine
eciphin
see: ephedrine
econopred
see: prednisolone acetate
ecoval 70
see: betamethasone valerate
ecovent
see: salbutamol
'ecstasy'
see: 3,4 methylenedioxymethamphetamine
ectosone
see: betamethasone valerate
ecural
see: mometasone furoate
ecylert
see: pemoline magnesium
edecril
see: etacrynic acid
edecrin
see: etacrynic acid
edemdal
see: chlortalidone
edemox
see: acetazolamide
edrul
see: muzolimine

efaproxiral

efaproxiral sodium
see: efaproxiral
efcorlin
see: hydrocortisone sodium succinate
ef cortelan
see: hydrocortisone
efcortelan
see: hydrocortisone
ef cortelan soluble
see: hydrocortisone sodium succinate
efcortelan soluble
see: hydrocortisone sodium succinate
efcortesol
see: hydrocortisone sodium phosphate
efedra orion
see: ephedrine
efedrin
see: ephedrine
efedrine
see: ephedrine
efektolol
see: propranolol
efektolol retard
see: propranolol
effectin
see: bitolterol mesilate
efflumidex
see: fluorometholone
effontil
see: etilefrine
effortil
see: etilefrine
effroxine
see: methamphetamine

efidrin
see: ephedrine
eformoterol
see: formoterol
eformoterol fumarate
see: formoterol fumarate
efortil
see: etilefrine
efroxin
see: methamphetamine
efroxine
see: methamphetamine
eggophedrin
see: ephedrine
egibren
see: selegiline
egis 5650
see: panomifene
egis5650
see: panomifene
egocort
see: hydrocortisone
eksalb
see: hydrocortisone
el 10
see: prasterone
el10
see: prasterone
el 737
see: ractopamine
el737
see: ractopamine
elastonin
see: amphetamine
elastonon
see: amphetamine
elbrol
see: propranolol
eldecort
see: hydrocortisone
eldeprine
see: selegiline
eldepryl
see: selegiline
eleagol
see: seric gonadotropin
electrocortin
see: aldosterone
elektrocortin
see: aldosterone
elfanex
see: dihydralazine plus hydrochlorothiazide plus reserpine
eligard
see: leuprorelin
elipten
see: aminoglutethimide
eliptin
see: aminoglutethimide
elitone
see: nikethamide
elkapin
see: etozolin
elocom
see: mometasone furoate
elocon
see: mometasone furoate
elohast
see: hetastarch
elohes
see: hetastarch
em 139
see: n butyl 11 (16alpha chloro 3,17beta dihydroxyestra 1,3,5(10) trien 7alpha yl) n methylundecanamide
em139
see: n butyl 11 (16alpha chloro 3,17beta dihydroxyestra 1,3,5(10) trien 7alpha yl) n methylundecanamide
em 343
see: 3 (4 hydroxyphenyl) 4 methyl 2 [4 [2 (1 piperidinyl)ethoxy]phenyl] 2h 1 benzopyran 7 ol
em343
see: 3 (4 hydroxyphenyl) 4 methyl 2 [4 [2 (1 piperidinyl)ethoxy]phenyl] 2h 1 benzopyran 7 ol
em 651
see: 3 (4 hydroxyphenyl) 4 methyl 2 [4 [2 (1 piperidinyl)ethoxy]phenyl] 2h 1 benzopyran 7 ol
em651
see: 3 (4 hydroxyphenyl) 4 methyl 2 [4 [2 (1 piperidinyl)ethoxy]phenyl] 2h 1 benzopyran 7 ol
em 652
see: 3 (4 hydroxyphenyl) 4 methyl 2 [4 [2 (1 piperidinyl)ethoxy]phenyl] 2h 1 benzopyran 7 ol
em652
see: 3 (4 hydroxyphenyl) 4 methyl 2 [4 [2 (1 piperidinyl)ethoxy]phenyl] 2h 1 benzopyran 7 ol
em 776
see: 4 [4 methyl 2 [4 [2 (1 piperidinyl)ethoxy]phenyl] 7 pivaloyloxy 2h 1 benzopyran 3 ylphenyl] pivalate
em776
see: 4 [4 methyl 2 [4 [2 (1 piperidinyl)ethoxy]phenyl] 7 pivaloyloxy 2h 1 benzopyran 3 ylphenyl] pivalate

em 800
see: 4 [4 methyl 2 [4 [2 (1 piperidinyl)ethoxy]phenyl] 7 pivaloyloxy 2h 1 benzopyran 3 ylphenyl] pivalate
em800
see: 4 [4 methyl 2 [4 [2 (1 piperidinyl)ethoxy]phenyl] 7 pivaloyloxy 2h 1 benzopyran 3 ylphenyl] pivalate
embryo hemoglobin
see: hemoglobin F
embryonic hemoglobin
see: hemoglobin F
emconcor
see: bisoprolol fumarate
emcor
see: bisoprolol fumarate
emcortina
see: fluprednidene acetate
emd 33512
see: bisoprolol fumarate
emd33512
see: bisoprolol fumarate
emi corlin
see: hydrocortisone sodium succinate
emiran
see: etamivan
emivan
see: etamivan
emovate
see: clobetasone butyrate
emsam
see: selegiline

enalapril plus hydrochlorothiazide

enanton
see: leuprorelin
enantone
see: leuprorelin
enarmon
see: testosterone propionate

enclomifene

enclomifene citrate

en clomiphene
see: enclomifene
enclomiphene
see: enclomifene
enclomiphene citrate
see: enclomifene citrate
encortelon
see: prednisolone
encortelone
see: prednisolone
encortolon
see: prednisolone
encorton
see: prednisone
encortone
see: prednisone
endabuse
see: ibogaine
endak
see: carteolol
endak mite
see: carteolol
endecril
see: etacrynic acid
endocorion
see: chorionic gonadotropin
endolate
see: pethidine
endone
see: oxycodone
endopancrine
see: neutral insulin
enduron
see: methyclothiazide
enduronum
see: methyclothiazide
energital
see: deoxycorticosterone phenpropionate plus nandrolone phenpropionate
enkorton
see: prednisone
entestil
see: testosterone propionate
entestil m
see: methyltestosterone
entocort
see: budesonide
entocort ec
see: budesonide
eoden
see: heptaminol
ep 23905
see: hexarelin
ep23905
see: hexarelin

epanolol

epaq
see: salbutamol sulfate
ephadrosan
see: ephedrine
ephalone
see: ephedrine
ephedral
see: ephedrine
ephedra orion
see: ephedrine
ephedrin
see: ephedrine

ephedrine

ephedrine,4 hydroxy
see: oxilofrine
ephedrine hydrochloride
see: ephedrine
ephedron
see: racephedrine
ephedrone
see: methcathinone
ephedrosan
see: ephedrine
ephedrosst
see: ephedrine
ephetonin
see: racephedrine

epiandrosterone

epicortisol
see: epihydrocortisone
11 epicortisol
see: epihydrocortisone
epifoam
see: hydrocortisone acetate
epifrin
see: dipivefrine
epiglaufrin
see: adrenalin

epihydrocortisone

11 epihydrocortisone
see: epihydrocortisone
epimephrine
see: adrenalin

epimestrol

epimorph
see: morphine
epinefrina
see: adrenalin
epinephran
see: adrenalin
epinephrin
see: adrenalin
epinephrine
see: adrenalin
epinephrine chloride
see: adrenalin
epinephrine dipivalate
see: dipivefrine
epinephrine hydrochloride
see: adrenalin
epinephrine isopropyl homolog
see: isoprenaline

epinine

epinine hydrochloride
see: epinine
epipen
see: adrenalin
epirenamine
see: adrenalin
epirenan
see: adrenalin
epitens
see: triamterene plus xipamide

epitestosterone

17 epitestosterone
see: epitestosterone
epithiazide
see: epitizide

epitizide

epitopic
see: difluprednate
epitrenbolone
see: 17alpha trenbolone

eplerenone

epoch
see: recombinant erythropoietin

Index

epoconn
see: recombinant erythropoietin
epoetin
see: recombinant erythropoietin
epoetin alfa
see: recombinant erythropoietin
epoetin beta
see: recombinant erythropoietin
epoetin delta
see: recombinant erythropoietin
epogen
see: recombinant erythropoietin
epogin
see: recombinant erythropoietin
epoietin
see: recombinant erythropoietin
epoietin alfa
see: recombinant erythropoietin
epoietin alpha
see: recombinant erythropoietin
epoietin beta
see: recombinant erythropoietin
epoxitin
see: recombinant erythropoietin
eprex
see: recombinant erythropoietin
equibold
see: boldenone undecenoate
equine gonadotrophin
see: seric gonadotropin
equinex
see: seric gonadotropin
equipois
see: boldenone undecenoate
equipoise
see: boldenone undecenoate
equoman
see: seric gonadotropin
era 923
see: pipendoxifene
era923
see: pipendoxifene
eraldin
see: practolol
eraldin inj.
see: practolol
erantin
see: recombinant erythropoietin
ermalone
see: mestanolone
erthropoietin
see: erythropoietin
erydin
see: isoprenaline
erypo
see: recombinant erythropoietin

erythrocruorin

erythrocruorins
see: erythrocruorin
erythropoietic factor
see: erythropoietin

erythropoietin

erythropoietin, recombinant
see: recombinant erythropoietin
erythroprocaterol
see: procaterol
erythroxylin
see: cocaine
esacortene
see: dexamethasone
escort
see: prednicarbate
esiclene
see: formebolone
esidrex
see: hydrochlorothiazide
esidrex apresoline
see: hydralazine plus hydrochlorothiazide
esidrex ismelin
see: guanethidine plus hydrochlorothiazide
esidrex k
see: hydrochlorothiazide
esidrex k forte
see: hydrochlorothiazide
esidrex plus apresoline
see: hydralazine plus hydrochlorothiazide
esidri
see: hydralazine plus hydrochlorothiazide plus reserpine
esidrix
see: hydrochlorothiazide
esimil
see: guanethidine plus hydrochlorothiazide
esiteren
see: hydrochlorothiazide plus triamterene
esjaydiol
see: methandriol
esmarin
see: trichlormethiazide

esmolol

esmolol hydrochloride
see: esmolol
esophan
see: methamphetamine
esperson
see: desoximetasone
espesil
see: acebutolol
espo
see: recombinant erythropoietin
estimulex
see: methamphetamine
estr 4 en 17beta ol 3 one
see: nandrolone
estr 4 en 3 one,17beta hydroxy
see: nandrolone

estr 4 ene 3,17 dione

estr 4 ene 3beta,17beta diol
see: bolandiol
estra 4 ene 3,17 dione
see: estr 4 ene 3,17 dione
estradiol antagonists
see: antiestrogen
estradiol plus drospirenone
see: drospirenone plus estradiol

estratest

4 estren 17beta ol 3 one
see: nandrolone
4 estrene 3,17 dione
see: estr 4 ene 3,17 dione
estrimex
see: toremifene
estrogen antagonist
see: antiestrogen
estrogen antagonists
see: antiestrogen
estrogen conjugated equine
see: seric gonadotropin
estrogen suppression
see: antiestrogen
estrogen synthetase inhibitor
see: aromatase inhibitor
etacortin
see: fluprednidene acetate
etacrinic acid
see: etacrynic acid
etacrynate
see: etacrynic acid

etacrynic acid

etafedrine

etafedrine hydrochloride
see: etafedrine
etamivam
see: etamivan

etamivan

etamivanum
see: etamivan

etanterol

etazolin
see: etozolin
ethacrinic acid
see: etacrynic acid
ethacrynate
see: etacrynic acid
ethacrynic acid
see: etacrynic acid
ethacryonic acid
see: etacrynic acid
ethamivan
see: etamivan

ethamoxytriphetol

ethamoxy triphetol
see: ethamoxytriphetol
ethanol
see: alcohol
ethanol solution
see: alcohol
ethanoxytriphetol
see: ethamoxytriphetol

ethiazide

ethimizol
see: ethimizole

Index

ethimizole

ethinylestradiol plus drospirenone
see: drospirenone plus ethinylestradiol

ethinylestradiol plus methyltestosterone

ethiocholanone
see: etiocholanone
ethocrynic acid
see: etacrynic acid
ethoxazolamide
see: ethoxzolamide

2beta ethoxy 3alpha hydroxy 11alpha isopentylamino 5alpha androstane 17beta carboxylic acid methyl ester

ethoxyzolamide
see: ethoxzolamide

ethoxzolamide

ethycrynic acid
see: etacrynic acid

13beta ethyl 17beta hydroxygon 4 en 3 one

17 ethyl 19 nor testosterone
see: norethandrolone
17 ethyl 19 nortestosterone
see: norethandrolone
19 ethyl 19 nortestosterone
see: norethandrolone

n ethyl 3,4 methylenedioxyamphetamine

3 ethyl 3 methylglutarimide
see: bemegride

5 ethyl 5 (3 methyl 2 butenyl)barbituric acid

4 ethyl 6,7 dimethoxy beta carboline 3 carboxylic acid methyl ester

ethyl adrianol
see: etilefrine
ethyladrianol
see: etilefrine
ethyladrianol hydrochloride
see: etilefrine
ethyl alcohol
see: alcohol
ethylalcohol
see: alcohol
ethyl amphetamine
see: n ethylamphetamine
ethylamphetamine
see: n ethylamphetamine

n ethylamphetamine

ethylcocaine
see: homococaine
ethylephedrine
see: etafedrine
ethylephrine
see: etafedrine
ethylestranol
see: ethylestrenol
ethylestrenal
see: ethylestrenol

ethylestrenol

ethyl estrenol
see: ethylestrenol
ethylestrenole
see: ethylestrenol
ethylnandrol
see: ethylestrenol
ethyl norphenylephrine
see: etilefrine
ethylnorphenyl ephrine
see: etilefrine
ethylnorphenylephrine
see: etilefrine
ethyloestrenol
see: ethylestrenol

1 (2 ethylphenoxy) 3 (1,2,3,4 tetrahydro 1 naphthylamino) 2 propanol oxalate

ethylphenylephrine
see: etilefrine
ethymisol
see: ethimizole
ethymizol
see: ethimizole
etilamphetamine
see: n ethylamphetamine

etilefrine

etilefrine acetate
see: etilefrine
etilefrine butyrate
see: etilefrine
etilefrine hydrochloride
see: etilefrine

etilefrine pivalate

etilefrine propionate
see: etilefrine
etilefrine sulfate
see: etilefrine
etilphrine
see: etafedrine
etimizol
see: ethimizole
etimizole
see: ethimizole
etiocholan 17beta ol 3 one
see: 5beta androstanolone

etiocholanone

etipuren
see: etilefrine
etnesol
see: betamethasone sodium phosphate
etoscol
see: hexoprenaline
etoxzolamide
see: ethoxzolamide

etozolin

etozoline
see: etozolin
etyprenaline
see: isoetarine
eu 4891
see: diacetolol
eu4891
see: diacetolol
eubine
see: oxycodone
eucannabinolide
see: cannabis derivative
eucardic
see: carvedilol
eucodal
see: oxycodone
eucodale
see: oxycodone
eucoran
see: nikethamide
eudin
see: oxycodone
eufodrin
see: methamphetamine
eufodrinal
see: methamphetamine
eukdin
see: oxycodone
eukodal
see: oxycodone
eukraton
see: bemegride
eumicton
see: acetazolamide
eumorphal
see: oxycodone
eumovate
see: clobetasone butyrate
eunephran
see: butizide
eunepran
see: butizide
euphobine
see: amphetamine
euphodine
see: amphetamine
euphodyn
see: amphetamine
eurax hc
see: crotamiton plus hydrocortisone
eurax hydrocortisone
see: crotamiton plus hydrocortisone
eurelix
see: piretanide
eurinol
see: trichlormethiazide
eurodamine
see: oxycodone
euspiran
see: isoprenaline
eutagen
see: oxycodone
eutensin
see: furosemide
eutensine
see: furosemide
euvaderm
see: betamethasone benzoate

Index

euvitol
see: adrenalin
eventin
see: propylhexedrine
everone
see: testosterone enantate
evista
see: raloxifene
evrodex
see: dexamphetamine
exactin
see: corticotropin
exadion
see: dexamethasone
exadione
see: dexamethasone
ex adipos
see: phentermine
exadipos
see: phentermine
exadrin
see: adrenalin
examorelin
see: hexarelin

exaprolol

exemestane

exirel
see: pirbuterol
exna
see: benzthiazide
exosalt
see: benzthiazide
expandex
see: dextran
expansolin
see: tretoquinol
exponcit
see: norpseudoephedrine
exprex
see: recombinant erythropoietin
ex s1
see: dexamethasone
f 1983
see: pyrovalerone
f1983
see: pyrovalerone
f 6060
see: bis(4 hydroxyphenyl)cyclohexylidenemethane
f6060
see: bis(4 hydroxyphenyl)cyclohexylidenemethane
f 6066
see: cyclofenil
f6066
see: cyclofenil
f 66e
see: bis(perfluorohexyl)ethylene
f66e
see: bis(perfluorohexyl)ethylene
fabedrine
see: amphetamine
factrel
see: gonadorelin

fadrozole

fadrozole hydrochloride
see: fadrozole
fagolipo
see: mazindol

falintolol

falintolol oxalate

fareston
see: toremifene
faslodex
see: fulvestrant
fastin
see: phentermine
fba 1500
see: mefruside
fba1500
see: mefruside
fc 1157 a
see: toremifene
fc 1157a
see: toremifene
fc1157a
see: toremifene
fc 1271a
see: ospemifene
fc1271a
see: ospemifene
fc 43
see: perfluorotributylamine
fc43
see: perfluorotributylamine
fc 47
see: perfluorotributylamine

Index

fc47
see: perfluorotributylamine
fc 80
see: perfluorobutyltetrahydrofuran
fc80
see: perfluorobutyltetrahydrofuran
fce 24304
see: exemestane
fce24304
see: exemestane
fce 24918
see: androsta 4,6,8(9) triene 3,17 dione
fce24918
see: androsta 4,6,8(9) triene 3,17 dione
fce 24928
see: minamestane
fce24928
see: minamestane
f cortef
see: fludrocortisone
f cortef acetate
see: fludrocortisone acetate
fedrin
see: ephedrine

felodipine plus metoprolol

femar
see: letrozole
femara
see: letrozole
fenacamfamine
see: fencamfamin
fenadon
see: methadone
fenam
see: isoxsuprine
fenamide
see: diclofenamide
fenamizol
see: amiphenazole
fenara
see: amphetamine

fencamfamin

fencamfamine
see: fencamfamin
fencamfamine hydrochloride
see: fencamfamin
fencamfamin hydrochloride
see: fencamfamin
fendimetrazine
see: phendimetrazine
fenedrin
see: amphetamine
fenethylline
see: fenetylline
fenethylline hydrochloride
see: fenetylline
fenetyllin
see: fenetylline

fenetylline

fenfluramide
see: fenfluramine
fenfluramin
see: fenfluramine

fenfluramine

fenfluramine,dextro
see: dexfenfluramine
fenfluramine hydrochloride
see: fenfluramine
fenicort
see: prednisolone sodium tetrahydrophthalate
fenmetralin
see: phenmetrazine
fenmetrazine
see: phenmetrazine

fenoldopam

fenoldopam 7,8 bis(n ethylcarbamate)

fenoldopam mesilate

fenoldopam mesylate
see: fenoldopam mesilate

fenoterol

fenoterol hydrobromide
see: fenoterol

fenoterol plus ipratropium bromide

fenoxazol
see: pemoline

fenproporex

fenquizone

fenured
see: fenfluramine
ferric hemoglobin
see: methemoglobin
ferrihemoglobin
see: methemoglobin
ferrohemoglobin
see: hemoglobin
ferrosan
see: prednisone acetate
fertagyl
see: gonadorelin
fertiline
see: follitropin
fertinex
see: urofollitropin
fertinom p
see: follitropin
fertinorm
see: urofollitropin
fertiral
see: gonadorelin
fertodur
see: cyclofenil
fertyl
see: clomifene citrate
fetal hb
see: hemoglobin F
fetal hemoglobin
see: hemoglobin F
fetanol
see: etilefrine
fetanyl
see: etilefrine
fetus hemoglobin
see: hemoglobin F
fi 5852
see: oxabolone cipionate
fi5852
see: oxabolone cipionate
ficortil
see: hydrocortisone acetate
ficortril
see: hydrocortisone
finajet
see: trenbolone acetate
finaplix
see: trenbolone acetate
finibron
see: buprenorphine

finrozole

firmalone
see: dexamethasone
fish insulin
see: insulin
fk 435
see: droloxifene
fk435
see: droloxifene
fl 75
see: perfluorotributylamine
fl75
see: perfluorotributylamine
fl 80
see: perfluorotributylamine
fl80
see: perfluorotributylamine
fla 365
see: 2,6 dichloro 4 dimethylaminoamphetamine
fla365
see: 2,6 dichloro 4 dimethylaminoamphetamine
flantadin
see: deflazacort
flebocortid
see: hydrocortisone sodium succinate

flerobuterol

flestolol

flestolol sulfate
see: flestolol
flixonase
see: fluticasone propionate
flixotide
see: fluticasone propionate
flonase
see: fluticasone propionate
florinef
see: fludrocortisone
florinef acetate
see: fludrocortisone acetate
florone
see: diflorasone diacetate
flovent
see: fluticasone propionate
fluandrenalone
see: fludroxycortide

fluandrenolide
see: fludroxycortide
fluandrenolone
see: fludroxycortide
fluandrenolone acetonide
see: fludroxycortide
fluaton
see: fluorometholone
fluazacort,defluoro
see: deflazacort
flubason
see: desoximetasone
flubenisolone
see: betamethasone
flucinar
see: fluocinonide
flucinolone
see: fluocinolone
flucinolone acetonide
see: fluocinolone acetonide

fluclorolone

fluclorolone acetonide

flucloronide
see: fluclorolone acetonide
flucon
see: fluorometholone
flucort
see: flumetasone acetate
flucort cream
see: flumetasone acetate
flucortin butyl
see: fluocortin butyl
flucortolon
see: fluocortolone
flucortolon caproate
see: fluocortolone caproate
flucortolon capronate
see: fluocortolone caproate
flucortolone
see: fluocortolone
flucortolone caproate
see: fluocortolone caproate
flucortolone capronate
see: fluocortolone caproate
flucortolone hexanoate
see: fluocortolone caproate
flucortolone trimethyl acetate
see: fluocortolone pivalate
flucortolonetrimethyl acetate
see: fluocortolone pivalate
fluderma
see: formocortal
fludestrin
see: testolactone
fludex
see: indapamide
fludrocortisate
see: fludrocortisone acetate
fludrocortisol
see: fludrocortisone

fludrocortisone

fludrocortisone 21 acetate
see: fludrocortisone acetate

fludrocortisone acetate

fludrocortone
see: fludrocortisone
fludrohydrocortisone
see: fludrocortisone
fludrone
see: fludrocortisone
fludronef
see: fludrocortisone
fludroxycordide
see: fludroxycortide

fludroxycortide

fludroxy cortide
see: fludroxycortide
fluidema
see: indapamide
fluidil
see: cyclothiazide
fluitran
see: trichlormethiazide
flumen
see: chlorothiazide

flumetasone

flumetasone 21 pivalate
see: flumetasone pivalate

flumetasone acetate

Index

flumetasone pivalate

flumetasone pivalate plus salicylic acid

flumetasone pivalate plus triclosan

flumetasone trimethylacetate
see: flumetasone pivalate
flumetazone pivalate
see: flumetasone pivalate
flumethason
see: flumetasone
flumethasone
see: flumetasone
flumethasone 21 acetate
see: flumetasone acetate
flumethasone acetate
see: flumetasone acetate
flumethasone pivalate
see: flumetasone pivalate
flumethazone pivalate
see: flumetasone pivalate
flumetholon
see: fluorometholone
flumethone
see: paramethasone acetate
flumil
see: buphenine
flumilar
see: flumetasone

flumoxonide

flunase
see: fluticasone propionate

flunisolide

flunisolide acetate

flunisolide hemihydrate
see: flunisolide
fluobate
see: betamethasone benzoate
fluocinolide
see: fluocinonide
fluocinolon
see: fluocinolone
fluocinolon acetonid
see: fluocinolone acetonide

fluocinolone

fluocinolone 16,17 acetonide
see: fluocinolone acetonide

fluocinolone acetonide

fluocinolone acetonide acetate
see: fluocinonide

fluocinonide

fluocortin

fluocortin butyl

fluocortin butyl ester
see: fluocortin butyl
fluocortolon caproate
see: fluocortolone caproate

fluocortolone

fluocortolone 21 caproate
see: fluocortolone caproate
fluocortolone 21 hexanoate
see: fluocortolone caproate

fluocortolone caproate

fluocortolone capronate
see: fluocortolone caproate
fluocortolone hexanoate
see: fluocortolone caproate
fluocortolone monohydrate
see: fluocortolone

fluocortolone pivalate

fluocortolone trimethylacetate
see: fluocortolone pivalate
fluohydrisone
see: fludrocortisone
fluohydrisone acetate
see: fludrocortisone acetate
fluohydrocortisone
see: fludrocortisone
fluohydrocortisone acetate
see: fludrocortisone acetate

fluolar
see: fluocinolone acetonide
fluometholone
see: fluorometholone
fluonid
see: fluocinolone acetonide
fluonide
see: fluocinolone acetonide
fluoprednilidene
see: fluprednidene
fluoprednilidene 21 acetate
see: fluprednidene acetate
fluoprednylidene 21 acetate
see: fluprednidene acetate
fluoprednylidene acetate
see: fluprednidene acetate
fluorandrenolone
see: fludroxycortide
fluorcortolone 21 capronate
see: fluocortolone caproate
fluor cortolone caproate
see: fluocortolone caproate
fluorhydrocortisone actetate
see: fludrocortisone acetate
fluorhydrocortisonum
see: fludrocortisone
fluorlon
see: fluorometholone
fluorlon lavsan
see: fluorometholone
fluormetholon
see: fluorometholone
fluormethylprednisolon
see: dexamethasone
fluormethyl prednisolone
see: dexamethasone
fluormethylprednisolone
see: dexamethasone
fluormone
see: dexamethasone
fluormone 17 valerate
see: dexamethasone 17 valerate
fluorobate
see: betamethasone benzoate
fluorocarbon 43
see: perfluorotributylamine
fluorocarbon fc 43
see: perfluorotributylamine
fluorocarbon fc43
see: perfluorotributylamine
fluorocarbon fc 80
see: perfluorobutyltetrahydrofuran
fluorocort
see: dexamethasone
fluorocortin butyl ester
see: fluocortin butyl
fluorocortisone
see: fludrocortisone
fluorocortolone
see: fluocortolone
fluorocortolone caproate
see: fluocortolone caproate
fluorodelta
see: dexamethasone
fluorofarmilone
see: formocortal
fluorohydrocortisone
see: fludrocortisone
fluorohydrocortisone acetate
see: fludrocortisone acetate
fluoromethalone
see: fluorometholone

fluorometholone

fluoromethylprednisolone
see: dexamethasone

2 [2 (4 fluorophenoxy)ethyl]phenol

[2 [2 (4 fluorophenoxy)ethyl]phenyl] sulfate

fluoroprednilidene
see: fluprednidene acetate
9 fluoroprednisolone
see: isoflupredone
fluoroprednylidene 21 acetate
see: fluprednidene acetate
fluorothyl
see: flurothyl
fluoroxymesterone
see: fluoxymesterone
fluorprednylidene
see: fluprednidene

fluosol

fluosol 43
see: perfluorotributylamine

Index

fluosol da

fluosol da 20
see: fluosol da
fluosol fc 43
see: perfluorotributylamine
fluosol fc43
see: perfluorotributylamine
fluosterone
see: fluoxymesterone
fluotestin
see: fluoxymesterone
fluotrex
see: fluocinolone acetonide
fluoximesterone
see: fluoxymesterone
fluoxiprednisolone
see: triamcinolone
fluoxiprednisolone acetonide
see: triamcinolone acetonide
fluoxymesteron
see: fluoxymesterone

fluoxymesterone

fluoxymestrone
see: fluoxymesterone
fluoxyprednisolone
see: triamcinolone

fluprednidene

fluprednidene 21 acetate
see: fluprednidene acetate

fluprednidene acetate

fluprednilene 21 acetate
see: fluprednidene acetate
flupredniliden acetate
see: fluprednidene acetate
fluprednilidene
see: fluprednidene
fluprednilidene 21 acetate
see: fluprednidene acetate
fluprednilidene acetate
see: fluprednidene acetate

fluprednisolone

fluprednylen 21 acetate
see: fluprednidene acetate
fluprednyliden 21 acetate
see: fluprednidene acetate
fluprednylidene
see: fluprednidene
fluprednylidene 21 acetate
see: fluprednidene acetate
fluprednylidene acetate
see: fluprednidene acetate
fluprednylidene acetate cream
see: fluprednidene acetate
flurandrenolide
see: fludroxycortide
flurandrenolon
see: fludroxycortide
flurandrenolone
see: fludroxycortide
flurandrenolone acetonide
see: fludroxycortide
flurinef
see: fludrocortisone
flurobate
see: betamethasone benzoate
flurohydrocortisone
see: fludrocortisone
flurosemide
see: furosemide
flurothil
see: flurothyl

flurothyl

flurotyl
see: flurothyl

flusoxolol

fluspiral
see: fluticasone propionate
flutec pp5
see: perfluorodecalin

fluticasone

fluticasone propionate

fluticasone propionate plus salmeterol

flutide
see: fluticasone propionate
flutide nasal
see: fluticasone propionate

Index

flutinase
see: fluticasone propionate
flutivate
see: fluticasone propionate
flutone
see: triamcinolone acetonide
flutra
see: trichlormethiazide
fluvin
see: hydrochlorothiazide
fluxonal
see: fluticasone propionate
fm 24
see: bornaprolol
fm24
see: bornaprolol
fml forte
see: fluorometholone
fml liquifilm
see: fluorometholone
focalin
see: dexmethylphenidate
foetal haemoglobin
see: hemoglobin F
foetal hemoglobin
see: hemoglobin F
folistiman
see: gonadotropin
follegon
see: urofollitropin
follicle stimulating hormone
see: follitropin
follicotropin
see: follitropin
folliculostimulating hormone
see: follitropin

folligen

folligon
see: seric gonadotropin
follistim
see: recombinant follitropin
follitrophin
see: follitropin

follitropin

follitropin alfa
see: recombinant follitropin
follitropin beta
see: recombinant follitropin
follitropin beta fragment
see: follitropin beta subunit

follitropin beta subunit

follitropin derivative

follitropine
see: follitropin

follitropin receptor binding inhibitor

follitropin release factor
see: follitropin releasing factor

follitropin releasing factor

folltropin
see: follitropin
follutein
see: chorionic gonadotropin

fominoben

fonurit
see: acetazolamide
foradil
see: formoterol fumarate
fordilen
see: formoterol fumarate
fordiuran
see: bumetanide

formebolone

formestane

formetamide
see: formetorex

formetorex

formocortal

formocortral
see: formocortal
formoftil
see: formocortal

Index

formoterol

formoterol fumarate

formoterol hemifumarate
see: formoterol fumarate
formoterol plus budesonide
see: budesonide plus formoterol
19 formylandrostenedione
see: 19 oxoandrostenedione
formyldienolone
see: formebolone
fortadex
see: nandrolone laurate
fortal
see: pentazocine
fortalgesic
see: pentazocine
fortecortin
see: dexamethasone
fortecortin 17 valerate
see: dexamethasone 17 valerate
fortigel
see: testosterone
fortral
see: pentazocine
fortraline
see: pentazocine
fortwin
see: pentazocine
fostimon
see: urofollitropin
fougera
see: triamcinolone acetonide
fovane
see: benzthiazide
fpdfpa
see: prenylamine
fpl 60278
see: dopexamine
fpl60278
see: dopexamine
fpl 60278 ar
see: dopexamine
fpl 60278ar
see: dopexamine
fpl60278ar
see: dopexamine
fpl 68397
see: 4 hydroxy 7 [2 [2 [3 (2 phenylethoxy)propylsulfonyl]ethylamino]ethyl]benzothiazol 2(3h) one
fpl68397
see: 4 hydroxy 7 [2 [2 [3 (2 phenylethoxy)propylsulfonyl]ethylamino]ethyl]benzothiazol 2(3h) one
free hemoglobin
see: hemoglobin
free testosterone
see: testosterone
frekven
see: propranolol

fresh frozen plasma

frespire
see: salbutamol
frideron
see: zeranol
fringanor
see: phendimetrazine embonate
frugalan
see: furfenorex

frumil

frusamil
see: frumil
frusemide
see: furosemide
frusene
see: furosemide plus triamterene
fruzex
see: furosemide
FSH
see: follitropin
FSH beta fragment
see: follitropin beta subunit
FSH beta subunit
see: follitropin beta subunit
fsh derivative
see: follitropin derivative
fsh nosticon
see: follitropin
fsh receptor binding inhibitor
see: follitropin receptor binding inhibitor
fsh releasing factor
see: follitropin releasing factor
fsh releasing hormone
see: follitropin releasing factor
fsh rf
see: follitropin releasing factor
fsh rh
see: follitropin releasing factor

ft 19
see: nandrolone phenpropionate
ft19
see: nandrolone phenpropionate
ft 81
see: bendroflumethiazide
ft81
see: bendroflumethiazide
ftorocort
see: triamcinolone acetonide

fulvestrant

fumarenid
see: furosemide
fumide
see: furosemide
furanthril
see: furosemide
furantril
see: furosemide
furasemide
see: furosemide

furazabol

furesis
see: furosemide

furfenorex

furfurylamphetamine

furfurylmethylamphetamine
see: furfenorex
furix
see: furosemide
furobasan
see: furosemide
furomide
see: furosemide
furo puren
see: furosemide
furopuren
see: furosemide
furorese
see: furosemide
furosamide
see: furosemide
furose
see: furosemide
furosemid
see: furosemide

furosemide

furosemide plus amiloride
see: frumil

furosemide plus triamterene

furosemide with triamterene
see: furosemide plus triamterene
furosemix
see: furosemide
furosimide
see: furosemide
fursemide
see: furosemide
fusid
see: furosemide
fx 80
see: perfluorobutyltetrahydrofuran
fx80
see: perfluorobutyltetrahydrofuran
g 33128
see: chlortalidone
g33128
see: chlortalidone
g 33 182
see: chlortalidone
g 33182
see: chlortalidone
g33 182
see: chlortalidone
g33182
see: chlortalidone
g 5668
see: prethcamide
g5668
see: prethcamide
gamma chain,hemoglobin
see: hemoglobin gamma chain
gammacorten
see: dexamethasone
gammacorten 17 valerate
see: dexamethasone 17 valerate
gammacortene
see: dexamethasone
gangesol
see: trichlormethiazide
ganja
see: cannabis

Index

ganjah
see: cannabis
geabol
see: metandienone

gelatinol

gelatin succinate

gelatin succinic anhydride
see: gelatin succinate
gelifundol
see: oxypolygelatin
gelofusine
see: gelatin succinate

gelonida

gelonida na
see: gelonida
genabol
see: norboletone
geno cristaux
see: testosterone
genotonorm
see: somatrem
genotropin
see: human growth hormone
gentran
see: dextran
gentran 40
see: dextran 40
gentran 70
see: dextran 70
gepefrin
see: gepefrine

gepefrine

gepefrine tartrate

geref
see: sermorelin
gerohormetten
see: growth hormone
gerovit
see: methamphetamine
gestasol dry
see: chorionic gonadotropin

gestrinone

gestyl
see: seric gonadotropin
gewazol
see: pentetrazole
GH
see: growth hormone
gh releasing factor
see: growth hormone releasing factor
gh rf
see: growth hormone releasing factor
GHRF
see: growth hormone releasing factor
ghrf 1-29
see: growth hormone releasing factor[1-29]
ghrf derivative
see: growth hormone releasing factor derivative
GHRH
see: growth hormone releasing factor
ghrh[1-29] amide
see: sermorelin
GHRP 2
see: pralmorelin
GHRP 6
see: histidyl dextro tryptophylalanyltryptophyl dextro phenylalanyllysinamide
gilucor
see: sotalol
giludop
see: dopamine
ginecrin
see: leuprorelin
ginecrin depot
see: leuprorelin

giractide

gl 701
see: prasterone
gl701
see: prasterone
glargine insulin
see: insulin glargine
glaucomide
see: acetazolamide
glaucon
see: adrenalin
glauconex
see: befunolol
glaucosan
see: adrenalin

Index

glaucothil
see: dipivefrine
glauco visken
see: pindolol
glaukonex
see: befunolol
glauline
see: metipranolol
glaupax
see: acetazolamide
glin epin
see: adrenalin
glistelone
see: prednisolone
globin alpha chain
see: hemoglobin alpha chain
globin beta chain
see: hemoglobin beta chain
globin delta chain
see: hemoglobin delta chain
globin gamma chain
see: hemoglobin gamma chain
globuren
see: recombinant erythropoietin
glosso sterandryl
see: methyltestosterone
glossosterandryl
see: methyltestosterone
glucitol
see: sorbitol

glucocorticoid

glucocorticoid drug
see: glucocorticoid
glucocorticoid hormone
see: glucocorticoid
glucocorticoids
see: glucocorticoid
glucocorticoids, synthetic
see: glucocorticoid
glucocorticoid steroid
see: glucocorticoid
glucocorticoidsteroid
see: glucocorticoid
glucocorticoids, topical
see: glucocorticoid
glucocorticosteroid
see: glucocorticoid
glucocortoid
see: glucocorticoid
glucoenergan
see: fencamfamin
glucohexitol
see: sorbitol
5 glutamine alpha 1-19 acth
see: corticotropin derivative
glycated hemoglobin
see: glycosylated hemoglobin
glycated hemoglobin A1c
see: hemoglobin A1c
glycerol 2 arachidonate
see: 2 arachidonoylglycerol
glycirenan
see: adrenalin
glycitol
see: sorbitol
glycocorticoid
see: glucocorticoid
glycocorticosteroid
see: glucocorticoid
glycohemoglobin
see: glycosylated hemoglobin

glycosylated hemoglobin

glycosylated hemoglobin A1c
see: hemoglobin A1c
glycosyl hemoglobin
see: glycosylated hemoglobin
glycosylhemoglobin
see: glycosylated hemoglobin
glycosylized hemoglobin
see: glycosylated hemoglobin
glypolix
see: dexfenfluramine
gn rh
see: gonadorelin
gnrh
see: gonadorelin
gnrh agonist
see: gonadorelin agonist
gnrh derivative
see: gonadorelin derivative
gnrh serono
see: gonadorelin
go 3282
see: ozolinone
go3282
see: ozolinone
go 687
see: etozolin
go687
see: etozolin
goe 3282
see: ozolinone

goe3282
see: ozolinone
goe 687
see: etozolin
goe687
see: etozolin
goedecke 3282
see: ozolinone
goldline
see: betamethasone valerate
gonabion
see: chorionic gonadotropin
gonadex
see: chorionic gonadotropin
gonadin
see: seric gonadotropin
gonadogen
see: seric gonadotropin
gonadoliberin
see: gonadorelin
gonadoliberin analog
see: gonadorelin derivative
gonadoliberin derivative
see: gonadorelin derivative

gonadorelin

gonadorelin[1-9][6 dextro alanine]

gonadorelin[1-9] ethylamide[6 dextro alanine]

gonadorelin[1-9] ethylamide[6 dextro tryptophan]

gonadorelin[6 dextro [3 (2 naphthyl)alanine] 10 azaglycine]

gonadorelin[6 dextro lysine] 2 pyrrolinodoxorubicin

gonadorelin[6 dextro lysine] doxorubicin

gonadorelin[6 medphalan]

gonadorelin acetate

gonadorelin agonist

gonadorelin analog
see: gonadorelin derivative

gonadorelin associated peptide

gonadorelin associated peptide derivative

gonadorelin associated protein
see: gonadorelin associated peptide

gonadorelin derivative

gonadorelin diacetate
see: gonadorelin acetate
gonadoryl
see: human menopausal gonadotropin
gonadotraphon f.s.h.
see: seric gonadotropin
gonadotraphon fsh
see: seric gonadotropin
gonadotraphon l.h.
see: chorionic gonadotropin
gonadotrophic hormone
see: gonadotropin
gonadotrophin
see: gonadotropin
gonadotrophin derivative
see: gonadotropin derivative
gonadotrophin,menopause
see: human menopausal gonadotropin
gonadotrophin releasing factor
see: gonadorelin
gonadotrophon
see: chorionic gonadotropin
gonadotropic hormone
see: gonadotropin

gonadotropin

gonadotropin derivative

gonadotropine
see: gonadotropin
gonadotropin,human chorionic
see: chorionic gonadotropin

gonadotropin,menopausal
see: human menopausal gonadotropin
gonadotropin,pituitary
see: gonadotropin
gonadotropin release factor
see: gonadorelin
gonadotropin releasing factor
see: gonadorelin
gonadotropin releasing hormone
see: gonadorelin
gonadotropins
see: gonadotropin
gonadotropins, chorionic
see: chorionic gonadotropin
gonadotropins, equine
see: seric gonadotropin
gonadotropins, pituitary
see: gonadotropin
gonadrone
see: testosterone propionate
gonad stimulating hormone
see: gonadotropin
gonad stimulatory hormone
see: gonadotropin
gonadyl seric
see: seric gonadotropin
gonal f
see: recombinant follitropin
gonan
see: gonadotropin
gormon
see: seric gonadotropin

goserelin

goserelin acetate
see: goserelin
gr 114297a
see: picumeterol
gr 18781
see: fluticasone propionate
gr18781
see: fluticasone propionate
gr 2 1214
see: clobetasone butyrate
gr 2-1214
see: clobetasone butyrate
gr 21214
see: clobetasone butyrate
gr2-1214
see: clobetasone butyrate
gr 2 925
see: clobetasol propionate
gr 2-925
see: clobetasol propionate
gr 2925
see: clobetasol propionate
gr2 925
see: clobetasol propionate
gr2-925
see: clobetasol propionate
gr2925
see: clobetasol propionate
gr 33343
see: salmeterol xinafoate
gr 33343x
see: salmeterol
gr 62
see: isoxsuprine
gr62
see: isoxsuprine
gr 63411
see: picumeterol
gr 63411b
see: picumeterol
gr 81706
see: 1 (1 naphthyloxy) 3 [6 [2 (2 pyridyl)ethoxy]hexylamino] 2 propanol
gracidin
see: phenmetrazine
gravosan
see: clomifene citrate
GRF
see: growth hormone releasing factor
groliberin
see: sermorelin
groliverin
see: sermorelin
grorm
see: growth hormone
grosodexon
see: dexamethasone
grosodexone
see: dexamethasone
growth factor ii,insulin like
see: somatomedin B
growth factor,insulin
see: somatomedin

growth hormone

growth hormone analog
see: growth hormone derivative
growth hormone,biosynthetic
see: recombinant growth hormone

growth hormone derivative

growth hormone fraction
see: growth hormone

growth hormone,human
see: human growth hormone

growth hormone,hypophysis
see: growth hormone

growth hormone,methionyl
see: somatrem

growth hormone release factor
see: growth hormone releasing factor

growth hormone releasing factor

growth hormone releasing factor[1-29]

growth hormone releasing factor derivative

growth hormone treatment
see: growth hormone

guabenxan plus bemetizide
see: tensigradyl

guanamprazine
see: amiloride

guanethidine plus hydrochlorothiazide

guaranine
see: caffeine

guarin
see: caffeine

gubernal
see: alprenolol

guinethazone
see: quinethazone

gulitole
see: sorbitol

gutron
see: midodrine

gyki 13504
see: panomifene

gyki13504
see: panomifene

gyki 41099
see: cloranolol

gynepral
see: hexoprenaline

gynipral
see: hexoprenaline

h 104-08
see: pamatolol

h 119-66
see: alpha hydroxymetoprolol

h 1285
see: 4 (2 diethylaminoethoxy) alpha' ethyl alpha (4 hydroxyphenyl) 4' methoxystilbene

h 133 22
see: prenalterol

h 133-22
see: prenalterol

h 13322
see: prenalterol

h 133-80
see: prenalterol

h 142 08
see: n [2 [2 hydroxy 3 [4 (2 isobutoxyethoxy)phenoxy]propylamino]ethyl] 4 morpholinecarboxamide

h 201 70
see: 4 hydroxy n [2 [2 hydroxy 3 [4 [2 (isobutoxy)ethoxy]phenoxy]propylamino]ethyl] 1 piperidinecarboxamide

h 216 44
see: n [2 [3 [4 [2 (2 cyclopropylmethoxyethoxy)ethyl]phenoxy] 2 hydroxypropylamino]ethyl] 4 hydroxy 1 piperidinecarboxamide

h 3452
see: cyclofenil

h3452
see: cyclofenil

h 35 25
see: 2 isopropylamino 1 (4 tolyl)propanol

h 35-25
see: 2 isopropylamino 1 (4 tolyl)propanol

h35 25
see: 2 isopropylamino 1 (4 tolyl)propanol

h 56-23
see: alprenolol

h 56-26
see: alprenolol

h 56 28
see: alprenolol

h 56-28
see: alprenolol

h 610
see: fencamfamin

h 66 37
see: hydroxyamphetamine

h 66-37
see: hydroxyamphetamine

h 80-62
see: prenalterol

h 835
see: cafedrine plus theodrenaline
h835
see: cafedrine plus theodrenaline
h 87-07
see: 1 isopropylamino 3 [4 (2 methoxyethoxy)phenoxy] 2 propanol
h 93-26
see: metoprolol
haelan
see: fludroxycortide
haemaccel
see: polygeline
haemaccel 35
see: polygeline
haemacel
see: polygeline
haemiglobin
see: methemoglobin
haemodan
see: adrenalone
haemoglobin
see: hemoglobin
haemoglobin a
see: hemoglobin A
haemoglobin alpha chain
see: hemoglobin alpha chain
haemoglobin beta chain
see: hemoglobin beta chain
haemoglobin c
see: hemoglobin C
haemoglobin chain
see: hemoglobin chain
haemoglobin e
see: hemoglobin E
haemoglobin f
see: hemoglobin F
haemoglobin gamma chain
see: hemoglobin gamma chain
haemoglobin h
see: hemoglobin H
haemoglobin j
see: hemoglobin J
haemoglobin m
see: hemoglobin M
haemoglobin s
see: hemoglobin S
haemostatin
see: adrenalin
haes steril
see: hetastarch
halciderm
see: halcinonide
halcimat
see: halcinonide

halcinonide

halcort
see: halcinonide
haldrate
see: paramethasone acetate
haldrone
see: paramethasone acetate
haloart
see: halopredone acetate
halobetasol propionate
see: ulobetasol propionate
halocrinic acid
see: brocrinat
halog
see: halcinonide

halometasone

halopredone

halopredone 17,21 diacetate
see: halopredone acetate

halopredone acetate

halotensin
see: fluoxymesterone
halotestin
see: fluoxymesterone
hashish
see: cannabis
Hb
see: hemoglobin
Hb A
see: hemoglobin A
hb a 1
see: glycosylated hemoglobin
hb a1
see: glycosylated hemoglobin
hb a(1c)
see: hemoglobin A1c
Hb A1c
see: hemoglobin A1c
hba 1c
see: hemoglobin A1c
hba1c
see: hemoglobin A1c

hb a 2
see: hemoglobin A2
Hb A2
see: hemoglobin A2
hb alpha chain
see: hemoglobin alpha chain
hb beta chain
see: hemoglobin beta chain
Hb C
see: hemoglobin C
HbCO
see: carboxyhemoglobin
Hb E
see: hemoglobin E
hb f
see: hemoglobin F
HbF
see: hemoglobin F
hb gamma chain
see: hemoglobin gamma chain
Hb H
see: hemoglobin H
Hb J
see: hemoglobin J
Hb M
see: hemoglobin M
hboc 201
see: polymerized hemoglobin
hboc-201
see: polymerized hemoglobin
Hb S
see: hemoglobin S
h.c.g.
see: chorionic gonadotropin
hCG
see: chorionic gonadotropin
hCG alpha subunit
see: chorionic gonadotropin alpha subunit
hCG beta subunit
see: chorionic gonadotropin beta subunit
hcg endo
see: chorionic gonadotropin
he 111
see: dexamethasone isonicotinate
hebcort
see: hydrocortisone
hebcort v
see: hydrocortisone
helfergin
see: meclofenoxate
hemaccel
see: polygeline
hemacel
see: polygeline
hemacell
see: polygeline
hemagel
see: polygeline
hemassist
see: diaspirin crosslinked hemoglobin
hematopoietin
see: erythropoietin
hemax
see: recombinant erythropoietin
hemiglobin
see: methemoglobin
hemisine
see: adrenalin
hemoantine
see: seric gonadotropin
hemodex
see: dextran
hemodex 40
see: dextran 40
hemodex 70
see: dextran 70

hemodialysis fluid

hemodialysis solutions
see: hemodialysis fluid

hemoglobin

hemoglobin A

hemoglobin a 1
see: glycosylated hemoglobin
hemoglobin A1
see: glycosylated hemoglobin

hemoglobin A1c

hemoglobin a 1c
see: hemoglobin A1c
hemoglobin a(1c)
see: hemoglobin A1c

hemoglobin A2

hemoglobin a 2
see: hemoglobin A2
hemoglobin a2 babinga
see: hemoglobin A2

hemoglobin a 2 indonesia
see: hemoglobin A2
hemoglobin a 2 melbourne
see: hemoglobin A2
hemoglobin a2 nyu
see: hemoglobin A2
hemoglobin a2 sphakia
see: hemoglobin A2
hemoglobin a, glycosylated
see: glycosylated hemoglobin
hemoglobin ai
see: glycosylated hemoglobin
hemoglobin aic
see: hemoglobin A1c
hemoglobin alpha
see: hemoglobin A
hemoglobin alpha 1
see: glycosylated hemoglobin
hemoglobin alpha 2
see: hemoglobin A2

hemoglobin alpha chain

hemoglobin beta chain

hemoglobin C

hemoglobin carbon monoxide
see: carboxyhemoglobin

hemoglobin chain

hemoglobin delta chain

hemoglobin derivative

hemoglobin E

hemoglobine
see: hemoglobin
hemoglobin e variant
see: hemoglobin E

hemoglobin F

hemoglobin f dammam
see: hemoglobin F
hemoglobin,fetal
see: hemoglobin F
hemoglobin gamma
see: hemoglobin C

hemoglobin gamma chain

hemoglobin glycoside
see: glycosylated hemoglobin
hemoglobin glycosylation
see: glycosylated hemoglobin

hemoglobin H

hemoglobin J

hemoglobin M

hemoglobinose m
see: hemoglobin M
hemoglobin polymer
see: polymerized hemoglobin
hemoglobin,pyridoxylated
see: pyridoxylhemoglobin

hemoglobin S

hemoglobins
see: hemoglobin
hemoglobins, abnormal
see: hemoglobin variant
hemoglobin, sickle
see: hemoglobin S
hemoglobin,sickle cell
see: hemoglobin S
hemoglobin subunit
see: hemoglobin chain

hemoglobin variant

hemoglobulin
see: hemoglobin
hemolink
see: hemoglobin
hemopoietin
see: erythropoietin
hemopure
see: polymerized hemoglobin
hemostasin
see: adrenalin

hemostatin
see: adrenalin
hemp
see: cannabis
heneicosafluorotripropylamine
see: perfluorotripropylamine
hepandrin
see: oxandrolone
hephentermine
see: mephentermine
heptacosafluorotributylamine
see: perfluorotributylamine
heptadon
see: methadone

heptaminol

heptaminol chlorhydrate
see: heptaminol
heptaminol hydrochloride
see: heptaminol
heptamyl
see: heptaminol
heptanon
see: methadone
heptonal
see: heptaminol
heptylon
see: heptaminol
herba cannabis
see: cannabis
hermalone gloset
see: mestanolone
heroin
see: diamorphine
heroine
see: diamorphine
heroine hydrochloride
see: diamorphine
heroin hydrochloride
see: diamorphine
hespan
see: hetastarch
hespander
see: hetastarch
hes steril
see: hetastarch
hetamine
see: dexamphetamine

hetastarch

hetastarch 120
see: hetastarch
hetastarch 200
see: hetastarch
hetastarch 40
see: hetastarch
hexadecadiol
see: dexamethasone
hexadecadrol
see: dexamethasone
hexadecadrol 17 valerate
see: dexamethasone 17 valerate
hexadiol
see: dexamethasone
hexadrol
see: dexamethasone
hexadrol 17 valerate
see: dexamethasone 17 valerate
hexadrol phosphate
see: dexamethasone sodium phosphate
hexafluorodiethyl ether
see: flurothyl
hexafluorodiethylether
see: flurothyl
hexahydrodesoxyephedrine
see: propylhexedrine
hexaprenaline
see: hexoprenaline

hexarelin

hexatrione
see: triamcinolone hexacetonide

hexoprenaline

hexoprenaline sulfate
see: hexoprenaline
hextend
see: hetastarch
hfe
see: flurothyl
h.g.h.
see: human growth hormone
hGH
see: human growth hormone
hgp 1
see: loteprednol etabonate
hgp1
see: loteprednol etabonate

hidril
see: hydrochlorothiazide
hidronal
see: chlortalidone
high ceiling diuretic
see: loop diuretic agent
high ceiling diuretic agent
see: loop diuretic agent
high molecular weight dextran
see: dextran
higroton
see: chlortalidone
higrotona
see: chlortalidone
hiropon
see: methamphetamine
hiserpin
see: hydroflumethiazide
histerelin
see: histrelin
histerone
see: testosterone

histidyl dextro tryptophylalanyltryptophyl dextro phenylalanyllysinamide

histrelin

histrelin acetate
see: histrelin
hizaar
see: hydrochlorothiazide plus losartan
hmd
see: oxymetholone
HMG
see: human menopausal gonadotropin
hmr 1964
see: insulin glulisine
hmr1964
see: insulin glulisine
hms liquifilm
see: medrysone
hoe 10820
see: methadone
hoe10820
see: methadone
hoe 118
see: piretanide
hoe118
see: piretanide
hoe 21 gh
see: neutral insulin
hoe 21 ph
see: neutral insulin
hoe 304
see: desoximetasone
hoe304
see: desoximetasone
hoe 39893d
see: penbutolol
hoe39893d
see: penbutolol
hoe 427
see: ebiratide
hoe 433
see: alsactide
hoe 471
see: gonadorelin
hoe471
see: gonadorelin
hoe 706
see: buserelin acetate
hoe 766
see: buserelin acetate
hoe 766 mp
see: buserelin acetate
hoe 777
see: prednicarbate
hoe777
see: prednicarbate
hoe 893d
see: penbutolol
hoe893d
see: penbutolol
hoe 901
see: insulin glargine
hoe901
see: insulin glargine
hoechst 471
see: gonadorelin
hokumalin
see: tulobuterol
homan
see: methyltestosterone
homandren
see: methyltestosterone
homandren amp
see: testosterone propionate
hombreol
see: androstanediol
homocaine
see: homococaine

Index

homococaine

homogonal
see: human menopausal gonadotropin
homosten
see: chorionic gonadotropin
homosteron
see: testosterone
hormale
see: methyltestosterone
hormandren
see: testosterone propionate
17 hormoforin
see: prasterone
17 hormoforin 3 sulfate
see: prasterone sulfate
hormoformin
see: prasterone
hormonabol
see: nandrolone phenpropionate
hormone,growth
see: growth hormone
hormone,human growth
see: human growth hormone
hormoteston
see: testosterone propionate
hostacortin
see: prednisone
hostacortin h
see: prednisolone
hostacortin h solubile
see: prednisolone sodium succinate
hostacortin h vet
see: prednisolone
hostaginan
see: prenylamine
howgan
see: amosulalol
hp 3522
see: brocrinat
hp 522
see: brocrinat
hp acthar gel
see: corticotropin
h tronin
see: human insulin
hu 210
see: dexanabinol
hu 211
see: dexanabinol
hubernol
see: boldenone undecenoate
hudorex
see: hydrochlorothiazide
humacthid
see: corticotropin
humactid
see: corticotropin
humalin r
see: recombinant human insulin
humalog
see: insulin[B28 lysine B29 proline]
humalog mix npl
see: insulin[B28 lysine B29 proline]
human choriogonadotropin
see: chorionic gonadotropin
human chorion gonadotrophin
see: chorionic gonadotropin
human chorion gonadotropin
see: chorionic gonadotropin
human chorionic gonadotrophin
see: chorionic gonadotropin
human chorionic gonadotropin
see: chorionic gonadotropin
human follitropin
see: follitropin
human fsh
see: follitropin
human gonadotrophin
see: chorionic gonadotropin
human gonadotropin
see: gonadotropin

human growth hormone

human insulin

humanized insulin
see: recombinant human insulin
human luteinizing hormone
see: luteinizing hormone
human menopausal gonadotrophin
see: human menopausal gonadotropin

human menopausal gonadotropin

human menopause gonadotropin
see: human menopausal gonadotropin
human monocomponent insulin
see: monocomponent insulin
human placental gonadotropin
see: chorionic gonadotropin
human proinsulin,biosynthetic
see: biosynthetic human proinsulin

human somatotropin
see: human growth hormone
humatrop
see: human growth hormone
humatrope
see: human growth hormone
humegon
see: human menopausal gonadotropin
humergon
see: human menopausal gonadotropin
humilin
see: insulin
huminsulin
see: recombinant human insulin
huminsulin normal
see: recombinant human insulin
humulin
see: human insulin
humulin i
see: isophane insulin
humulin n
see: isophane insulin
humulin r
see: isophane insulin
humulin regular
see: human insulin
humulin s
see: neutral insulin
hy 21011
see: practolol
hy21011
see: practolol
hybolin
see: nandrolone phenpropionate
hybolin decanoate
see: nandrolone decanoate
hybolin improved
see: nandrolone phenpropionate
hycorace
see: hydrocortisone sodium succinate
hycort
see: hydrocortisone
hydeltra
see: prednisolone
hydeltrasol
see: prednisolone sodium phosphate
hydeltrone
see: prednisolone
hydracort
see: hydrocortisone

hydralazine plus hydrochlorothiazide

hydralazine plus hydrochlorothiazide plus reserpine

hydrallostane

hydrargan
see: mersalyl
hydrasson
see: hydrocortisone
hydrelta
see: prednisolone
hydrenox
see: hydroflumethiazide
hydril
see: hydrochlorothiazide
hydro adreson
see: hydrocortisone sodium succinate
hydroadreson
see: hydrocortisone sodium succinate
hydro aquil
see: hydrochlorothiazide
hydroaquil
see: hydrochlorothiazide
hydrochlor
see: hydrochlorothiazide
hydrochlorothiamide
see: hydrochlorothiazide
hydrochlorothiazid
see: hydrochlorothiazide

hydrochlorothiazide

hydro chlorothiazide
see: hydrochlorothiazide
hydrochloro thiazide
see: hydrochlorothiazide

hydrochlorothiazide plus irbesartan

hydrochlorothiazide plus lisinopril

hydrochlorothiazide plus losartan

hydrochlorothiazide plus metoprolol

Index

hydrochlorothiazide plus metoprolol tartrate

hydrochlorothiazide plus propranolol

hydrochlorothiazide plus quinapril

hydrochlorothiazide plus telmisartan

hydrochlorothiazide plus triamterene

hydrochlorothiazide plus valsartan

hydrochlorothiazine
see: hydrochlorothiazide
hydrochlorthiazide
see: hydrochlorothiazide
hydrochlothiazide
see: hydrochlorothiazide
hydrocodal
see: oxycodone
hydrocort
see: hydrocortisone
hydrocortal
see: hydrocortisone acetate
hydrocortancyl
see: prednisolone
hydrocorticosteroid
see: hydrocortisone
hydrocortidelt
see: prednisolone
hydrocortisate
see: hydrocortisone
hydrocortison
see: hydrocortisone

hydrocortisone

hydrocortisone,11 epi
see: epihydrocortisone
hydrocortisone 17 butyrate
see: hydrocortisone butyrate

hydrocortisone 17 butyrate 21 propionate

hydrocortisone 17 valerate
see: hydrocortisone valerate
hydrocortisone,18 oxo
see: 18 oxohydrocortisone
hydrocortisone 21 acetate
see: hydrocortisone acetate
hydrocortisone 21 phosphate
see: hydrocortisone sodium phosphate
hydrocortisone 21 sodium succinate
see: hydrocortisone sodium succinate
hydrocortisone 21 succinate
see: hydrocortisone sodium succinate
hydrocortisone 21 thiol
see: tixocortol
hydrocortisone,6beta hydroxy
see: 6beta hydroxyhydrocortisone

hydrocortisone acetate

hydrocortisone acetonide
see: hydrocortisone
hydrocortisone buteprate
see: hydrocortisone 17 butyrate 21 propionate

hydrocortisone butyrate

hydrocortisone derivative

hydrocortisone dorsch
see: hydrocortisone acetate
hydrocortisone hemisuccinate
see: hydrocortisone sodium succinate
hydrocortisone intraveineux
see: hydrocortisone sodium succinate
hydrocortisone ointment
see: hydrocortisone
hydrocortisone phosphate
see: hydrocortisone sodium phosphate
hydrocortisone plus crotamiton
see: crotamiton plus hydrocortisone
hydrocortisone plus miconazole
see: daktacort
hydrocortisone plus saline
see: hydrocortisone

hydrocortisone plus urea

hydrocortisone probutate
see: hydrocortisone 17 butyrate 21 propionate

hydrocortisone sodium phosphate

Index

hydrocortisone sodium succinate

hydrocortisone steroid
see: hydrocortisone
hydrocortisone succinate
see: hydrocortisone sodium succinate
hydrocortisone, topical
see: hydrocortisone

hydrocortisone valerate

hydrocortisone with urea
see: hydrocortisone plus urea
hydrocortison sodium phosphate
see: hydrocortisone sodium phosphate
hydrocortistab
see: hydrocortisone acetate
hydrocortistab soluble
see: hydrocortisone sodium succinate
hydrocortisyl
see: hydrocortisone
hydrocortone
see: hydrocortisone
hydrocortone acetate
see: hydrocortisone acetate
hydrodeltalone
see: prednisolone
hydrodeltisone
see: prednisolone
hydroderm
see: hydrocortisone
hydrodexan
see: hydrocortisone plus urea
hydro diuril
see: hydrochlorothiazide
hydrodiuril
see: hydrochlorothiazide

hydroflumethiazide

hydro-long tablinen
see: chlortalidone
hydromal
see: hydrochlorothiazide
hydromedin
see: etacrynic acid
hydromorphinone hydrochloride
see: hydromorphone

hydromorphone

hydromorphone hydrochloride
see: hydromorphone
hydromox
see: quinethazone
hydronol
see: isosorbide
hydro rapid
see: furosemide
hydroretrocortin
see: prednisolone
hydroretrocortine
see: prednisolone
hydro ricortex
see: hydrocortisone
hydroronol
see: hydrochlorothiazide
hydro saluric
see: hydrochlorothiazide
hydrosaluric
see: hydrochlorothiazide
hydro saluric k
see: hydrochlorothiazide
hydrosaluric k
see: hydrochlorothiazide
hydrosone
see: hydrocortisone acetate
hydro t
see: hydrochlorothiazide
hydrothide
see: hydrochlorothiazide
hydro tonuron
see: hydrochlorothiazide
hydrotrichlorothiazide
see: trichlormethiazide
hydrotrix
see: furosemide plus triamterene
17 hydroxy 11 dehydrocortisone
see: cortisone
4 hydroxy 19 nortestosterone
see: oxabolone

17 hydroxy 15beta,16beta methylene 7alpha methylthio 3 oxo 17alpha pregna 1,4 diene 21 carboxylic acid gamma lactone

3 hydroxy 20 oxo 5 pregnene
see: pregnenolone

6 hydroxy 2 (4 hydroxyphenyl) 3 [4 [2 (1 pyrrolidinyl)ethoxy]benzoyl]benzo[b]thiophene

Index

4 [2 [(2 hydroxy 2 phenylethyl)amino]ethoxy]phenylacetic acid

4 [2 [(2 hydroxy 2 phenylethyl)amino]propyl]benzoic acid

4 [2 [(2 hydroxy 2 phenylethyl)amino]propyl]benzoic acid methyl ester

4 [2 [(2 hydroxy 2 phenylethyl)amino]propyl]benzoic acid methyl ester hydrogen maleate

4 [2 hydroxy 3 [(1 methyl 3 phenylpropyl)amino]propoxy]benzeneacetamide

5 [2 [[2 hydroxy 3 [4 (1 methyl 4 trifluoromethyl 2 imidazolyl)phenoxy]propyl]amino]ethoxy]salicylamide

n [2 [2 hydroxy 3 [4 (2 isobutoxyethoxy)phenoxy]propylamino]ethyl] 4 morpholinecarboxamide

n [4 [2 [[2 hydroxy 3 (4 hydroxyphenoxy)propyl]amino]ethyl] phenyl]benzenesulfonamide

n hydroxy 3,4 methylenedioxyamphetamine

4 (2 hydroxy 3 isopropylaminopropoxy)carbanilic acid propyl ester

3 [4 (2 hydroxy 3 isopropylaminopropoxy)phenyl]propionic acid

4 [2 [(2 hydroxy 3 phenoxypropyl)amino]ethoxy] n (2 methoxyethyl)phenoxyacetamide

4 [2 [(2 hydroxy 3 phenoxypropyl)amino]ethoxy]phenoxyacetic acid

8 hydroxy 5 [1 hydroxy 2 [n [2 (4 methoxyphenyl) 1 methylethyl]amino]ethyl]carbostyril

4 hydroxy 7 [2 [2 [3 (2 phenylethoxy)propylsulfonyl]ethylamino]ethyl]benzothiazol 2(3h) one

hydroxyamphetamine

4 hydroxyamphetamine
see: hydroxyamphetamine

hydroxyamphetamine bromide
see: hydroxyamphetamine

n hydroxyamphetamine

4 hydroxyandrostene 3,17 dione
see: formestane

11beta hydroxyandrostenedione

19 hydroxyandrostenedione

4 hydroxyandrostenedione
see: formestane

hydroxyandrostenone
see: testosterone

hydroxybenzylisoprenaline

hydroxybenzylisoproterenol
see: hydroxybenzylisoprenaline

hydroxybenzylpindolol

Index

8 hydroxycarteolol

hydroxychlorothiazide
see: chlorothiazide derivative
hydroxycodeinoma
see: oxycodone
17 hydroxycorticosterone
see: hydrocortisone
18 hydroxycortisol
see: 18 hydroxyhydrocortisone
17 hydroxycortisone
see: cortisone derivative

3' hydroxy delta9 tetrahydrocannabinol

3 hydroxydenopamine

14 hydroxydihydrocodeinone
see: oxycodone
hydroxydihydromorphinone
see: oxymorphone

11 hydroxydronabinol

4 hydroxyephedrine
see: oxilofrine
hydroxyethylamylopectin
see: hetastarch
2 hydroxyethyldimethylamine
see: deanol
hydroxy ethyl starch
see: hetastarch
hydroxyethyl starch
see: hetastarch
hydroxyethylstarch
see: hetastarch
2 hydroxyethyl starch
see: hetastarch
hydroxyethyl starch 60
see: hetastarch
3 hydroxyetioallocholan 17 one
see: prasterone
hydroxyfedrine
see: oxilofrine

18 hydroxyhydrocortisone

6beta hydroxyhydrocortisone

hydroxymesteron
see: medrysone
hydroxymesterone
see: medrysone
4 hydroxymethamphetamine
see: pholedrine
hydroxymethyl progesterone
see: medrysone
hydroxymethylprogesterone
see: medrysone

alpha hydroxymetoprolol

4 hydroxy n [2 [2 hydroxy 3 [4 [2 (isobutoxy)ethoxy]phenoxy]propylamino]ethyl] 1 piperidinecarboxamide

4 hydroxy n methylamphetamine
see: pholedrine

3 (4 hydroxyphenyl) 4 methyl 2 [4 [2 (1 piperidinyl)ethoxy]phenyl] 2h 1 benzopyran 7 ol

hydroxyphenylorciprenaline
see: fenoterol

16alpha hydroxyprednisolone

hydroxypregnenolone
see: pregnenolone derivative
hydroxypregnenone
see: pregnenolone
hydroxypregnenone sulfate
see: pregnenolone sulfate
21 hydroxyprogesterone
see: deoxycorticosterone

3 (2 hydroxypropylamino) 3 methyl n [2,3,4,5 tetrahydro 2 oxo 1 [[2' (1h tetrazol 5 yl) 1,1' biphenyl 4 yl]methyl] 1h 1 benzazepin 3 yl]butanamide

hydroxypropylaminopropoxyindol
see: pindolol

hydroxytamoxifen

3 hydroxytamoxifen
see: droloxifene

4 hydroxytamoxifen

Index

4 hydroxytestosterone

hydroxytestosterones
see: testosterone derivative

4 hydroxytoremifene

hydroxytyramine
see: dopamine
3 hydroxytyramine
see: dopamine
hydro z 50
see: hydrochlorothiazide
hydrozide 50
see: hydrochlorothiazide
hygroton
see: chlortalidone
hygroton k
see: chlortalidone
hygroton reserpine
see: chlortalidone plus reserpine
hymorphan
see: hydromorphone
hypadil
see: nipradilol
hypernephrin
see: adrenalin
hypertane
see: ethiazide
hypophyseal gonadotropin
see: gonadotropin
hypophysis gonadotropin
see: gonadotropin
hypophysis growth hormone
see: growth hormone
hypothalamic releasing factor
see: hypothalamus releasing factor
hypothalamus release factor
see: hypothalamus releasing factor

hypothalamus releasing factor

hypothiazid
see: hydrochlorothiazide
hypothiazide
see: hydrochlorothiazide
hyprenan
see: prenalterol
hyrex
see: phendimetrazine tartrate
hyskon
see: dextran 70
hysone
see: hydrocortisone
hysone a
see: hydrocortisone acetate
hyton
see: pemoline
hytone
see: hydrocortisone
hyzaar
see: hydrochlorothiazide plus losartan
iatropur
see: triamterene
ibaril
see: desoximetasone
ibidomide
see: labetalol
ibiozedrine
see: amphetamine
iboga
see: ibogaine

ibogaine

ibogine
see: ibogaine

ibopamine

ibopamine hydrochloride
see: ibopamine

ibutamoren

ibutamoren mesylate
see: ibutamoren

ibuterol

ici 118,551
see: 3 isopropylamino 1 (7 methyl 4 indanyloxy) 2 butanol
ici 118551
see: 3 isopropylamino 1 (7 methyl 4 indanyloxy) 2 butanol
ici 118587
see: xamoterol hydrogen fumarate
ici 118 630
see: goserelin
ici 118630
see: goserelin
ici118630
see: goserelin

Index

ici 118630 depot
see: goserelin
ici 141292
see: epanolol
ici 147,798
see: 3,5 diamino 6 chloro n [1 [n [2 [2 hydroxy 3 (1 naphthoxy)propylamino]ethyl]carbamoyl] 1 methylethyl]pyrazine 2 carboxamide
ici 147798
see: 3,5 diamino 6 chloro n [1 [n [2 [2 hydroxy 3 (1 naphthoxy)propylamino]ethyl]carbamoyl] 1 methylethyl]pyrazine 2 carboxamide
ici 164,384
see: n butyl 11 (3,17beta dihydroxyestra 1,3,5(10) trien 7alpha yl) n methylundecanamide
ici 164384
see: n butyl 11 (3,17beta dihydroxyestra 1,3,5(10) trien 7alpha yl) n methylundecanamide
ici 182780
see: fulvestrant
ici182780
see: fulvestrant
ici 188551
see: 3 isopropylamino 1 (7 methyl 4 indanyloxy) 2 butanol
ici 201651
see: 4 [2 [(2 hydroxy 3 phenoxypropyl)amino]ethoxy] n (2 methoxyethyl)phenoxyacetamide
ici 215001
see: 4 [2 [(2 hydroxy 3 phenoxypropyl)amino]ethoxy]phenoxyacetic acid
ici 33,828
see: methallibure
ici 33828
see: methallibure
ici33,828
see: methallibure
ici33828
see: methallibure
ici 38174
see: pronetalol
ici38174
see: pronetalol
ici 45520
see: propranolol
ici 45673
see: toliprolol
ici 45,763
see: toliprolol
ici 45763
see: toliprolol
ici 46 474
see: tamoxifen citrate
ici 46,474
see: tamoxifen citrate
ici 46474
see: tamoxifen citrate
i.c.i. 50172
see: practolol
ici 50,172
see: practolol
ici 50172
see: practolol
ici50172
see: practolol
ici 55548
see: nortamoxifen
ici 66,082
see: atenolol
ici 66082
see: atenolol
ici 72222
see: cetamolol
ici 79280
see: 4 hydroxytamoxifen
ici 88262
see: gonadorelin
ici88262
see: gonadorelin
ici 89,406
see: 1 (2 cyanophenoxy) 3 [2 (3 phenylureido)ethylamino] 2 propanol
ici 89406
see: 1 (2 cyanophenoxy) 3 [2 (3 phenylureido)ethylamino] 2 propanol
ici compound 33828
see: methallibure
ici d1033
see: anastrozole
icid1033
see: anastrozole
ici d 7114
see: 4 [2 [(2 hydroxy 3 phenoxypropyl)amino]ethoxy] n (2 methoxyethyl)phenoxyacetamide
ici d7114
see: 4 [2 [(2 hydroxy 3 phenoxypropyl)amino]ethoxy] n (2 methoxyethyl)phenoxyacetamide
icoralb
see: metaraminol
icsh
see: luteinizing hormone

idoxifene

idph 8032
see: 2,4 dihydro 6,8 dinitro 1,2,4 triazolo[3,4 c][1,4]benzoxazin 1 one
idrolone
see: fenquizone
igrolina
see: chlortalidone
igroton
see: chlortalidone
igroton lopresor
see: chlortalidone plus metoprolol
igroton reserpina
see: chlortalidone plus reserpine
ikaclomin
see: clomifene citrate
ikaklomin
see: clomifene citrate
ikapharm
see: phenmetrazine
ikopal
see: propranolol
il 17803a
see: acebutolol
il17803a
see: acebutolol
ildamen
see: oxyfedrine
iletin
see: insulin zinc suspension
iletin ii
see: insulin
iludrin
see: isoprenaline
iludrina
see: isoprenaline
iludrine
see: isoprenaline
immune reactive insulin
see: immunoreactive insulin
immunocorticotropin
see: immunocortin

immunocortin

immunoinsulin
see: insulin
immunoreactive growth hormone
see: growth hormone

immunoreactive insulin

imoxiterol

impugan
see: furosemide
impulsin
see: palmidrol
incorlin
see: cortisone
incortin
see: cortisone
incortin h
see: hydrocortisone
indacrinic acid
see: indacrinone

indacrinone

indacrynic acid
see: indacrinone

indapamide

indenolol

indenolol hydrochloride
see: indenolol
inderal
see: propranolol
inderal la
see: propranolol
inderal retard
see: propranolol
inderex
see: propranolol
inderide
see: hydrochlorothiazide plus propranolol
indian bhang
see: cannabis
indian ganja
see: cannabis
indian hemp
see: cannabis
indobloc
see: propranolol
indoklon
see: flurothyl
indokolon
see: flurothyl

indopamide
see: indapamide
inflamase
see: prednisolone sodium phosphate
inflanefran
see: prednisolone
inflarest
see: prasterone sulfate
inflatine
see: lobeline
infucoll m 40
see: dextran 40
infukoll m 40
see: dextran 40
ingelan
see: isoprenaline
inhacort
see: flunisolide
inicardio
see: nikethamide
initard
see: insulin
innopran
see: propranolol
innopran xl
see: propranolol
inolin
see: tretoquinol
inopamil
see: ibopamine
inotres
see: dobutamine
inotrex
see: dobutamine
inotrop
see: dopamine
inovan
see: dopamine
INPEA
see: nifenalol
inpea hydrochloride
see: nifenalol
insolone
see: prednisolone
insone
see: prednisone
inspra
see: eplerenone
insulatard
see: isophane insulin
insulatard nph
see: isophane insulin

insulin

insulin actrapid
see: insulin
insulin analog
see: insulin derivative
insulin analogue
see: insulin derivative
insulina pronta lilly
see: insulin

insulin aspart

insulin, Asp(B28)
see: insulin aspart
insulin[B28 aspartic acid]
see: insulin aspart

insulin[B28 lysine B29 proline]

insulin,beef
see: bovine insulin
insulin,bovine
see: bovine insulin
insulin,chemically synthesized
see: synthetic insulin

insulin deoctapeptide

insulin derivative

insulin desoctapeptide
see: insulin deoctapeptide

insulin detemir

insuline
see: insulin

insulin glargine

insulin glulisine

insulin growth factor
see: somatomedin
insulin hnc
see: insulin
insulin,human
see: human insulin

Index

insulin,immunoreactive
see: immunoreactive insulin
insulin, isophane
see: isophane insulin
insulin lente
see: insulin zinc suspension
insulin, lente
see: insulin zinc suspension
insulin lente mc
see: monocomponent insulin
insulin like growth factor
see: somatomedin
insulin like growth factor 1
see: somatomedin C
insulin like growth factor 2
see: somatomedin B
insulin like growth factor I
see: somatomedin C
insulin-like growth factor i
see: somatomedin C
insulin like growth factor II
see: somatomedin B
insulin-like growth factor ii
see: somatomedin B
insulin lispro
see: insulin[B28 lysine B29 proline]
insulin lyspro
see: insulin[B28 lysine B29 proline]
insulin,monocomponent
see: monocomponent insulin
insulin novo actrapid
see: insulin
insulin novo lente
see: insulin zinc suspension
insulin novolente
see: insulin zinc suspension
insulin novo rapitard
see: biphasic insulin
insulin,pig
see: pig insulin
insulin plus protamine sulfate
see: isophane insulin
insulin precursor precursor
see: preproinsulin
insulin,pro
see: proinsulin
insulin, protamine zinc
see: isophane insulin
insulin semilente
see: insulin zinc suspension
insulin snc
see: insulin
insulin subtardum
see: insulin zinc suspension
insulin ultralente
see: insulin zinc suspension
insulinum
see: insulin
insulin zinc
see: insulin zinc suspension
insulin zinc protamine
see: isophane insulin

insulin zinc suspension

insuman
see: recombinant human insulin
intracort
see: hydrocortisone sodium succinate
intradex
see: dextran
intropin
see: dopamine
invamed
see: hydrochlorothiazide plus propranolol
iodinated insulin
see: insulin

4 iodo 2,5 dimethoxyamphetamine

4 iodoamphetamine

iodocyanopindolol
see: cyanoiodopindolol
4 iodo n isopropylamphetamine
see: iofetamine

iodopindolol

iofetamine

iomupren
see: isoprenaline
ionamin
see: phentermine resin
ionamine 15
see: phentermine resin
ionomin
see: phentermine resin
iopidine
see: apraclonidine
ip 751
see: ajulemic acid

ip751
see: ajulemic acid
ipa
see: isoprenaline

ipamorelin

ipradol
see: hexoprenaline
iprafen
see: fenoterol plus ipratropium bromide
ipran
see: propranolol
iprenol
see: isoprenaline

iprocrolol

ips 339
see: 9 (1 tert butylamino 3 hydroxy 2 propyloxyimino)fluorene
IRI
see: immunoreactive insulin
isadren
see: isoprenaline
isadrin
see: isoprenaline
isadrine
see: isoprenaline

isamoltane

isazotane
see: isamoltane
i sedrin
see: ephedrine
ismelin esidrex
see: guanethidine plus hydrochlorothiazide
ismelin navidrex
see: cyclopenthiazide plus guanethidine
ismotic
see: isosorbide
isnacort
see: dexamethasone
isoamin
see: amphetamine
isoamine
see: amphetamine
isoamyn
see: amphetamine
isoamyne
see: amphetamine
isoandrosterone
see: epiandrosterone
isoarinehydrochloride
see: isoetarine
iso autohaler
see: isoprenaline
isobide
see: isosorbide
iso bronchisan
see: isoprenaline
isobronchisan
see: isoprenaline
isobutylhydrochlorothiazide
see: butizide

isoetarine

isoetharine
see: isoetarine
isoetharine hydrochloride
see: isoetarine
isofane insulin
see: isophane insulin

isoflupredone

isoflupredone 21 acetate
see: isoflupredone acetate

isoflupredone acetate

iso glycirenan
see: isoprenaline
isoglycirenan
see: isoprenaline
isolin
see: isoprenaline
isomer a
see: zuclomifene
isomer b
see: enclomifene
isomeride
see: dexfenfluramine
isomyn
see: amphetamine
isonipecaine
see: pethidine
isonorin
see: isoprenaline
isonorin sulfate
see: isoprenaline
isophan
see: methamphetamine

isophane insulin

isophane insulin suspension
see: isophane insulin
isophane zinc insulin
see: isophane insulin
isophan insulin
see: isophane insulin
isophen
see: methamphetamine
isophenethanol
see: nifenalol
isophenethyl alcohol
see: nifenalol
isophenylephrine
see: metaraminol
isophone insulin
see: isophane insulin
isoprel
see: isoprenaline
isoprenalin
see: isoprenaline

isoprenaline

isoprenaline hydrochloride
see: isoprenaline
isoprenaline,hydroxybenzyl
see: hydroxybenzylisoprenaline
isoprenaline sulfate
see: isoprenaline
isoprenalin hydrochloride
see: isoprenaline
isoprenalinum
see: isoprenaline
isoprenol
see: isoprenaline
isopro
see: isoprenaline
isoprofenamine
see: clorprenaline
isoprophenamine
see: clorprenaline
isopropidin
see: isoprenaline
isopropydrin
see: isoprenaline
isopropydrine
see: isoprenaline
isopropydrinum
see: isoprenaline

2 isopropylamino 1 (4 tolyl)propanol

3 isopropylamino 1 (7 methyl 4 indanyloxy) 2 butanol

1 isopropylamino 3 [4 (2 methoxyethoxy)phenoxy] 2 propanol

isopropylarterenol
see: isoprenaline
isopropyl noradrenalin
see: isoprenaline
isopropylnoradrenalin
see: isoprenaline
isopropyl noradrenaline
see: isoprenaline
isopropylnoradrenaline
see: isoprenaline
isopropyl noradrenalin sulfate
see: isoprenaline
isopropylnorepinephrin
see: isoprenaline
isopropylnorepinephrine
see: isoprenaline
isopropylnorphenylephrine
see: isoprenaline
isoprotenol hydrochloride
see: isoprenaline
isoproterenol
see: isoprenaline
isoproterenol hydrochloride
see: isoprenaline
isoproterenol sulfate
see: isoprenaline
isoproterenol sulfaye dihydrate
see: isoprenaline
isoproterol
see: isoprenaline
isopto cetapred
see: prednisolone acetate
isopto dex
see: dexamethasone
isoptodex
see: dexamethasone
isopto epinal
see: adrenalin
isopto flucon
see: fluorometholone
isopto maxidex
see: dexamethasone

isoptomaxidex
see: dexamethasone
iso puren
see: isosorbide
isopuren
see: isosorbide
isoren
see: chlortalidone

isosorbide

isosorbide disodium
see: isosorbide
isosorbine
see: isosorbide
isotalol
see: sotalol

isoxaprolol

isoxozol
see: danazol
isoxsuprin
see: isoxsuprine

isoxsuprine

isoxsuprine hydrochloride
see: isoxsuprine
isoxuprine
see: isoxsuprine
ispranil
see: isoprenaline
istalol
see: timolol
isuprel
see: isoprenaline
isuprel iso
see: isoprenaline
isupren
see: isoprenaline
iszilin
see: insulin
ivaugan
see: hydrochlorothiazide
ixense
see: apomorphine
izadrin
see: isoprenaline
jatropur
see: triamterene
jdl 464
see: torasemide
jdl464
see: torasemide
jellin
see: fluocinolone acetonide
jetrium
see: dextromoramide
jo 1016
see: tixocortol pivalate
jumex
see: selegiline
jumexal
see: selegiline
k 060
see: droloxifene
k060
see: droloxifene
k 21060e
see: droloxifene
k21060e
see: droloxifene
k 30 052
see: etilefrine pivalate
k 30052
see: etilefrine pivalate
k 30081
see: dipivefrine
k 351
see: nipradilol
kabolin
see: nandrolone decanoate
kadian
see: morphine sulfate

kadiur

kalgut
see: denopamine
kanrenol
see: canrenoate potassium
kapanol
see: morphine sulfate
kapodine
see: metoprolol tartrate
kardonyl
see: nikethamide
karfedon
see: carphedon
kargut
see: denopamine
karion
see: sorbitol
karphedon
see: carphedon

karvezide
see: hydrochlorothiazide plus irbesartan
kataline
see: fenfluramine
kathine
see: norpseudoephedrine
katine
see: norpseudoephedrine
katonil
see: chlormerodrin
katovit
see: prolintane
kemodrin
see: methamphetamine
kenac
see: triamcinolone acetonide
kenacomb
see: mycolog
kenacombin
see: mycolog
kenacort
see: triamcinolone
kenacort a
see: triamcinolone acetonide
kenacort e
see: triamcinolone acetonide
kenacort retard
see: triamcinolone
kena log
see: triamcinolone acetonide
kenalog
see: triamcinolone acetonide
kenalog 10
see: triamcinolone acetonide
kenalog 40
see: triamcinolone acetonide
kenalog a 40
see: triamcinolone acetonide
kenalog suspensoid
see: triamcinolone acetonide
kenalone
see: triamcinolone acetonide
kendall compound e
see: cortisone
kendall deoxy compound b
see: deoxycorticosterone
kenlog
see: triamcinolone acetonide
kenocort diacetate syrup
see: triamcinolone diacetate
keoxifene
see: raloxifene
kephrin
see: adrenalone
kephrine
see: adrenalone
kerlon
see: betaxolol
kerlone
see: betaxolol
kessar
see: tamoxifen
ketalgin
see: methadone
ketastarch
see: hetastarch
keteocort h
see: prednisolone
kethamed
see: pemoline
11 ketotestosterone
see: 11 oxotestosterone
key pred
see: prednisolone acetate
kf 4317
see: 4 [2 hydroxy 3 [(1 methyl 3 phenylpropyl)amino]propoxy]benzeneacetamide
kf 868
see: mabuterol
kidney erythropoietic factor
see: erythropoietin
kindavate
see: clobetasone butyrate
kinetazone
see: quinethazone
kl 105
see: 1 tert butylamino 3 (2 chlorophenoxy) 2 propanol
kl 255
see: bupranolol
kl255
see: bupranolol
ko 1366
see: bunitrolol
ko 592
see: toliprolol
komed hc
see: hydrocortisone acetate
kontexin
see: phenylpropanolamine
korazole
see: pentetrazole
korazoli
see: pentetrazole

Index

kordiamin
see: nikethamide
kortikoid ratiopharm
see: triamcinolone acetonide
kp 102
see: pralmorelin
kratedyn
see: ephedrine
kredex
see: carvedilol
krinocort
see: deoxycorticosterone
kristepin
see: briserin
krn 5702
see: recombinant erythropoietin
kryptocur
see: gonadorelin
kt 210
see: nipradilol
kwd 2019
see: terbutaline sulfate
kwd2019
see: terbutaline sulfate
kyliformin
see: clomifene
l 163540
see: 1 [2 (2 amino 2 methylpropionylamino) 3 (1h indol 3 yl)propionyl] 3 benzyl 3 piperidinecarboxylic acid ethyl ester
l 20025
see: clorprenaline
l20025
see: clorprenaline
l 20522
see: dichlorisoprenaline
l 32379
see: drostanolone propionate
l 33379
see: fludroxycortide
l 35483
see: cyclothiazide
l35483
see: cyclothiazide
l 644969
see: 6 amino alpha [[(1 methyl 3 phenylpropyl)amino]methyl] 3 pyridinemethanol
l 692428
see: 3 amino 3 methyl n [2,3,4,5 tetrahydro 2 oxo 1 [[2' (1h tetrazol 5 yl) 1,1' biphenyl 4 yl]methyl] 1h 1 benzazepin 3 yl]butanamide
l 692429
see: 3 amino 3 methyl n [2,3,4,5 tetrahydro 2 oxo 1 [[2' (1h tetrazol 5 yl) 1,1' biphenyl 4 yl]methyl] 1h 1 benzazepin 3 yl]butanamide
l 692585
see: 3 (2 hydroxypropylamino) 3 methyl n [2,3,4,5 tetrahydro 2 oxo 1 [[2' (1h tetrazol 5 yl) 1,1' biphenyl 4 yl]methyl] 1h 1 benzazepin 3 yl]butanamide
l 714465
see: timolol
l714465
see: timolol
l 739574
see: n [4 [2 [[2 hydroxy 3 (4 hydroxyphenoxy)propyl]amino]ethyl]phenyl]benzenesulfonamide
la 956
see: pemoline
labeline
see: lobeline

labetalol

l adrenalin
see: adrenalin
l adrenaline
see: adrenalin
lafax
see: piretanide
l aldosterone
see: aldosterone
l alprenolol
see: alprenolol
lamitol
see: labetalol
l amphetamine
see: amphetamine

landiolol

landiolol hydrochloride
see: landiolol
lantus
see: insulin glargine
lapidine
see: apraclonidine
lasiletten
see: furosemide
lasilix
see: furosemide
lasix
see: furosemide
lasix retard
see: furosemide

Index

lasofoxifene

lasofoxifene tartrate
see: lasofoxifene
laticort
see: hydrocortisone butyrate
laudaconum
see: hydromorphone
laurabolin
see: nandrolone laurate
laurobolin
see: nandrolone laurate
laxis
see: furosemide
lb 46
see: pindolol
lb46
see: pindolol
lb 4675
see: pindolol
lb 502
see: furosemide
lb502
see: furosemide
l benzphetamine
see: benzphetamine
l bunolol hydrochloride
see: levobunolol
l cocaine
see: cocaine
l deprenyl
see: selegiline
l dopamine
see: dopamine
ledercort
see: triamcinolone
ledercort d
see: triamcinolone acetonide
lederlon
see: triamcinolone hexacetonide
lederpronol
see: propranolol
lederspan
see: triamcinolone hexacetonide

leghemoglobin

legoglobin
see: leghemoglobin
leguminous hemoglobin
see: leghemoglobin
lentard
see: insulin zinc suspension
lentard mc
see: insulin zinc suspension
lentaron
see: formestane
lente iletin
see: insulin zinc suspension
lente insulin
see: insulin zinc suspension
leocortol
see: prednisolone
leodrin
see: hydroflumethiazide
leodrine
see: hydroflumethiazide
lepetan
see: buprenorphine
l ephedrine
see: ephedrine
l epinephrine
see: adrenalin
leptamin
see: nikethamide
leptazol
see: pentetrazole
leptazole
see: pentetrazole
leptidrol
see: pipradol

letrozole

7 leucyl alpha 1 24 acth
see: corticotropin derivative
leuplin
see: leuprorelin
leuprogel
see: leuprorelin
leuprolid
see: leuprorelin
leuprolide
see: leuprorelin
leuprolide acetate
see: leuprorelin
leupron
see: leuprorelin

leuprorelin

leuprorelin acetate
see: leuprorelin
leutrophin
see: growth hormone

levadil
see: dilevalol
levadone
see: levomethadone

levalbuterol

levalbuterol hydrochloride
see: levalbuterol
levamfetamine
see: amphetamine
levamphetamine
see: amphetamine
levarterenol
see: noradrenalin
levarterenol bitartrate
see: noradrenalin bitartrate
levatol
see: penbutolol
levedrine
see: amphetamine
levicor
see: metaraminol
levo adrenalin
see: adrenalin
levoadrenalin
see: adrenalin
levo adrenaline
see: adrenalin
levoadrenaline
see: adrenalin
levo adrenalin hydrochloride
see: adrenalin
levo aldosterone
see: aldosterone
levo amphetamine
see: amphetamine
levoamphetamine
see: amphetamine
levo amphetamine sulphate
see: amphetamine
levo benzphetamine
see: benzphetamine

levobunolol

levo bunolol
see: levobunolol
levo cocaine
see: cocaine
levo deprenyl
see: selegiline
levo dextro alprenolol
see: alprenolol
levo dopamine
see: dopamine
levo ephedrine
see: ephedrine
levo epinephrine
see: adrenalin
levoepinephrine
see: adrenalin

levofacetoperane

levo inpea
see: nifenalol
levo isoprenaline
see: isoprenaline
levoisoprenaline
see: isoprenaline
levo isoprenaline sulfate
see: isoprenaline
levo isoproterenol sulfate
see: isoprenaline
levo lobeline
see: lobeline
levo metaraminol
see: metaraminol
levo metaraminol bitartrate
see: metaraminol

levomethadone

levo methadone
see: levomethadone

levomoprolol

levo moprolol
see: levomoprolol

levonantradol

levo nantradol
see: levonantradol
levonantradol,deacetyl
see: deacetyllevonantradol
levonantradol hydrochloride
see: levonantradol
levo n ethylephedrine
see: etafedrine
levonor
see: noradrenalin

Index

levo noradrenalin
see: noradrenalin
levo noradrenalin bitartrate
see: noradrenalin bitartrate
levo noradrenaline
see: noradrenalin
levo norepinephrine
see: noradrenalin
levo norpseudoephedrine
see: norpseudoephedrine
levo oxprenolol
see: oxprenolol
levo oxyprenolol
see: oxprenolol
levo para chloroamphetamine
see: chloramphetamine
levophacetoperan
see: levofacetoperane
levophacetoperane
see: levofacetoperane
levophed
see: noradrenalin
levo pipradol
see: pipradol
levo propranolol
see: propranolol
levopropranolol
see: propranolol
levorenin
see: adrenalin
levorenine
see: adrenalin
levormeloxifene
see: centchroman
levo sotalol
see: sotalol
levosotalol
see: sotalol
levotensin
see: levomoprolol
levo tetrazol
see: pentetrazole
levo tretoquinol
see: tretoquinol
levo trimetoquinol
see: tretoquinol
l fenylfluramine
see: fenfluramine
lg 152
see: androstanolone
LH
see: luteinizing hormone
lhadi
see: recombinant luteinizing hormone
LH beta subunit
see: luteinizing hormone beta subunit
lh derivative
see: luteinizing hormone derivative
lh releasing hormone
see: gonadorelin
lh releasing hormone analog
see: gonadorelin derivative
lhrf
see: gonadorelin
LHRH
see: gonadorelin
lhrh[6 dextro tryptophan]
see: triptorelin
lhrh a
see: gonadorelin derivative
LHRH agonist
see: gonadorelin agonist
lhrh analog
see: gonadorelin derivative
LHRH derivative
see: gonadorelin derivative
lhrh (d trp 6)
see: triptorelin
lhrh t
see: deslorelin
li 32 468
see: spirendolol
li 32-468
see: spirendolol
li 32468
see: spirendolol

liarozole

liarozole fumarate

liarozole hydrochloride
see: liarozole
liazal
see: liarozole fumarate
liazol
see: liarozole fumarate
libigen
see: chorionic gonadotropin
lidepran
see: levofacetoperane
lidex
see: fluocinonide

Index

lidex e
see: fluocinonide
lidol
see: pethidine
lilly 410001
see: recombinant human insulin
linampheta
see: amphetamine
l inpea
see: nifenalol
linyl
see: phentermine resin
liprolog
see: insulin[B28 lysine B29 proline]
liquivent
see: perfluorooctyl bromide
l isoprenaline
see: isoprenaline
l isoproterenol
see: isoprenaline
l isoproterenol sulfate
see: isoprenaline
lispro
see: insulin[B28 lysine B29 proline]
lispro insulin
see: insulin[B28 lysine B29 proline]
liticon
see: pentazocine
litraderm
see: hydrocortisone acetate
livial
see: tibolone
liviella
see: tibolone
lixil
see: bumetanide
lmd
see: dextran 40
l mefruside
see: mefruside
l metaraminol bitartrate
see: metaraminol
l methadone
see: levomethadone
l methamphetamine
see: methamphetamine
l moprolol
see: levomoprolol
lmwd
see: dextran 40
lmw dextran
see: dextran
l nantradol
see: levonantradol
l noradrenalin
see: noradrenalin
l noradrenalin bitartrate
see: noradrenalin bitartrate
l noradrenaline
see: noradrenalin
l noradrenaline acid tartrate
see: noradrenalin bitartrate
l noradrenaline bitartrate
see: noradrenalin bitartrate
l noradrenalin hydrochloride
see: noradrenalin
l norepinephrine
see: noradrenalin
l norpseudoephedrine
see: norpseudoephedrine
lobatox
see: lobeline
lobelidine
see: lobeline
lobelin
see: lobeline

lobeline

lobeline hydrochloride
see: lobeline
lobeline sandoz
see: lobeline
lobeline sulfate
see: lobeline
lobeton
see: lobeline
lobidan
see: lobeline
lobivon
see: nebivolol
lobulantina
see: seric gonadotropin
locacorten
see: flumetasone pivalate
locacorten tar
see: flumetasone pivalate
locacorten vioform
see: clioquinol plus flumetasone pivalate
localyn
see: fluocinolone acetonide
localyn glicole
see: fluocinolone acetonide
locapred
see: desonide

Index

locasalen
see: flumetasone pivalate plus salicylic acid
locasyn
see: flunisolide
locoid
see: hydrocortisone butyrate
locorten
see: flumetasone pivalate
locorten vioform
see: clioquinol plus flumetasone pivalate
locosalen
see: flumetasone pivalate plus salicylic acid
locosthetic
see: cocaine
loftan
see: salbutamol
logamel
see: flumetasone pivalate plus triclosan
logimax
see: felodipine plus metoprolol
logoderm
see: alclometasone dipropionate
logotron
see: chlortalidone plus metoprolol
logroton
see: chlortalidone plus metoprolol
lokalison f
see: dexamethasone
lokilan
see: flunisolide
longasteril
see: dextran
longasteril 40
see: dextran 40
lonovar
see: oxandrolone
loop diuretic
see: loop diuretic agent

loop diuretic agent

lopresor
see: metoprolol tartrate
lopresoretic
see: chlortalidone plus metoprolol
lopresor igroton
see: chlortalidone plus metoprolol
lopresor oros
see: metoprolol fumarate
lopresor sr
see: metoprolol tartrate
lopresside
see: hydrochlorothiazide plus metoprolol
lopressor
see: metoprolol tartrate
lopressor hct
see: hydrochlorothiazide plus metoprolol
lopressor retard
see: metoprolol tartrate
lorinden
see: flumetasone pivalate

lorinden a

lorinden t

lorvas
see: indapamide
lorzaar plus
see: hydrochlorothiazide plus losartan
losalen
see: flumetasone pivalate plus salicylic acid
lotemax
see: loteprednol etabonate
lotensin HCT
see: benazepril plus hydrochlorothiazide

loteprednol etabonate

loterox
see: loteprednol etabonate
loticort
see: fluorometholone

lotricomb

lotrisone
see: betamethasone dipropionate
lowgan
see: amosulalol
low molecular dextran
see: dextran
low molecular weight dextran
see: dextran
loxifen
see: raloxifene
l oxyprenolol
see: oxprenolol
lozol
see: indapamide
l pentazocine
see: pentazocine
l pethidine
see: pethidine

Index

l polamidon
see: levomethadone
l propranolol
see: propranolol
lrh
see: gonadorelin
l sotalol
see: sotalol
lt 31200
see: bopindolol
lt31200
see: bopindolol
l theodrenaline hydrochloride
see: theodrenaline
lucidril
see: meclofenoxate
lucofen
see: chlorphentermine
lucofene
see: chlorphentermine
lucrin
see: leuprorelin
ludonal
see: oxycodone
luf iso
see: isoprenaline
luforan
see: gonadorelin
lukrutor
see: fluprednisolone
luliberin
see: gonadorelin
luliberin analog
see: gonadorelin derivative
luliberin derivative
see: gonadorelin derivative
luliberine
see: gonadorelin
lumitens
see: xipamide
lunetoron
see: bumetanide
lunis
see: flunisolide
lupron
see: leuprorelin
lupron depot
see: leuprorelin
luramide
see: furosemide
luret
see: azosemide
lutal
see: gonadorelin
lutamin
see: gonadorelin
luteinising hormone
see: luteinizing hormone

luteinizing hormone

luteinizing hormone beta subunit

luteinizing hormone derivative

lutotropin
see: luteinizing hormone
lutrelef
see: gonadorelin acetate

lutrelin

lutrepulse
see: gonadorelin acetate
lutropin
see: luteinizing hormone
lutropin beta subunit
see: luteinizing hormone beta subunit
lutropin derivative
see: luteinizing hormone derivative
luveris
see: recombinant luteinizing hormone
luvion
see: canrenone
luxazone
see: dexamethasone
luxazone 17 valerate
see: dexamethasone 17 valerate
lvd
see: dextran 40
ly 031537
see: ractopamine
ly031537
see: ractopamine
ly 10074
see: 6 hydroxy 2 (4 hydroxyphenyl) 3 [4 [2 (1 pyrrolidinyl)ethoxy]benzoyl]benzo[b]thiophene
ly 113174
see: 8 chloro 5 (4 chlorophenyl) 5h indeno[1,2 d]pyrimidine
ly 117018
see: 6 hydroxy 2 (4 hydroxyphenyl) 3 [4 [2 (1 pyrrolidinyl)ethoxy]benzoyl]benzo[b]thiophene

Index

ly 139481
see: raloxifene
ly139481
see: raloxifene
ly 156758
see: raloxifene
ly156758
see: raloxifene
ly 275585
see: insulin[B28 lysine B29 proline]
ly275585
see: insulin[B28 lysine B29 proline]
ly 31537
see: ractopamine
ly31537
see: ractopamine
ly 353381
see: arzoxifene
ly353381
see: arzoxifene
lydex
see: fluocinonide
lydex e
see: fluocinonide
lydol
see: pethidine
lyovac diuril
see: chlorothiazide
lyovac saluric
see: chlorothiazide
lyovac saluril
see: chlorothiazide
lyspro
see: insulin[B28 lysine B29 proline]
lyspro insulin
see: insulin[B28 lysine B29 proline]
m 1 36
see: etilefrine
m (2 aminopropyl)phenol
see: gepefrine

mabuterol

mabuterol hydrochloride
see: mabuterol
macrobin
see: clostebol acetate
macrodex
see: dextran
macrodex 500
see: dextran
macrose
see: dextran
madiol
see: methandriol
magnesium pemolate
see: pemoline magnesium
magnesium pemolinate
see: pemoline magnesium
magnesium pemoline
see: pemoline magnesium
magrene
see: amfepramone
maintate
see: bisoprolol fumarate
malestrone
see: methyltestosterone
malogen
see: methyltestosterone
malogen cyp 200
see: testosterone cipionate
malogene
see: methyltestosterone
malogen la 200
see: testosterone enantate
malogex
see: testosterone enantate
malysol
see: bemegride
m and b 16 942
see: diacetolol
m and b 16942
see: diacetolol
m and b 16942 a
see: diacetolol
m and b 16942a
see: diacetolol
m and b 17803 a
see: acebutolol
m and b 17803a
see: acebutolol
mandrin
see: ephedrine
manitol
see: mannitol
mannit
see: mannitol
mannite
see: mannitol

mannitol

mannitol hydrochloride
see: mannitol
manzindol
see: mazindol

marazide
see: benzthiazide
marihuana
see: cannabis
marihuana derivative
see: cannabis derivative
marijuana
see: cannabis
marinol
see: dronabinol
marogen
see: recombinant erythropoietin
marsin
see: phenmetrazine
marvidione
see: dexamethasone
masacin
see: procaterol
masdiol
see: methandriol
masenate
see: testosterone propionate
masenone
see: methyltestosterone
masterid
see: drostanolone propionate
masteril
see: drostanolone propionate
masteron
see: drostanolone propionate
masterone
see: drostanolone propionate
mastodanatrol
see: danazol
matenon
see: mibolerone
maxair
see: pirbuterol acetate
maxibolin
see: ethylestrenol
maxide
see: hydrochlorothiazide plus triamterene
maxidex
see: dexamethasone
maxidex ointment
see: dexamethasone sodium phosphate
maxiflor
see: diflorasone diacetate
maxirapid
see: insulin
maxsoten
see: bisoprolol fumarate plus hydrochlorothiazide
maxzide
see: hydrochlorothiazide plus triamterene
mazanor
see: mazindol

mazindol

mazindole
see: mazindol

mazipredone

MCDF
see: 1,3,8 trichloro 6 methyldibenzofuran
mcm 822
see: 4 methylaminorex
mcn 6186
see: n (3,5 dimethoxyphenethyl) 5 methoxy 2 (phenylethynyl)amphetamine
mcn 742
see: aminorex
md 39 am
see: 4 anilino 2 methylthiopyrido[2,3 d]pyrimidine
mda
see: 3,4 methylenedioxyamphetamine
MDEA
see: n ethyl 3,4 methylenedioxyamphetamine
mdi 193
see: cyclothiazide
mdi193
see: cyclothiazide
mdl 16289f
see: enclomifene citrate
mdl 17330 a
see: medroxalol
mdl 17330a
see: medroxalol
mdl 18962
see: 10 propargylestr 4 ene 3,17 dione
mdl 3978g
see: perhexiline
MDMA
see: 3,4 methylenedioxymethamphetamine
mecasermin
see: recombinant somatomedin C

meclofenoxate

meclofenoxate hydrochloride
see: meclofenoxate
meclophenoxate
see: meclofenoxate

mecnazone
see: methadone
mecodrin
see: amphetamine
mediamethasone
see: dexamethasone
mediamid
see: nikethamide
mediasolone
see: prednisolone
medicodal
see: oxycodone
medihaler cort
see: hydrocortisone
medihaler duo
see: hydrocortisone
medihaler iso
see: isoprenaline
medihaler isoforte
see: isoprenaline
medrisone
see: medrysone
medrocort
see: medrysone
medrol
see: methylprednisolone
medrol adt pak
see: methylprednisolone
medrol compositum
see: methylprednisolone
medrol dosepak
see: methylprednisolone
medrol enpak
see: methylprednisolone acetate
medrone
see: methylprednisolone
medrosol
see: methylprednisolone suleptanate

medroxalol

medroxalol hydrochloride
see: medroxalol

medrysone

mefedina
see: pethidine

mefenorex

mefenorex hydrochloride
see: mefenorex
mefentermine
see: mephentermine
mefeprol
see: buphenine

mefexamide

mefruside

megabion
see: methandriol
megacortin
see: dexamethasone
megagrisevit
see: clostebol acetate
megimide
see: bemegride
melfiat
see: phendimetrazine tartrate
men 935
see: adimolol
menaderm
see: isoflupredone acetate
menandron
see: methyltestosterone
menethyl
see: etafedrine
menetyl
see: etafedrine
menocil
see: aminorex
menogon
see: human menopausal gonadotropin
menopausal gonadotrophin
see: human menopausal gonadotropin
menopausal gonadotropin
see: human menopausal gonadotropin
menopausal human gonadotropin
see: human menopausal gonadotropin
menopause gonadotrophin
see: human menopausal gonadotropin
menopause gonadotropin
see: human menopausal gonadotropin
menotropin
see: human menopausal gonadotropin
menotropins
see: human menopausal gonadotropin
MENT
see: trestolone
mepadin
see: pethidine

Index

mepecton
see: methadone
meperiden
see: pethidine
meperidin
see: pethidine
meperidine
see: pethidine
meperidine hydrobromide
see: pethidine
meperidine hydrochloride
see: pethidine
mephameson
see: dexamethasone
mephamesone
see: dexamethasone
mephedine
see: pethidine
mephenon
see: methadone

mephentermine

mephentermine sulfate
see: mephentermine
mephetedrine
see: mephentermine
mephine
see: mephentermine

mepindolol

mepindolol sulfate
see: mepindolol
mepiridine
see: pethidine

mepitiostane

mepred
see: methylprednisolone acetate
meprednisolone
see: methylprednisolone

meprednisone

meprisolon
see: prednisolone
meprisolone
see: prednisolone
meprison
see: prednisone
meptin
see: procaterol
mepyrapone
see: metyrapone
mer 25
see: ethamoxytriphetol
mer 41
see: clomifene citrate
meratan
see: pipradol
meratonic
see: pipradol
meratran
see: pipradol
mercardox
see: chlormerodrin
mercloran
see: chlormerodrin
mercoral
see: chlormerodrin

mercuderamide

mercugan
see: mersalyl
merculest
see: chlormerodrin
mercuramide
see: mersalyl
mercurial diuretic
see: diuretic agent
mercurosalyl
see: mersalyl
mercury diuretic
see: diuretic agent
mercury diuretic agent
see: diuretic agent
mercuryluree
see: chlormerodrin
mercusal
see: mersalyl
meretran
see: pipradol
merilid
see: chlormerodrin
merphilin
see: mersalyl
merphyllin
see: mersalyl
mersalic acid
see: mersalyl
mersalin
see: mersalyl

Index

mersalyl

mersalyl acid
see: mersalyl
mersalyn
see: mersalyl
mertestate
see: testosterone
mesocarb
see: sydnocarb
mesopren
see: methylprednisolone

mespirenone

mestalonone
see: mestanolone

mestanolone

mestenediol
see: methandriol

mesterolone

mesteron
see: methyltestosterone
mesterone
see: methyltestosterone
mestoranum
see: mesterolone
meta (2 aminopropyl)phenol
see: gepefrine
metabolina
see: metandienone
metacortalon
see: prednisolone
metacortalone
see: prednisolone
metacortandracin
see: prednisone
metacortandralon
see: prednisolone
metacortandralone
see: prednisolone
metacortelone
see: prednisolone
metadate
see: methylphenidate
metaderm
see: betamethasone valerate
metadienone
see: metandienone
metadin sodium
see: pipradol
metahaemoglobin
see: methemoglobin
metahemoglobin
see: methemoglobin
metahydrin
see: trichlormethiazide
meta hydroxyamphetamine
see: gepefrine
meta hydroxynorephedrine
see: metaraminol
metalazone
see: metolazone
metallibure
see: methallibure
metamphetamine
see: methamphetamine
metanabol
see: methandriol
metandienon
see: metandienone

metandienone

metandienone,4 chloro
see: 4 chloro 17beta hydroxy 17 methylandrosta 1,4 dien 3 one
metandiol
see: methandriol
metandren
see: methyltestosterone
metandrene
see: methyltestosterone
metandrostenediol
see: methandriol
metandrostenolone
see: metandienone
metapiron
see: metyrapone
metapirone
see: metyrapone
metaprel
see: orciprenaline
meta proterenol
see: orciprenaline
metaproterenol
see: orciprenaline
metaproterenol sulfate
see: orciprenaline
metapyrone
see: metyrapone

Index

metaradrine
see: metaraminol

metaraminol

metaraminol bitartrate
see: metaraminol
metaril
see: metaraminol
metasedin
see: methadone
metasolon
see: dexamethasone
metasolone
see: dexamethasone
metazolamide
see: methazolamide
metendiol
see: methandriol
metenix
see: metolazone

metenolone

metenolone acetate

metenolone enantate

metenolone enanthate
see: metenolone enantate
metenolone heptanoate
see: metenolone enantate
metenolone heptanonate
see: metenolone enantate
meterdos iso
see: isoprenaline
meterdos iso forte
see: isoprenaline
metestine
see: methyltestosterone
metexterona
see: methyltestosterone
metflorylthiadiazine
see: hydroflumethiazide
methadon
see: methadone

methadone

methadone base
see: methadone
methadone hydrobromide
see: methadone
methadone hydrochloride
see: methadone
methadose
see: methadone
methaemoglobin
see: methemoglobin
methagon
see: flumetasone acetate
methahydrin
see: trichlormethiazide

methallibure

methamine
see: methamphetamine
methampex
see: methamphetamine
methamphetamin
see: methamphetamine

methamphetamine

methamphetamine,2 methoxy
see: 2 methoxymethamphetamine
methamphetamine,3 methoxy
see: 3 methoxymethamphetamine
methamphetamine,4 methoxy
see: 4 methoxymethamphetamine
methamphetamine hcl
see: methamphetamine
methamphetamine hydrochloride
see: methamphetamine
methamphetamine,n furfuryl
see: furfenorex
methamphetamine sulfate
see: methamphetamine
methamphetaminium chloride
see: methamphetamine
methamphin
see: methamphetamine
methanabol
see: methandriol

methanandamide

methandienone
see: metandienone
methandiol
see: methandriol

methandriol

methandriol dipropionate

methandrostenolone
see: metandienone
metharaminol
see: metaraminol
methasite
see: fluorometholone
methasone
see: betamethasone

methazolamide

methazone ion
see: dexamethasone
methazon ion
see: dexamethasone
methazonion
see: dexamethasone
methazonione
see: dexamethasone
methbipyranone
see: metyrapone
methbipyrapone
see: metyrapone

methcathinone

methedrine
see: methamphetamine

methemoglobin

methenolon
see: metenolone
methenolone
see: metenolone
methenolone acetate
see: metenolone acetate
methenolone enanthate
see: metenolone enantate
methenolone oenanthate
see: metenolone enantate
methephedrine
see: methylephedrine
methetharimide
see: bemegride
methiclothiazide
see: methyclothiazide
methionyl growth hormone
see: somatrem
methionylgrowth hormone
see: somatrem
methionylgrowth hormone 20k
see: somatrem
methionylgrowth hormone 22k
see: somatrem
methionyl somatotropin
see: somatrem
methionylsomatotropin
see: somatrem
methocryst
see: methandriol
metholone
see: drostanolone propionate
methopyrapone
see: metyrapone
methopyrone
see: metyrapone
methosarb
see: calusterone
methostan
see: methandriol
methoxamedrine
see: methoxamine

methoxamine

methoxamine hydrochloride
see: methoxamine
methoxiphenadrin
see: methoxyphenamine
3 methoxy 17 epiestriol
see: epimestrol

4 methoxyamphetamine

12 methoxyibogamine
see: ibogaine

2 methoxymethamphetamine

3 methoxymethamphetamine

4 methoxymethamphetamine

methoxyn
see: methamphetamine
2 methoxy n methylamphetamine
see: 2 methoxymethamphetamine

Index

3 methoxy n methylamphetamine
see: 3 methoxymethamphetamine
4 methoxy n methylamphetamine
see: 4 methoxymethamphetamine

methoxyphenamine

methoxyphenamine hydrochloride
see: methoxyphenamine
methybol
see: mestanolone

methyclothiazide

4 [4 methyl 2 [4 [2 (1 piperidinyl)ethoxy]phenyl] 7 pivaloyloxy 2h 1 benzopyran 3 ylphenyl] pivalate

6 methyl 2 amino 6 heptanol
see: heptaminol
3 methyl 2 phenylmorpholine
see: phenmetrazine
2 methyl 6 amino 2 heptanol
see: heptaminol
2 methylamino 1 phenylpropane
see: methamphetamine
methylaminoethanolcatechol
see: adrenalin
2 methylaminopropiophenone
see: methcathinone

4 methylaminorex

methyl amphetamine
see: methamphetamine
methylamphetamine
see: methamphetamine

4 methylamphetamine

17 methylandrostanolone
see: mestanolone
methylandrostanopyrazole
see: stanozolol
methylandrostendiole
see: methandriol
methylandrostenediol
see: methandriol
methylandrostenediole
see: methandriol
methylandrostenolone
see: metenolone
methylarterenol
see: adrenalin
methylbenzedrine
see: methamphetamine
17 methyl b nortestosterone
see: benorterone
methylchlorothiazide
see: methyclothiazide
methylclothiazide
see: methyclothiazide
methyl d
see: methyldienolone
methyl dien
see: methyldienolone
methyldien
see: methyldienolone
1 methyl delta1 androstenolone
see: metenolone
methyldihydrotestosterone
see: methandriol

methyldienolone

2 methyldihydrotestosterone
see: drostanolone
methylene dioxyamphetamine
see: 3,4 methylenedioxyamphetamine
methylenedioxyamphetamine
see: 3,4 methylenedioxyamphetamine

3,4 methylenedioxyamphetamine

3,4-methylenedioxyamphetamine
see: 3,4 methylenedioxyamphetamine

3,4 methylenedioxyamphetamine derivative

methylenedioxymethamphetamine
see: 3,4 methylenedioxymethamphetamine

3,4 methylenedioxymethamphetamine

15beta,16beta methylenemexrenone

methylene prednisolone
see: prednylidene
methyleneprednisolone
see: prednylidene

Index

16 methylene prednisolone
see: prednylidene
16 methyleneprednisolone
see: prednylidene
16 methylenprednisolone
see: prednylidene

methylephedrine

methylets
see: methyltestosterone
methylfenidate
see: methylphenidate
methylin
see: methylphenidate
methylisamin
see: methamphetamine
methylisomyn
see: methamphetamine
methylmydriatin
see: racephedrine
18 methylnandrolone
see: 13beta ethyl 17beta hydroxygon 4 en 3 one

3 methylnaringenin

methylphenidate

methyl phenidate
see: methylphenidate
methylphenidate hydrochloride
see: methylphenidate
methylphenidylacetate
see: methylphenidate
methylphenindate
see: methylphenidate
methylphenydate
see: methylphenidate
(4 methylphenyl)isopropylamine
see: 4 methylamphetamine
methyl prednisolon acetate
see: methylprednisolone acetate

methylprednisolone

methyl prednisolone
see: methylprednisolone
16 methylprednisolone
see: 16beta methylprednisolone

16beta methylprednisolone

2 methylprednisolone
see: methylprednisolone
5 methylprednisolone
see: methylprednisolone
6 methyl prednisolone
see: methylprednisolone
6 methylprednisolone
see: methylprednisolone

methylprednisolone aceponate

methylprednisolone acetate

methyl prednisolone acetate
see: methylprednisolone acetate
6 methylprednisolone acetate
see: methylprednisolone acetate

methylprednisolone sodium succinate

methylprednisolone succinate
see: methylprednisolone sodium succinate

methylprednisolone suleptanate

methylprednisone
see: meprednisone
methylpropamine
see: methamphetamine
methylpropion
see: methcathinone
methylstanazole
see: stanozolol
methylsterolone
see: methylprednisolone
methylsympathol
see: oxilofrine
methyltesterone
see: methyltestosterone
methyltestosteron
see: methyltestosterone

methyltestosterone

methyl testosterone
see: methyltestosterone
17 methyl testosterone
see: methyltestosterone
17 methyltestosterone
see: methyltestosterone

Index

methyltheobromine
see: caffeine
methylthiocarbamoylinsulin
see: insulin derivative
methylthiocarbamylinsulin
see: insulin derivative

4' methylthiopropranolol

methyltrienolone
see: metribolone
methypatch
see: methylphenidate
methypranol
see: metipranolol
methyrapone
see: metyrapone
meticortelone
see: prednisolone
meticortelone acetate
see: prednisolone acetate
meticorten
see: prednisone
meticortine
see: prednisone
meti derm
see: prednisolone
metiderm
see: prednisolone
metidione
see: methandriol
metilar
see: paramethasone
metildiolo
see: methandriol

metipranolol

metipranolol,deacetyl
see: deacetylmetipranolol
metipranolol hydrochloride
see: metipranolol
metipranolol plus butizide
see: torrat
metisone lafi
see: dexamethasone
metocryst
see: methandriol
metolazon
see: metolazone

metolazone

metopiron
see: metyrapone
metopirone
see: metyrapone
metopirone ditartrate
see: metyrapone

metoprolol

metoprolol,alpha hydroxy
see: alpha hydroxymetoprolol
metoprolol durules
see: metoprolol

metoprolol fumarate

metoprolol oros
see: metoprolol
metoprolol plus chlortalidone
see: chlortalidone plus metoprolol
metoprolol plus felodipine
see: felodipine plus metoprolol

metoprolol succinate

metoprolol tartrate

metopyrone
see: metyrapone
metoros
see: metoprolol fumarate
metosyn
see: fluocinonide
metoxamine
see: methoxamine
metra
see: phendimetrazine tartrate
metrazol
see: pentetrazole
metrazole
see: pentetrazole
metreton
see: prednisolone sodium phosphate

metribolone

metrisone
see: methylprednisolone
metrodin
see: urofollitropin

Index

metrodine
see: urofollitropin
metrodin high purity
see: urofollitropin
metrodin hp
see: urofollitropin
metromin
see: dimetamfetamine
metropolol
see: metoprolol
metroprione
see: metyrapone
metypresol
see: methylprednisolone
metyrapon
see: metyrapone

metyrapone

metyrapone 637
see: metyrapone
metyrapone hydrochloride
see: metyrapone
metyrapone tartrate
see: metyrapone
mexan
see: methoxamine
mexane
see: methoxamine
mexican marihuana
see: cannabis
mexrenoate
see: mexrenoic acid

mexrenoate potassium

mexrenoic acid

mexrenoic acid lactone
see: mexrenone

mexrenone

mexrenone,9,11alpha epoxy
see: eplerenone
mexyphamine
see: methoxyphenamine
mf 125
see: actovegin
mf 465 a
see: canrenoate potassium
mf 465a
see: canrenoate potassium
mf465a
see: canrenoate potassium
mg 13054
see: fenquizone
mg 8823
see: exaprolol
miadone
see: methadone
mialgin
see: pethidine

mibolerone

micardisplus
see: hydrochlorothiazide plus telmisartan
miclox
see: metolazone
miconazole plus hydrocortisone
see: daktacort
micoren
see: prethcamide
microx
see: metolazone
microzide
see: hydrochlorothiazide
mictrin
see: hydrochlorothiazide
midamor
see: amiloride
midodrin
see: midodrine

midodrine

midon
see: midodrine
mikedimide
see: bemegride
mikelan
see: carteolol
mildison lipocream
see: hydrocortisone
'millibar'
see: indapamide
millicorten
see: dexamethasone
millicorten 17 valerate
see: dexamethasone 17 valerate
millicortenol
see: dexamethasone

millicortenol vioform
see: clioquinol plus dexamethasone
millicorten vioform
see: clioquinol plus dexamethasone
mimetina
see: amphetamine

minamestane

minifage
see: fenfluramine
miocardina
see: nikethamide
miolene
see: ritodrine
miotolon
see: furazabol

miproxifene phosphate

miracorten
see: ulobetasol propionate
mirapront
see: phentermine resin
mirfat
see: furosemide
miro
see: morphine
misodrine
see: midodrine
mistaprel
see: isoprenaline
miten plus
see: hydrochlorothiazide plus valsartan
mitodrine
see: midodrine
mixogen
see: ethinylestradiol plus methyltestosterone
mixtard
see: isophane insulin
mj 13105
see: bucindolol
mj 13,105 1
see: bucindolol
mj 13105 1
see: bucindolol
mj 1992
see: soterenol
mj 1999
see: sotalol
mj 5763 1
see: sotalol
mj 9184 1
see: zinterol
mj 91841
see: zinterol
mjf 10,938
see: xipamide
mjf 10938
see: xipamide
mk 0677
see: ibutamoren
mk 125
see: dexamethasone
mk 188
see: zeranol
mk188
see: zeranol
mk 196
see: indacrinone
mk 447
see: 2 aminomethyl 4 tert butyl 6 iodophenol
mk 595
see: etacrynic acid
mk 677
see: ibutamoren
mk 870
see: amiloride
mk 950
see: timolol maleate
mk950
see: timolol maleate
mobloc
see: felodipine plus metoprolol

modafinil

modamide
see: amiloride
modasomil
see: modafinil
modenol
see: butizide
moderatan
see: amfepramone
moderex
see: fenfluramine
modiodal
see: modafinil
modrasone
see: alclometasone dipropionate
moducren
see: timolol
moduret
see: amiloride plus hydrochlorothiazide

moduretic
see: amiloride plus hydrochlorothiazide
moheptan
see: methadone
moludar
see: amfepramone
mometasone 17 (2 furoate)
see: mometasone furoate
mometasone 17 furoate
see: mometasone furoate

mometasone furoate

monetamin
see: amphetamine
6 monoacetylmorphine
see: morphine 6 acetate
monocomponent human insulin
see: monocomponent insulin

monocomponent insulin

monocor
see: bisoprolol fumarate
monocortin
see: paramethasone acetate
monohydroxytamoxifen
see: hydroxytamoxifen
4 monohydroxytamoxifen
see: 4 hydroxytamoxifen
mononitroinsulin
see: insulin derivative
monophos
see: amphetamine
monores
see: clenbuterol
monotard
see: insulin zinc suspension
monotard hm
see: insulin zinc suspension
monotard human
see: insulin
monotard insulin
see: insulin
monydrin
see: phenylpropanolamine

moprolol

moprolol,levo
see: levomoprolol
moramide
see: dextromoramide
moraxen
see: morphine sulfate

morazone

morfin
see: morphine
morfine
see: morphine
morlone
see: prednisolone
morphacetin
see: diamorphine
morphia
see: morphine
morphidex
see: dextromethorphan plus morphine
morphin
see: morphine

morphine

morphine,14beta bromoacetamido
see: 14beta bromoacetamidomorphine
morphine 3,6 diacetate
see: diamorphine
morphine 3,6 dinicotinate
see: nicomorphine
morphine 3 ethereal sulfate
see: morphine sulfate
morphine 3 sulfate
see: morphine sulfate

morphine 6 acetate

morphine 6 sulfate
see: morphine sulfate
morphine alkaloid
see: morphine
morphine chlorhydrate
see: morphine
morphine chloride
see: morphine
morphine hydrochloride
see: morphine
morphine plus dextromethorphan
see: dextromethorphan plus morphine

morphine sulfate

morphinesulfate
see: morphine sulfate

morphine sulfate pentahydrate
see: morphine sulfate
morphine suspension
see: morphine
morphinium
see: morphine
morphium
see: morphine
moscontin
see: morphine sulfate
movergan
see: selegiline
mpv 2213ad
see: finrozole
mpv2213ad
see: finrozole
mrd 108
see: pipradol
mrl 41
see: clomifene citrate
ms 1112
see: betamethasone benzoate
ms contin
see: morphine sulfate
msir
see: morphine sulfate
mst
see: morphine sulfate
mst 100
see: morphine sulfate
mst 60
see: morphine sulfate
mst continus
see: morphine sulfate
mst mundipharma
see: morphine sulfate
mucidrina
see: adrenalin
mucodine
see: procaterol
mucosolvan compositum
see: ambroxol plus clenbuterol
munitren
see: hydrocortisone
musolimino
see: muzolimine

muzolimine

mxl
see: morphine sulfate
my 1997
see: soterenol
myagen
see: bolasterone

mycolog

mycoren
see: prethcamide
mydrapred
see: prednisolone
mydriatin
see: phenylpropanolamine
mykrox
see: metolazone
mylis
see: prasterone sulfate
myosthenine
see: adrenalin
myotrophin
see: recombinant somatomedin C
myser
see: difluprednate
mytrex
see: mycolog
n (2 chlorobenzyl)amphetamine
see: clobenzorex
n (2 cyanoethyl)amphetamine
see: fenproporex
n (2 hydroxyethyl)palmitamide
see: palmidrol
n (3 chloropropyl)amphetamine
see: mefenorex
n 610
see: fencamfamin
n 696
see: tilisolol
nab 365
see: clenbuterol
nabadial
see: methandriol
nabolin
see: metandienone
naclex
see: hydroflumethiazide
naclex glaxo
see: hydroflumethiazide
naclex robins
see: benzthiazide

nadolol

nadosterone
see: methyltestosterone

Index

nafarelin

nafarelin acetate

nafoxidine

nafoxidine hydrochloride
see: nafoxidine
n alderlin
see: pronetalol
nalide
see: buphenine

naminterol

nandrobolic
see: nandrolone phenpropionate
nandrobolic la
see: nandrolone decanoate
nandrolin
see: nandrolone phenpropionate
nandrolondecanoate
see: nandrolone decanoate

nandrolone

nandrolone 17beta undecanoate
see: nandrolone undecanoate
nandrolone 17beta undecylate
see: nandrolone undecanoate
nandrolone 17 decanoate
see: nandrolone decanoate

nandrolone 4 hexyloxyhydrocinnamate

nandrolone,7alpha,17 dimethyl
see: mibolerone

nandrolone cyclohexylpropionate

nandrolone decanoate

nandrolone derivative

nandrolone dodecanoate
see: nandrolone laurate

nandrolone furylpropionate

nandrolone laurate

nandrolone laurinate
see: nandrolone laurate

nandrolone phenpropionate

nandrolone phenylpropionate
see: nandrolone phenpropionate
nandrolonephenylpropionate
see: nandrolone phenpropionate

nandrolone undecanoate

nandrolone undecylate
see: nandrolone undecanoate
nanormon
see: growth hormone

nantradol

nantradol,dextro
see: dextronantradol
nantradol hydrochloride
see: nantradol
nantradol,levo
see: levonantradol
napharelin acetate
see: nafarelin acetate

1 (1 naphthyloxy) 3 [6 [2 (2 pyridyl)ethoxy]hexylamino] 2 propanol

napionate
see: testosterone propionate
napriline
see: propranolol
naqua
see: trichlormethiazide
naquasone
see: trichlormethiazide
narbivolol
see: nebivolol
narcobasina
see: oxycodone
narcobasine
see: oxycodone
narcosin
see: oxycodone
narcotic analgesic
see: narcotic analgesic agent

narcotic analgesic agent

narcotic analgetic agent
see: narcotic analgesic agent
nargenol
see: oxycodone
narodal
see: oxycodone
nasacort
see: triamcinolone acetonide
nasal fluocinolone acetonide
see: fluocinolone acetonide
nasalide
see: flunisolide
nasal synalar
see: fluocinolone acetonide
nasarel
see: flunisolide
nasdol
see: testosterone propionate
nasonex
see: mometasone furoate
nastenon
see: oxymetholone
natolone
see: pregnenolone
natrilix
see: indapamide
natrionex
see: acetazolamide
natriuran
see: chlortalidone
naturetin
see: bendroflumethiazide
naturetin k
see: bendroflumethiazide
naturine
see: bendroflumethiazide
naurazol
see: pentetrazole
navidex k
see: cyclopenthiazide
navidrex
see: cyclopenthiazide
navidrex ismelin
see: cyclopenthiazide plus guanethidine
navidrex k
see: cyclopenthiazide
navidrex serpasil k
see: cyclopenthiazide
navidrix
see: cyclopenthiazide
navispare
see: amiloride plus cyclopenthiazide
nazlin
see: human insulin
n benzylmethamphetamine
see: benzphetamine
n benzyl n methylamphetamine
see: benzphetamine
nbl
see: metandienone
nc 1400
see: bevantolol
nc1400
see: bevantolol
nd 1966
see: aminoglutethimide
n demethyltamoxifen
see: nortamoxifen
n desmethyltamoxifen
see: nortamoxifen
nebilet
see: nebivolol
nebilox
see: nebivolol

nebivolol

nebivolol hydrochloride
see: nebivolol
nefenalol
see: nifenalol
nefrix
see: hydrochlorothiazide
nekethamide
see: nikethamide
nemestran
see: gestrinone
neoasman
see: isoprenaline
neocardol
see: pentetrazole
neoclym
see: cyclofenil
neo codema
see: hydrochlorothiazide
neocordial
see: nikethamide
neo cortef
see: hydrocortisone
neocortef
see: hydrocortisone
neodecadron ophthalmic
see: dexamethasone sodium phosphate

neo delta
see: prednisolone
neodrenal
see: isoprenaline
neodrenol
see: isoprenaline
neodrol
see: androstanolone
neo durabolic
see: nandrolone decanoate
neoepine
see: isoprenaline
neoepinephrine
see: isoprenaline
neo epinine
see: isoprenaline
neoepinine
see: isoprenaline
neofanal
see: isoprenaline
neo fedrin
see: ephedrine
neo flumen
see: hydrochlorothiazide
neoflumen
see: hydrochlorothiazide
neo hambreol m
see: methyltestosterone
neo hombreol
see: testosterone propionate
neo-hombreol
see: testosterone propionate
neohombreol
see: testosterone propionate
neo hombreol m
see: methyltestosterone
neohombreol m
see: methyltestosterone
neohydrin
see: chlormerodrin
neoisuprel
see: isoetarine
neomedrone
see: methylprednisolone
neomelubrin
see: noradrenalin
neomersyl
see: mersalyl
neo naclex
see: bendroflumethiazide
neonaclex k
see: bendroflumethiazide
neo nadex k
see: bendroflumethiazide
neonadex k
see: bendroflumethiazide
neonatal hemoglobin f
see: hemoglobin F
neopergonal
see: human menopausal gonadotropin
neopharmedrine
see: methamphetamine
neoplasmafusin
see: dextran
neorecormon
see: recombinant erythropoietin
neoschiwadex
see: dextran
neosorb
see: sorbitol
neostene
see: methandriol
neosteron
see: methandriol
neosterone
see: methandriol
neosynalar
see: fluocinolone acetonide
neotenol
see: atenolol
neotestis
see: testosterone
neotri
see: triamterene plus xipamide
neotril
see: triamterene plus xipamide
neo zine
see: phenmetrazine
nephenal
see: isoprenaline
nephenalin
see: isoprenaline
nephral
see: hydrochlorothiazide plus triamterene
nephramid
see: acetazolamide
nephridine
see: adrenalin
nephril
see: polythiazide
neptal
see: mercuderamide
neptall
see: acebutolol

neptazane
see: methazolamide
nerabol
see: metandienone
neriforte
see: diflucortolone valerate
nerisona
see: diflucortolone valerate
nerisona forte
see: diflucortolone valerate
nerisone
see: diflucortolone valerate
nerobol
see: metandienone
neroboletta
see: metandienone
nerobolil
see: nandrolone phenpropionate
nerobolyl
see: nandrolone phenpropionate
NESP
see: novel erythropoiesis stimulating protein
nespo
see: novel erythropoiesis stimulating protein
nethalide
see: pronetalol
nethamine
see: etafedrine
n ethyl amphetamine
see: n ethylamphetamine
n ethylephedrine
see: etafedrine
1 n ethylephedrine
see: etafedrine
netilar
see: paramethasone acetate
neurocaine
see: cocaine
neurogenic noradrenalin
see: noradrenalin
neusulin
see: insulin

neutral insulin

neutropin
see: human growth hormone
neutrormone
see: methandriol
neutrosteron
see: methandriol
n formylamphetamine
see: formetorex
n furfurylmethamphetamine
see: furfenorex
n furfuryl n methylamphetamine
see: furfenorex
niagar
see: hydrochlorothiazide
nibal
see: metenolone acetate
nibal injection
see: metenolone enantate
nicaethamidum
see: nikethamide
nicamide
see: nikethamide
nicardin
see: nikethamide
nicerase
see: lobeline
nicetamid
see: nikethamide
nicetamide
see: nikethamide
nicethamide
see: nikethamide
nicholin
see: citicoline
nickethamide
see: nikethamide

nicocortonide

nicomorphine

nicomorphine hydrochloride
see: nicomorphine
ni cor
see: nikethamide
nicor
see: nikethamide
nicordamin
see: nikethamide
nicorine
see: nikethamide
nicorine latema
see: nikethamide
nicoryl
see: nikethamide
4 nicotinamidobutyric acid
see: picamilon
nicotinic acid diethylamide
see: nikethamide

4 nicotinoylaminobutyric acid
see: picamilon
nieraline
see: adrenalin
nifedipine plus atenolol
see: atenolol plus nifedipine

nifenalol

niften
see: atenolol plus nifedipine
nih 10567
see: ibogaine
nih10567
see: ibogaine
nih 7958
see: pentazocine
nih 8805
see: buprenorphine
nih8805
see: buprenorphine
nikardin
see: nikethamide

nikethamide

nikethamine
see: nikethamide
niketharol
see: nikethamide
nikethyl
see: nikethamide
nikidess
see: exemestane
nikoban
see: lobeline
nikorin
see: nikethamide
nilevar
see: norethandrolone
nilidrine
see: buphenine
nilvitam
see: buphenine

nipradilol

nipradolol
see: nipradilol

niravoline

nisisco
see: hydrochlorothiazide plus valsartan
nisolon
see: prednisolone
nisolone
see: prednisolone
nisomethasona
see: dexamethasone
nisone
see: prednisone acetate
n isopropyl 4 iodoamphetamine
see: iofetamine
n isopropylnoradrenalin
see: isoprenaline
n isopropylnoradrenaline
see: isoprenaline
nitoman
see: tetrabenazine
2 nitrilophenoxypropanolamine
see: bunitrolol

nitromifene

nitromiphene
see: nitromifene

nivacortol

nivazol
see: nivacortol
nivitin
see: sorbitol
n methyl amphetamine
see: methamphetamine
n methylamphetamine
see: methamphetamine
n methyldopamine
see: epinine
n methyldopamine diisobutyrate
see: ibopamine
n methyl ephedrine
see: methylephedrine
n methylephedrine
see: methylephedrine
nn 304
see: insulin detemir
nn304
see: insulin detemir
nn 703
see: tabimorelin

nn703
see: tabimorelin
nnc 26 0161
see: ipamorelin
n,n diethylnicotinamide
see: nikethamide
n,n diethylvanillamide
see: etamivan
n,n dimethylamphetamine
see: dimetamfetamine
n,n dimethylethanolamine
see: deanol
n nortamoxifen
see: nortamoxifen
nobese
see: phenylpropanolamine
noceptin
see: morphine sulfate
noclon
see: amphetamine
no doz
see: caffeine
nodoz
see: caffeine
no kotin
see: lobeline
nolvadex
see: tamoxifen citrate
19 nor 4 androstene 3,17 dione
see: estr 4 ene 3,17 dione
19 nor 4 androstenediol
see: bolandiol
19 nor 4 androstenedione
see: estr 4 ene 3,17 dione
norabol
see: nandrolone phenpropionate
noradrec
see: noradrenalin

noradrenalin

noradrenalin acid tartrate
see: noradrenalin bitartrate

noradrenalin bitartrate

noradrenaline
see: noradrenalin
noradrenaline bitartrate
see: noradrenalin bitartrate
noradrenalin ethyltheophylline
see: theodrenaline
noradrenalin hydrochloride
see: noradrenalin
noradrenalin hydrotartrate
see: noradrenalin bitartrate
noradrenalin tartrate
see: noradrenalin bitartrate
noradrenalin theophylline
see: theodrenaline
noradrine
see: noradrenalin
noranat
see: indapamide
19 norandrodiol
see: bolandiol
norandrol
see: nandrolone phenpropionate
19 norandrost 4 enedione
see: estr 4 ene 3,17 dione
19 norandrostenedione
see: estr 4 ene 3,17 dione
norandrostenedione
see: estr 4 ene 3,17 dione
norandrostenolonedecanoate
see: nandrolone decanoate
19 norandrostenediol
see: bolandiol
norandrostenolone
see: nandrolone
19 norandrostenolone
see: nandrolone
norandrostenolone decanoate
see: nandrolone decanoate
norandrostenolone derivative
see: nandrolone derivative
norandrostenolone laurinate
see: nandrolone laurate
norartrinal
see: noradrenalin bitartrate
noratrinal
see: noradrenalin bitartrate
norbalin
see: nandrolone phenpropionate
norbolethane
see: norboletone
norbolethone
see: norboletone

norboletone

norclostebol

norclostebol acetate

norcocaine

nordexfenfluramine
see: dexnorfenfluramine
19 nor d homosterone
see: nandrolone
nordicort
see: hydrocortisone sodium succinate
19 nordiol
see: bolandiol
norditropin
see: human growth hormone
nordrin
see: noradrenalin bitartrate
norephedrane
see: amphetamine
norepinephrin
see: noradrenalin
norepinephrine
see: noradrenalin
norepinephrine bitartrate
see: noradrenalin bitartrate
norepinephrine hydrochloride
see: noradrenalin
norethandrolon
see: norethandrolone

norethandrolone

norexadrin
see: noradrenalin

norfenfluramine

noridyl
see: triamterene
norisedrin
see: isoprenaline
norisodine
see: isoprenaline
norisodrine
see: isoprenaline
norisodrine aerotrol
see: isoprenaline
norisoephedrine
see: norpseudoephedrine
norisophedrine
see: norpseudoephedrine
normadrine
see: methamphetamine
normegon
see: human menopausal gonadotropin
normiten
see: atenolol
normodyne
see: labetalol
norodin
see: methamphetamine
norodrin
see: methamphetamine
norphedrane
see: amphetamine
norpholedrine
see: hydroxyamphetamine

norpseudoephedrine

norstenol
see: nandrolone phenpropionate

nortamoxifen

19 nortesterone
see: nandrolone
nortesterone derivative
see: nandrolone derivative
19 nortesterone derivative
see: nandrolone derivative
nortestonate
see: nandrolone
nortestosterone
see: nandrolone
17 nortestosterone
see: nandrolone
19 nortestosterone
see: nandrolone
nortestosterone decanoate
see: nandrolone decanoate
19 nortestosterone decanoate
see: nandrolone decanoate
nortestosterone derivative
see: nandrolone derivative
19 nortestosterone derivative
see: nandrolone derivative
19 nortestosterone enantiomer
see: nandrolone
nortestosterone ester
see: nandrolone
nortestosterone hydrocinnamate
see: nandrolone phenpropionate
nortestosterone laurate
see: nandrolone laurate

19 nortestosterone laurate
see: nandrolone laurate
nortestosterone laurinate
see: nandrolone laurate
19 nortestosterone laurinate
see: nandrolone laurate
nortestosterone undecanoate
see: nandrolone undecanoate
nortestosterone undecylate
see: nandrolone undecanoate
nortestosterone undecylenate
see: nandrolone undecanoate
nor tpp
see: nandrolone phenpropionate
notandron
see: methandriol
novadex
see: tamoxifen citrate
novadren
see: isoprenaline
novaldex
see: tamoxifen citrate
novartrina
see: morazone
novazyd
see: hydrochlorothiazide plus lisinopril
novedrin
see: etafedrine
novegan
see: clenbuterol

novel erythropoiesis stimulating protein

novo actrapid
see: neutral insulin
novoactrapid insulin
see: neutral insulin
novocort
see: dexamethasone
novodrin
see: isoprenaline
novodrine
see: isoprenaline
novohydrocort
see: hydrocortisone
novolaudon
see: hydromorphone
novo lente
see: insulin zinc suspension
novolente
see: insulin zinc suspension
novolin
see: insulin
novolin l
see: insulin zinc suspension
novolin lente
see: insulin zinc suspension
novolin n
see: isophane insulin
novolin nph
see: isophane insulin
novolog
see: insulin aspart
novomix
see: insulin aspart
novomix 30
see: insulin aspart
novopen
see: neutral insulin
novorapid
see: insulin aspart
novorapide
see: insulin aspart
novotriamzide
see: hydrochlorothiazide plus triamterene
novotropin
see: human growth hormone
novozolamide
see: acetazolamide
novydrine
see: amphetamine
np 13
see: bemegride
n palmitoylethanolamine
see: palmidrol
nph
see: isophane insulin
nph iletin
see: isophane insulin
nph insulin
see: isophane insulin
nph umuline
see: isophane insulin
nsc 10023
see: prednisone
nsc10023
see: prednisone
nsc 100638
see: amfonelic acid
nsc 101791
see: fluocinonide
nsc101791
see: fluocinonide
nsc 10483
see: hydrocortisone

Index

nsc10483
see: hydrocortisone
nsc 106565
see: butoxamine
nsc106565
see: butoxamine
nsc 107430
see: pentazocine
nsc 107680
see: flumetasone pivalate
nsc107680
see: flumetasone pivalate
nsc 108161
see: polythiazide
nsc 108164
see: epitizide
nsc 11319
see: deoxycorticosterone
nsc 114650
see: dimefline
nsc114650
see: dimefline
nsc 12165
see: fluoxymesterone
nsc12165
see: fluoxymesterone
nsc 12173
see: testolactone
nsc 12198
see: drostanolone propionate
nsc 180973
see: tamoxifen
nsc 19043
see: oxycodone
nsc 19987
see: methylprednisolone
nsc 23162
see: nandrolone phenpropionate
nsc23162
see: nandrolone phenpropionate
nsc 25159
see: pemoline
nsc 25259
see: pemoline
nsc 26198
see: oxymetholone
nsc26198
see: oxymetholone
nsc 34521
see: dexamethasone
nsc 35770
see: clomifene
nsc 39470
see: betamethasone
nsc 406087
see: etamivan
nsc406087
see: etamivan
nsc 42722
see: metandienone
nsc 43193
see: stanozolol
nsc 47439
see: fluprednisolone
nsc47439
see: fluprednisolone
nsc 526062
see: dexoxadrol
nsc 54702
see: flumetasone
nsc54702
see: flumetasone
nsc 55975
see: epimestrol
nsc55975
see: epimestrol
nsc 63278
see: medrysone
nsc 6365
see: trometamol
nsc 64967
see: metenolone enantate
nsc 66233
see: bolasterone
nsc 66952
see: aminorex
nsc 69536
see: methallibure
nsc69536
see: methallibure
nsc 70735
see: nafoxidine
nsc 73713
see: dexamphetamine
nsc 741
see: hydrocortisone
nsc 74226
see: metenolone acetate
nsc 75054
see: mesterolone
nsc 77625
see: triamterene
nsc77625
see: triamterene

nsc 80998
see: cortivazol
nsc80998
see: cortivazol
nsc 85791
see: etacrynic acid
nsc 88536
see: calusterone
nsc 9120
see: prednisolone
nsc 91523
see: propranolol
nsc 9166
see: testosterone propionate
nsc9166
see: testosterone propionate
nsc 9700
see: testosterone
nsc 9701
see: methyltestosterone
nsc 9703
see: cortisone
nucodan
see: oxycodone
nu man
see: methyltestosterone
numan
see: methyltestosterone
numorphan
see: oxymorphone
numotac
see: isoetarine
numotac tablets
see: isoetarine
nuralin
see: neutral insulin
nutracort
see: hydrocortisone
nutropin
see: human growth hormone
nutropin aq
see: human growth hormone
nutropin depot
see: human growth hormone
nuvacthen
see: tetracosactide
nuvacthen depot
see: tetracosactide
nyderal
see: buphenine
nylhydrine
see: buphenine
nylidrin
see: buphenine
nylidrine
see: buphenine
nylidrin hydrochloride
see: buphenine
nylin
see: buphenine
6 o acetylmorphine
see: morphine 6 acetate
obermine black and yellow
see: phentermine
obesedrin
see: dexamphetamine
obesin
see: propylhexedrine
obesin andromacro
see: amphetamine
obesitex
see: amfepramone
obesonil
see: dexamphetamine
obetrol
see: amphetamine
oblioser
see: morphine sulfate
obsidan
see: propranolol
obsin
see: propranolol
obzidan
see: propranolol
oceprenalin
see: orciprenaline
ociprenaline
see: orciprenaline
ocriten
see: deoxycorticosterone acetate
ocupress
see: carteolol
oedemase
see: furosemide
oedemex
see: furosemide
oftan timolol
see: timolol maleate
okasa mascul
see: testosterone propionate
oktedrin
see: amphetamine
olfex
see: budesonide

olfex bucal
see: budesonide
olmifon
see: adrafinil
olux
see: clobetasol propionate
omcilon
see: triamcinolone
o methylcannabidiol
see: cannabidiol methyl ether
omifin
see: clomifene citrate
omnifen
see: clomifene
omnisterin
see: oxandrolone
6 o monoacetylmorphine
see: morphine 6 acetate
oncovertin
see: dextran
ondogyne
see: cyclofenil
onkohaes
see: hetastarch
onkohas
see: hetastarch
onkotin
see: dextran
onkovertin
see: dextran
ono 1101
see: landiolol
ono1101
see: landiolol
onoact
see: landiolol
onsuki
see: procaterol
onsukil
see: procaterol
opc 1085
see: carteolol
opc 2009
see: procaterol
opc2009
see: procaterol
ophthocort
see: medrysone
ophthocortin
see: medrysone
ophtiole
see: metipranolol
ophtocortin
see: medrysone
ophtorenin
see: bupranolol
opso
see: morphine
opticor
see: pentetrazole
opticorten
see: dexamethasone
opticortinol
see: dexamethasone
optipranolol
see: metipranolol
optisulin
see: insulin glargine
opton
see: oxycodone
optro
see: recombinant hemoglobin
optruma
see: raloxifene
orabolin
see: ethylestrenol
oradexan
see: dexamethasone
oradexon
see: dexamethasone
oradexon 17 valerate
see: dexamethasone 17 valerate
oradexone
see: dexamethasone
oralcon
see: diclofenamide
oraldrina
see: amphetamine
oralin
see: insulin
oral turinabol
see: 4 chloro 17beta hydroxy 17 methylandrosta 1,4 dien 3 one
oramercur
see: chlormerodrin
oramorph
see: morphine sulfate
oranabol
see: oxymesterone
orasone
see: prednisone
oratestin
see: fluoxymesterone
ora testryl
see: fluoxymesterone

oratrol
see: diclofenamide
oraviron
see: methyltestosterone
oravirone
see: methyltestosterone
orchiol
see: testosterone propionate
orchiormon
see: testosterone propionate
orchiprenaline sulfate
see: orciprenaline
orchisteron
see: methyltestosterone
orchisterone
see: testosterone propionate
orchisterone m
see: methyltestosterone
orchisterone p
see: testosterone propionate
orchistin
see: testosterone propionate
orciprenalin
see: orciprenaline

orciprenaline

orciprenaline sulfate
see: orciprenaline
oreon methyl
see: methyltestosterone
oretic
see: hydrochlorothiazide
oreton
see: testosterone propionate
oretone
see: testosterone propionate
oreton f
see: testosterone
oreton m
see: methyltestosterone
oreton methyl
see: methyltestosterone
oreton propionate
see: testosterone propionate
orf 17070
see: histrelin
orf17070
see: histrelin
org 2766
see: 2 amino 4 (methylsulfonyl)butyrylglutamylhistidylphenylalanyl dextro lysylphenylalanine
org 32489
see: recombinant follitropin
org32489
see: recombinant follitropin
org 6001
see: amafolone
org 6216
see: rimexolone
org6216
see: rimexolone
org 817
see: epimestrol
org817
see: epimestrol
orgabolin
see: ethylestrenol
orgadrone
see: dexamethasone
organomercurial diuretic
see: diuretic agent
orgasuline
see: neutral insulin
orgasuline nph
see: isophane insulin
org od 14
see: tibolone
org od14
see: tibolone
oricur
see: chlormerodrin
orimercur
see: chlormerodrin
orimeten
see: aminoglutethimide
orimetene
see: aminoglutethimide
orisane
see: prednisone
ormeloxifene
see: centchroman
ormidol
see: atenolol
oro insulin
see: insulin

oropivalone

oropivalone bacitracin
see: oropivalone
oropivalone bacitracine
see: oropivalone
orquisteron
see: testosterone

orquisterone p
see: testosterone propionate
orquisteron p
see: testosterone propionate
ortedrine
see: amphetamine
orthoxine
see: methoxyphenamine
ortodrinex
see: methoxyphenamine
osiren
see: spironolactone
osmitrol
see: mannitol
osmofundin
see: mannitol
osmosal
see: mannitol
osmosteril
see: mannitol
osmotic diuretic
see: osmotic diuretic agent

osmotic diuretic agent

ospemifene

ossicodone
see: oxycodone
ossiprenol
see: isoprenaline
osyrol
see: spironolactone
osyrol 50 100
see: spironolactone
otosone f
see: hydrocortisone
otosporin
see: cortisporin
ovagen
see: follitropin
ovarelin
see: gonadorelin acetate
ovidrel
see: recombinant chorionic gonadotropin
ovidrelle
see: recombinant chorionic gonadotropin
ovine fsh
see: follitropin
ovine growth hormone
see: growth hormone
ovine icsh
see: luteinizing hormone
ovitrelle
see: recombinant chorionic gonadotropin
ovulating hormone
see: luteinizing hormone

ovurelin

oxabol
see: oxabolone

oxabolone

oxabolone cipionate

oxabolone cypionate
see: oxabolone cipionate
oxamphetamine
see: hydroxyamphetamine
oxandrine
see: oxandrolone

oxandrolone

oxanest
see: oxycodone
oxicone
see: oxycodone
oxiconum
see: oxycodone
oxikon
see: oxycodone
oxilofrin
see: oxilofrine

oxilofrine

oxis
see: formoterol
3 oxo 4 estren 17beta ol
see: nandrolone
17 oxo 5 androsten 3beta ol
see: prasterone
11 oxoandrost 4 enedione
see: adrenosterone

19 oxoandrostenedione

18 oxocorticosterone
see: aldosterone

Index

18 oxocortisol
see: 18 oxohydrocortisone
11 oxo delta 4 androstenedione
see: adrenosterone
oxodolin
see: chlortalidone

18 oxohydrocortisone

11 oxotestosterone

oxprenoate potassium

oxprenol
see: oxprenolol

oxprenolol

oxprenolol hydrochloride
see: oxprenolol
oxprenolol plus chlortalidone
see: trasitensin
oxprenolol plus dihydralazine
see: dihydralazine plus oxprenolol
oxtrenolol
see: oxprenolol

oxyamal

oxycodeinonhydrochloride
see: oxycodone

oxycodone

oxycodone hydrochloride
see: oxycodone
oxycodonhydrochlorid
see: oxycodone
oxycodyl
see: oxycodone
oxycone
see: oxycodone
oxycontin
see: oxycodone
oxydess
see: methamphetamine
oxydrene
see: methamphetamine
oxyfed
see: methamphetamine
oxyfedrin
see: oxyfedrine

oxyfedrine

oxyfedrine hydrochloride
see: oxyfedrine
oxyferol
see: perfluorotributylamine
oxygent
see: perfluorooctyl bromide
oxygent ht
see: perfluorooctyl bromide
oxygesic
see: oxycodone
oxyhaemoglobin
see: oxyhemoglobin

oxyhemoglobin

oxyhemoglobin a
see: oxyhemoglobin
oxyhemoglobins
see: oxyhemoglobin
oxykon
see: oxycodone
oxylone
see: fluorometholone

oxymesterone

oxymestrone
see: oxymesterone
oxymethalone
see: oxymetholone
oxymethemoglobin
see: methemoglobin

oxymetholone

oxymetolone
see: oxymetholone

oxymorphone

oxymorphone hydrochloride
see: oxymorphone
oxyphedrin
see: oxyfedrine
oxyphedrine
see: oxyfedrine

oxyphedrine hydrochloride
see: oxyfedrine
oxypherol
see: perfluorotributylamine

oxypolygelatin

oxyprenolol
see: oxprenolol
oxyprenolol hydrochloride
see: oxprenolol

ozolinone

ozolinone ethyl ester
see: etozolin
p 1393
see: benzthiazide
p1393
see: benzthiazide
p 1496
see: zeranol
p1496
see: zeranol
p16cm
see: 11beta,17alpha,21 trihydroxy 3,20 dioxopregna 1,4 diene 16alpha carboxylic acid methyl ester
p 1779
see: altizide
p 2105
see: epitizide
p 2525
see: polythiazide
p (2 aminopropyl)phenol
see: hydroxyamphetamine
p 5369
see: clenbuterol
p 5604
see: loteprednol etabonate
p5604
see: loteprednol etabonate
pabracort
see: hydrocortisone acetate
pac compound
see: caffeine
pafadrin
see: isoprenaline

pafenolol

paginol
see: penbutolol
palfium
see: dextromoramide
palladon
see: hydromorphone
palladone
see: hydromorphone
palladone xl
see: hydromorphone

palmidrol

palmitoylethanolamide
see: palmidrol
palphium
see: dextromoramide

pamatolol

panafcortolone
see: prednisolone
panafort
see: prednisolone
panalog
see: triamcinolone acetonide
panbesy
see: phentermine
pancodine
see: oxycodone
pandel
see: hydrocortisone 17 butyrate 21 propionate
panimit
see: bupranolol

panomifene

pantalgin
see: pethidine
pantestin
see: testosterone propionate
pantestin oral
see: methyltestosterone
pantestone
see: testosterone undecanoate
para (2 aminopropyl)phenol
see: hydroxyamphetamine
para aminoclonidine
see: apraclonidine
parabolan
see: trenbolone
para chloramphetamine
see: chloramphetamine
para chloroamphetamine
see: chloramphetamine

para chloromethamphetamine
see: 4 chloromethamphetamine
para chloro methylamphetamine
see: 4 chloromethamphetamine
para chloromethylamphetamine
see: 4 chloromethamphetamine
para chloro n methamphetamine
see: 4 chloromethamphetamine
para chlorophenoxyacetate 235
see: meclofenoxate
paracort
see: prednisone
paracortol
see: prednisolone
paradrine
see: hydroxyamphetamine
para hydroxyamphetamine
see: hydroxyamphetamine
parahydroxyamphetamine
see: hydroxyamphetamine
para hydroxyephedrine
see: oxilofrine
para hydroxymethamphetamine
see: pholedrine
para iodoamphetamine
see: 4 iodoamphetamine
paramesone
see: paramethasone
parametazon
see: paramethasone
paramethason
see: paramethasone

paramethasone

para methasone
see: paramethasone
paramethasone 21 acetate
see: paramethasone acetate
paramethasone acetat
see: paramethasone acetate

paramethasone acetate

paramethazone
see: paramethasone
paramethazone acetate
see: paramethasone acetate
para methoxyamphetamine
see: 4 methoxyamphetamine
para methylamphetamine
see: 4 methylamphetamine
paramezone
see: paramethasone
paramol 118
see: codydramol
paranephrin
see: adrenalin
1 para tolyl 2 propylamine
see: 4 methylamphetamine
paredrine
see: hydroxyamphetamine
paredrinea
see: hydroxyamphetamine
paredrinex
see: hydroxyamphetamine
paredrinol
see: pholedrine
parenabol
see: boldenone undecenoate
parkryl
see: selegiline
partusisten
see: fenoterol
partusisten perlongets
see: fenoterol
pavinal
see: oxycodone
pb 005
see: prasterone
pb005
see: prasterone
pb 868 cl
see: mabuterol
pb 89
see: fominoben
pb89
see: fominoben
p-chloroamphetamine
see: chloramphetamine
p chloroamphetamine
see: chloramphetamine
pectobloc
see: pindolol
pectoblock mite
see: pindolol
pedrolone
see: hydroxyamphetamine
peha norm
see: trometamol
pehanorm
see: trometamol
peltazon
see: pentazocine

pemetesan
see: pentetrazole
pemolate magnesium
see: pemoline magnesium
pemolin
see: pemoline
pemolinate magnesium
see: pemoline magnesium

pemoline

pemoline magnesium

pemoline magnesiumchelate
see: pemoline magnesium
pemoline magnesium hydroxide
see: pemoline magnesium
penandren
see: testosterone propionate
penbutalol
see: penbutolol

penbutolol

penbutolol sulfate
see: penbutolol
penecort
see: hydrocortisone
penitardon
see: buphenine
pentacard
see: pentetrazole
pentacozine
see: pentazocine
pentafen
see: pentazocine

11 [4 [[5 [(4,4,5,5,5 pentafluoropentyl)sulfonyl]pentyl]oxy]phenyl]estradiol

pentafraction
see: hetastarch
pentagin
see: pentazocine
pentalgina
see: pentazocine
pentamethazol
see: pentetrazole
pentamethylene 1,5 tetrazole
see: pentetrazole
pentamethylenetetrazol
see: pentetrazole
pentamethylene tetrazole
see: pentetrazole
pentamethylenetetrazole
see: pentetrazole
1,5 pentamethylenetetrazole
see: pentetrazole
pentamethylenetrazol
see: pentetrazole
pentaspan
see: hetastarch
pentastarch
see: hetastarch
pentazocin
see: pentazocine

pentazocine

pentazocine hydrochloride
see: pentazocine
pentazocine isomer
see: pentazocine
pentazol
see: pentetrazole
pentazole
see: pentetrazole
pentemesan
see: pentetrazole
pentetrazol
see: pentetrazole

pentetrazole

penticort
see: amcinonide
pento adiparthrol
see: mazindol
pentozocine
see: pentazocine
pentrozol
see: pentetrazole
pentylene tetrazol
see: pentetrazole
pentylenetetrazol
see: pentetrazole
pentylene tetrazole
see: pentetrazole
pentylenetetrazole
see: pentetrazole
perandren
see: testosterone propionate

perandren amp
see: testosterone propionate
perandrone
see: testosterone propionate
perandrone amp
see: testosterone propionate
perbilen
see: piretanide
percapyl
see: chlormerodrin

percocet

percodan

percodan demi
see: percodan
percomon
see: amphetamine
percoral
see: nikethamide
percorten
see: deoxycorticosterone acetate
percorten acetate
see: deoxycorticosterone acetate
percutacrine androgenique
see: testosterone
percutacrine androgine
see: testosterone
perdilat
see: buphenine
perdilatal
see: buphenine
perfluamine
see: perfluorotripropylamine
perflubron
see: perfluorooctyl bromide
perflunafene
see: perfluorodecalin

perfluorobutyltetrahydrofuran

perfluorodecalin

perfluorooctyl bromide

perfluorooctylbromide
see: perfluorooctyl bromide

perfluoroperhydrofluoranthene

perfluorotributylamine

perfluorotri(n butyl)amine
see: perfluorotributylamine

perfluorotripropylamine

perfucol
see: fluosol da
pergonal
see: human menopausal gonadotropin
pergonal 500
see: human menopausal gonadotropin
pergotime
see: clomifene citrate
perhexilene hydrogen maleate
see: perhexiline maleate
perhexilene maleate
see: perhexiline maleate

perhexiline

perhexiline maleate

permastril
see: drostanolone propionate
permastryl
see: drostanolone propionate
pertestis
see: testosterone cipionate
perutagin
see: pentazocine
pervadil
see: buphenine
pervitin
see: methamphetamine
pesomax
see: androstanolone
pesos
see: fenfluramine
petadin
see: pethidine
petantin
see: pethidine
petantina
see: pethidine
pethanol
see: pethidine

pethedine
see: pethidine
pethidin
see: pethidine

pethidine

pethidine hydrobromide
see: pethidine
pethidine hydrochloride
see: pethidine
pethidine roche
see: pethidine
petibelle
see: drospirenone plus ethinylestradiol
petidin
see: pethidine
pexid
see: perhexiline maleate
pg 600
see: seric gonadotropin
phanurane
see: canrenone
pharmadil
see: buphenine
pharmamedrine
see: amphetamine
pharmanocarb
see: sydnocarb
pharmedrine
see: amphetamine
pharmodex
see: dextran
phemetrazine
see: phenmetrazine
phenadon
see: methadone
phenamin
see: amphetamine
phenamizole
see: amiphenazole

phendimetrazine

phendimetrazine bitartrate
see: phendimetrazine tartrate

phendimetrazine embonate

phendimetrazine pamoate
see: phendimetrazine embonate

phendimetrazine tartrate

phenedrine
see: amphetamine
phenetylline
see: fenetylline
phenfluoramine
see: fenfluramine
phenidylate
see: methylphenidate
phenidyl hydrochloride
see: methylphenidate
phenimethoxazine
see: phendimetrazine
phenmetrazin
see: phenmetrazine

phenmetrazine

phenmetrazine hydrochloride
see: phenmetrazine
phenoprominum
see: amphetamine
phenoterol
see: fenoterol
phenoxazole
see: pemoline
phenoxyisopropylnorsuprifen
see: isoxsuprine
phenpromin
see: amphetamine
phenproporex
see: fenproporex
phentermide
see: phentermine
phentermin
see: phentermine

phentermine

phentermine hydrochloride
see: phentermine

phentermine resin

phentermine resinate
see: phentermine resin
phentrol
see: phentermine
5 phenyl 2,4 thiazolediamine
see: amiphenazole
1 phenyl 2 aminopropane
see: amphetamine

1 phenyl 2 ethylaminopropane
see: n ethylamphetamine
1 phenyl 2 propanamine
see: amphetamine
1 phenyl 2 pyrrolidinopentane
see: prolintane
phenylaminopropane
see: amphetamine
phenylisohydantoin
see: pemoline
(phenylisopropyl) amine
see: amphetamine
(phenylisopropyl)amine
see: amphetamine
phenyl isopropylamine
see: amphetamine
phenylmethyltetrahydro oxazine
see: phenmetrazine
4 phenylpiracetam
see: carphedon
phenylpropanolamide
see: phenylpropanolamine

phenylpropanolamine

phenyl propanolamine
see: phenylpropanolamine
phenylpropylolamine
see: phenylpropanolamine
phenylpyrrolidine pentane
see: prolintane
phenylpyrrolidone pentane
see: prolintane
phenylsec.butylnorsuprifen
see: buphenine
phenzine
see: phendimetrazine tartrate
phepranon
see: amfepramone
phetadex
see: dexamphetamine
phetanol
see: etilefrine
phetanyl
see: etilefrine
phetidine
see: pethidine
philipon
see: methamphetamine
philopon
see: methamphetamine
phlogex
see: prednisolone

pholedrine

phortisolone
see: prednisolone sodium phosphate
phrenazol
see: pentetrazole
phthalamidine
see: chlortalidone
phthalamodine
see: chlortalidone
phthalamudine
see: chlortalidone
p-hydroxyamphetamine
see: hydroxyamphetamine
phyol
see: growth hormone
phyon
see: growth hormone
physepton
see: methadone
physeptone
see: methadone
physex
see: chorionic gonadotropin

picamilon

picrotoxin

picrotoxine
see: picrotoxin

picumeterol

picumeterol fumarate
see: picumeterol

pig insulin

pikamilon
see: picamilon
pinactizine
see: aldactazine

pindolol

pindolol analog
see: pindolol derivative

Index

pindolol derivative

pindolol,hydroxybenzyl
see: hydroxybenzylpindolol
pindolol,methyl
see: mepindolol
pindolol plus clopamide
see: viskaldix
pinolol lb 46
see: pindolol
pioxol
see: pemoline

pipendoxifene

pipendoxifene hydrochloride
see: pipendoxifene

2 [4 (2 piperidinoethoxy)phenyl] 3 phenyl 2h 1 benzopyran

pipradol

pipradol chloride
see: pipradol
pipradol hydrochloride
see: pipradol
pipradrol
see: pipradol
pipradrol chloride
see: pipradol
pipradrol hydrochloride
see: pipradol
piracetam,4 phenyl
see: carphedon

pirbuterol

pirbuterol acetate

pirem
see: carbuterol

piretanide

piridosal
see: pethidine
pituitary gonadotrophin
see: gonadotropin
pituitary gonadotropin
see: gonadotropin
pituitary growth hormone
see: growth hormone
pituitary hormones, anterior
see: adenohypophysis hormone
piurone
see: chlormerodrin
pivalephrine
see: dipivefrine
pivalone
see: tixocortol pivalate
plasmacair
see: dextran 40
plasmaclair
see: dextran
plasma expander
see: plasma substitute
plasma expanding agent
see: plasma substitute
plasma expansion
see: plasma substitute
plasma,fresh frozen
see: fresh frozen plasma
plasmafusin
see: hetastarch
plasmasteril
see: hetastarch
plasma substituent
see: plasma substitute

plasma substitute

plasma substitute agent
see: plasma substitute
plasma substitutes
see: plasma substitute
plasma substitution
see: plasma substitute
plasma volume expander
see: plasma substitute

plasmion

plasmodex
see: dextran 40
platelet concentrate
see: thrombocyte concentrate
plavolex
see: dextran
plazmozid
see: oxypolygelatin
ple 1053
see: azosemide

Index

plegine
see: phendimetrazine tartrate
plenastril
see: oxymetholone
plurimen
see: selegiline
pluryl
see: bendroflumethiazide
pluryle
see: bendroflumethiazide
PMSG
see: seric gonadotropin
pms gonadotrophin
see: seric gonadotropin
pms gonadotropin
see: seric gonadotropin
pnu 155971
see: exemestane
pnu155971
see: exemestane
pokkortolon
see: triamcinolone acetonide
polamidon
see: methadone
polamivet
see: methadone
polamivit
see: methadone
polcortolon
see: triamcinolone
policort
see: dexamethasone
policort 17 valerate
see: dexamethasone 17 valerate
polyalanylinsulin series
see: insulin derivative
polygelin
see: polygeline

polygeline

polyglucin
see: dextran
polyglucine
see: dextran
polyglucinum
see: dextran
polyglusol
see: dextran
polyglusole
see: dextran
polyheme
see: polymerized hemoglobin
polyhemoglobin,pyridoxylated
see: pyridoxylpolyhemoglobin
polyhydroxyamylopectin
see: hetastarch

polymerized hemoglobin

poly pred
see: prednisolone acetate
polythiaside
see: polythiazide

polythiazide

ponderal
see: fenfluramine
ponderax
see: fenfluramine
ponderex
see: fenfluramine
pondimin
see: fenfluramine
pondinil
see: mefenorex
ponflural
see: fenfluramine
ponflural retard
see: fenfluramine
porcine acth
see: corticotropin
porcine corticotropin
see: corticotropin
porcine insulin
see: pig insulin
porcine proinsulin
see: proinsulin
potassium canrenoate
see: canrenoate potassium
potassium mexrenoate
see: mexrenoate potassium
potassium sparing diuretic
see: potassium sparing diuretic agent

potassium sparing diuretic agent

practalol
see: practolol
practazin
see: aldactazine

practolol

practolole
see: practolol
practon
see: spironolactone
praedil
see: isoprenaline
praedyn
see: chorionic gonadotropin
praktolol
see: practolol

pralmorelin

prandol
see: propranolol
prano puren
see: propranolol
pranopuren
see: propranolol
pranturon
see: chorionic gonadotropin
prasterone 3 beta acetate
see: prasterone acetate

prasterone

prasterone acetate

prasterone sulfate

praxinor
see: cafedrine plus theodrenaline
precort
see: prednisone
precortal
see: prednisone
precortalon
see: prednisolone
precortancyl
see: prednisolone
pre cortisyl
see: prednisolone
precortisyl
see: prednisolone
predalon
see: chorionic gonadotropin
predartrina
see: prednisolone
predartrine
see: prednisolone
predef
see: isoflupredone acetate
predfoam
see: prednisolone 3 sulfobenzoate
pred forte
see: prednisolone acetate
predforte
see: prednisolone acetate
pred forte tm
see: prednisolone acetate
pred mild
see: prednisolone acetate
prednacinolone
see: desonide
predne dome
see: prednisolone
prednedome
see: prednisolone
prednelan
see: prednisolone
prednesol
see: prednisolone sodium phosphate

prednicarbate

predni coelin
see: prednisolone
prednicoelin
see: prednisolone
prednicort
see: prednisolone
prednicortelone
see: prednisolone
prednifor drops
see: prednisolone
predni f tablinen
see: dexamethasone
predni h
see: prednisolone acetate
predni h tablinen
see: prednisolone
prednilidene
see: prednylidene
predniment
see: prednisolone
predniretard
see: prednisolone
prednis
see: prednisolone
prednisol
see: prednisolone sodium succinate

Index

prednisol n
see: prednisolone sodium succinate
prednisolon
see: prednisolone

prednisolone

prednisolone,16alpha hydroxy
see: 16alpha hydroxyprednisolone
prednisolone 17 acetate
see: prednisolone acetate
prednisolone 21 acetate
see: prednisolone acetate
prednisolone 21 hemisuccinate
see: prednisolone hemisuccinate

prednisolone 21 phosphate

prednisolone 21 succinate
see: prednisolone hemisuccinate

prednisolone 3 sulfobenzoate

prednisolone acetate

prednisolone alcohol
see: prednisolone
prednisolone bisuccinate
see: prednisolone hemisuccinate

prednisolone derivative

prednisolone f
see: dexamethasone
prednisolone h
see: prednisolone

prednisolone hemisuccinate

prednisolone oleosae sr 82
see: prednisolone
prednisolone phosphate
see: prednisolone 21 phosphate
prednisolone phosphate sodium
see: prednisolone sodium phosphate

prednisolone pivalate

prednisolone sodium phosphate

prednisolone sodium succinate

prednisolone sodium tetrahydrophthalate

prednisolone succinate
see: prednisolone hemisuccinate
prednisolone succinate sodium
see: prednisolone sodium succinate
prednisolone, topical
see: prednisolone
prednisolone trimethylacetate
see: prednisolone pivalate
prednisolone valerate acetate
see: prednival acetate
prednisolut
see: prednisolone hemisuccinate
predniso n
see: prednisone

prednisone

prednisone acetate

prednisone alcohol
see: prednisone
prednisone test
see: prednisone

prednival acetate

prednivet
see: prednisolone
prednol
see: methylprednisolone
prednorsolon
see: prednisolone
prednorsolone
see: prednisolone

prednylidene

prednylidine
see: prednylidene
predonine
see: prednisolonc
predorgasolona
see: prednisolone
predorgasolone
see: prednisolone

Index

predsol
see: prednisolone sodium phosphate
preferid
see: budesonide
pregn 4 en 21 ol 3,20 dione
see: deoxycorticosterone
pregn 5 en 3 beta ol 20 one
see: pregnenolone
pregn 5 en 3beta ol 20 one
see: pregnenolone
pregnacol
see: seric gonadotropin
pregnant mare serum
see: seric gonadotropin
4 pregnen 20 ol 3 one
see: pregnenolone
4 pregnen 21 ol 3,20 dione
see: deoxycorticosterone
5 pregnen 3 beta ol 20 one
see: pregnenolone
5 pregnen 3beta ol 20 one
see: pregnenolone
5 pregnen 3 ol 20 one
see: pregnenolone
pregnenalone
see: pregnenolone

pregnenolone

pregnenolone 16 alpha nitrite
see: pregnenolone derivative
5 pregnenolone
see: pregnenolone
pregnenolone derivates
see: pregnenolone derivative

pregnenolone derivative

pregnenolone sulfate

pregnesin
see: chorionic gonadotropin
pregnyl
see: chorionic gonadotropin
pregonadotropin
see: gonadotropin
pregova
see: human menopausal gonadotropin
prelis
see: metoprolol tartrate
prelis comp
see: chlortalidone plus metoprolol
prelobane
see: seric gonadotropin
prelone
see: prednisolone
preludin
see: phenmetrazine
premodrin
see: methamphetamine
prempar
see: ritodrine
prenacid
see: desonide
prenalex
see: tertatolol

prenalterol

prenasma
see: isoprenaline
prenolon
see: pregnenolone
prenolone
see: prednisolone
prenomiser
see: isoprenaline
prenomiser forte
see: isoprenaline
prent
see: acebutolol
prenyl
see: prenylamine
prenylamin
see: prenylamine

prenylamine

prepar
see: ritodrine
prepcort
see: hydrocortisone

preproinsulin

presaril
see: torasemide
pre sate
see: chlorphentermine
presate
see: chlorphentermine
presdate
see: labetalol
pressedrine
see: phenylpropanolamine

pressionorm
see: gepefrine tartrate
pressomin
see: methoxamine
pressomin hydrochloride
see: methoxamine
pressonex
see: metaraminol
pressonex bitartrate
see: metaraminol
pressonol
see: metaraminol
pressural
see: indapamide
prestara
see: prasterone
prestole
see: hydrochlorothiazide plus triamterene
pretcamide
see: prethcamide

prethcamide

prethcamine
see: prethcamide
prezidilol
see: prizidilol
prezolon
see: prednisolone
priantin
see: seric gonadotropin
primantron
see: seric gonadotropin
primatene
see: ephedrine
primatene mist
see: adrenalin
primicort
see: deoxycorticosterone acetate

primidolol

primobolan
see: metenolone acetate
primobolan depot
see: metenolone enantate
primobolan s
see: metenolone acetate
primocorten
see: deoxycorticosterone acetate
primogonyl
see: chorionic gonadotropin
primoniat
see: testosterone propionate
primotest
see: testosterone
primoteston
see: testosterone
primoteston depot
see: testosterone
prinactizide
see: aldactazine
prindolol
see: pindolol
prinodolol
see: pindolol
prinzide
see: hydrochlorothiazide plus lisinopril
pritor plus
see: hydrochlorothiazide plus telmisartan
pritorplus
see: hydrochlorothiazide plus telmisartan

prizidilol

prizidilol hydrochloride
see: prizidilol
proair
see: procaterol
proamatine
see: midodrine
proaqua
see: benzthiazide
probalan
see: probenecid
probecid
see: probenecid
probemecid
see: probenecid

probenecid

probenecide
see: probenecid
probenicid
see: probenecid
probenid
see: probenecid
probolin
see: methandriol dipropionate
probose p
see: phenmetrazine
procadil
see: procaterol

procardin(e)
see: nikethamide

procaterol

procaterol,erythro
see: procaterol
procaterol hydrochloride
see: procaterol
procid
see: probenecid

procinolol

procinonide

procol
see: phenylpropanolamine
procorman
see: nikethamide
pro cort
see: hydrocortisone
procort
see: hydrocortisone
procortan
see: corticotropin
procortan forte
see: corticotropin
procrin
see: leuprorelin
procrit
see: recombinant erythropoietin
proctalol
see: practolol
proctocort
see: hydrocortisone
proctosone
see: hydrocortisone
prodexona
see: dexamethasone
prodexone
see: dexamethasone
profamina
see: amphetamine
profasi
see: chorionic gonadotropin
profetamine
see: amphetamine

proinsulin

pro insulin
see: proinsulin
proinsulin,bovine
see: proinsulin
proinsuline
see: proinsulin
proinsulin,human biosynthetic
see: biosynthetic human proinsulin
prolease
see: human growth hormone

prolintane

prolintane hydrochloride
see: prolintane
prolol
see: propranolol
prolongine
see: probenecid
promedrol
see: methylprednisolone suleptanate
promeran
see: chlormerodrin
promit
see: dextran
promiten
see: dextran
promogonyl
see: chorionic gonadotropin
promotil
see: prolintane
pronarcin
see: oxycodone
pronetal
see: pronetalol

pronetalol

pronetalol hydrochloride
see: pronetalol
pronethalol
see: pronetalol
pronethalol hydrochloride
see: pronetalol
pronison
see: prednisone
pronisone
see: prednisone
pronizone
see: prednisone

pronovan
see: propranolol
prontovent
see: clenbuterol
propabloc
see: propranolol
propaderm
see: beclometasone dipropionate
propaderm forte
see: beclometasone dipropionate
propadrine
see: phenylpropanolamine
propagest
see: phenylpropanolamine
propal
see: propranolol
propanolol derivative
see: propranolol derivative
propanolol hydrochloride
see: propranolol

10 propargylestr 4 ene 3,17 dione

propercuten
see: propranolol
prophasi
see: chorionic gonadotropin
prophylux
see: propranolol
propine
see: dipivefrine
propiokan
see: testosterone propionate
propisamine
see: amphetamine
propral
see: propranolol

propranolol

propranolol,4' methylthio
see: 4' methylthiopropranolol
propranolol analog
see: propranolol derivative

propranolol derivative

propranolol hydrochloride
see: propranolol
propranolol isomer
see: propranolol
propranolol quaternary analog
see: propranolol derivative

propranur
see: propranolol
propra ratiopharm
see: propranolol
proprasylyt
see: propranolol
proprasylyte
see: propranolol

propylhexedrine

7alpha propylspironolactone

propylon
see: isoprenaline
propynalin
see: isoprenaline
prostap
see: leuprorelin
prostap sr
see: leuprorelin
protamine insulin
see: isophane insulin
protamine zinc insulin
see: isophane insulin
protandren
see: methandriol
protanol
see: isoprenaline
protaphan
see: isophane insulin
protaphane
see: isophane insulin
proteina
see: androstanolone
proterenol
see: isoprenaline
protergine
see: mestanolone
proternol
see: isoprenaline
proternol l
see: isoprenaline
prothecamide
see: prethcamide
protona
see: androstanolone
protophane
see: isophane insulin
protophane hm
see: isophane insulin

Index

protropin
see: somatrem
proventil
see: salbutamol
proventil inhaler
see: salbutamol
proventil repetabs
see: salbutamol
provigil
see: modafinil
proviron
see: mesterolone

proxodolol

prymogonyl
see: chorionic gonadotropin
pseudonorephedrine
see: norpseudoephedrine
psicosterone
see: prasterone
psicosterone 3 sulfate
see: prasterone sulfate
psi norcocaine
see: norcocaine
psl 14 537
see: adrafinil
psl 14537
see: adrafinil
psl14 537
see: adrafinil
psl14537
see: adrafinil
psoranide
see: fluocinolone acetonide
psorcon
see: diflorasone diacetate
psp iv
see: prednisolone sodium phosphate
psychamine
see: phenmetrazine
psychamine a 66
see: phenmetrazine
psychedrin
see: amphetamine
psychedrine
see: amphetamine
psychoanaleptic agent
see: central stimulant agent
psychostimulant
see: psychostimulant agent

psychostimulant agent

psychostimulating agent
see: psychostimulant agent
psychoton
see: amphetamine
psykoton
see: methamphetamine
pterofen
see: triamterene
pterophene
see: triamterene
1 (p tolyl) 2 propylamine
see: 4 methylamphetamine
puberogen
see: chorionic gonadotropin
pulmadil
see: rimiterol
pulmaxan
see: budesonide
pulmicort
see: budesonide
pulmicort respules
see: budesonide
pulmicort turbuhaler
see: budesonide
pulsan
see: indenolol
pulsoton
see: hydroxyamphetamine
pulsotyl
see: pholedrine
pulstim
see: gonadorelin
purantix
see: clocortolone pivalate
puregon
see: recombinant follitropin
pvtd
see: dextran
pw-135
see: pemoline
pyricardyl
see: nikethamide

pyridoglutethimide

pyridoxylated hemoglobin
see: pyridoxylhemoglobin
pyridoxylated polyhemoglobin
see: pyridoxylpolyhemoglobin

pyridoxylhemoglobin

pyridoxylpolyhemoglobin

pyrocardyl
see: nikethamide

pyrovalerone

pyrovalerone hydrochloride
see: pyrovalerone
pyrrolamidole
see: dextromoramide
pyrrolidino 4 iodotamoxifen
see: idoxifene
pyrroloamidol
see: dextromoramide
qcd 84924
see: dronabinol
querto
see: carvedilol

quinbolone

quinethazon
see: quinethazone

quinethazone

quinoprenaline
see: quinprenaline

quinprenaline

quinterenol
see: quinprenaline
quinterenol dihydrochloride
see: quinprenaline
qvar
see: beclometasone dipropionate
r 067555
see: nebivolol
r 1697
see: trenbolone acetate
r1697
see: trenbolone acetate
r 17 desoxy dexamethasone
see: desoximetasone
r 1881
see: metribolone
r 2113
see: desoximetasone
r2113
see: desoximetasone
r 2323
see: gestrinone
r2323
see: gestrinone
r 2580
see: trenbolone
r2580
see: trenbolone
r 65824
see: nebivolol
r 67138
see: nebivolol
r 67145
see: nebivolol
r 67555
see: nebivolol
r 720 11
see: fenetylline
r 75251
see: liarozole
r 76713
see: vorozole
r 798
see: rimiterol
r798
see: rimiterol
r 812
see: prednisolone 3 sulfobenzoate
r 83839
see: vorozole
r 83842
see: vorozole
r 85246
see: liarozole fumarate
r 875
see: dextromoramide
racedrine
see: racephedrine
racemic adrenalin
see: adrenalin
racemic desoxy nor ephedrine
see: amphetamine
racemic desoxy norephedrine
see: amphetamine
racemic ephedrine
see: racephedrine

racephedrine

racephedrine hydrochloride
see: racephedrine

Index

racephen
see: amphetamine

ractopamine

ractopamine hydrochloride
see: ractopamine
ralabol
see: zeranol
ralgro
see: zeranol

raloxifene

raloxifene hydrochloride
see: raloxifene
ranestol
see: bevantolol
raphetamine
see: amphetamine
rapitard
see: biphasic insulin
rapitard insulin
see: biphasic insulin
rapitard mc
see: biphasic insulin
rat follitropin
see: follitropin
rat fsh
see: follitropin
rat growth hormone
see: growth hormone
reacthin
see: corticotropin
reactivan
see: fencamfamin
rec 7 0267
see: dimefline
rec 7-0267
see: dimefline
rec 70267
see: dimefline
rec7 0267
see: dimefline
rec7-0267
see: dimefline
rec70267
see: dimefline
recagon
see: recombinant follitropin
receptal
see: buserelin

recombinant chorionic gonadotropin

recombinant DNA insulin
see: recombinant human insulin

recombinant erythropoietin

recombinant follitropin

recombinant fsh
see: recombinant follitropin

recombinant growth hormone

recombinant hemoglobin

recombinant human follitropin
see: recombinant follitropin

recombinant human insulin

recombinant insulin
see: recombinant human insulin

recombinant luteinizing hormone

recombinant somatomedin B

recombinant somatomedin C

recombinant somatotropin
see: recombinant growth hormone
recombinant somatropin
see: human growth hormone
recormon
see: recombinant erythropoietin
recormone
see: recombinant erythropoietin
recrein
see: deanol
recthormone
see: testosterone propionate
recthormone testosterone
see: testosterone propionate
rectocort
see: hydrocortisone
rectodelt
see: prednisone

rectomenaderm
see: isoflupredone acetate
rectovalone
see: tixocortol pivalate
reducyl
see: phentermine
redux
see: dexfenfluramine
regenon
see: amfepramone
regenon retard
see: amfepramone
regnosone
see: pregnenolone
regroton
see: chlortalidone plus reserpine
reichstein substance fa
see: cortisone
reichstein substance g
see: adrenosterone
reichstein substance q
see: deoxycorticosterone
relane
see: dexoxadrol
release factor,corticotropin
see: corticotropin releasing factor

relefact

relisorm
see: gonadorelin
remeflin
see: dimefline
renacor
see: enalapril plus hydrochlorothiazide
renaglandin
see: adrenalin
renaleptine
see: adrenalin
renal erythropoietic factor
see: erythropoietin
renalina
see: adrenalin
renaline
see: adrenalin
renese
see: polythiazide
renidur
see: enalapril plus hydrochlorothiazide
renoform
see: adrenalin
renon
see: chlortalidone
renostypticin
see: adrenalin
renostyptin
see: adrenalin
rentibloc
see: sotalol
reomax
see: etacrynic acid
repetabs
see: salbutamol
repicin
see: bendroflumethiazide

reproterol

reproterol hydrochloride
see: reproterol
resectisol
see: mannitol
reserpine hygroton
see: chlortalidone plus reserpine
reserpine plus chlortalidone
see: chlortalidone plus reserpine
respicort
see: budesonide
respifral
see: isoprenaline
respocort
see: beclometasone dipropionate
respolin
see: salbutamol
restandol
see: testosterone undecanoate
retabolil
see: nandrolone decanoate
retandrol
see: testosterone phenylpropionate
retarbolin
see: nandrolone cyclohexylpropionate
retef
see: hydrocortisone acetate
retenema
see: betamethasone valerate
retisert
see: fluocinolone acetonide
rev 5320
see: celiprolol
rev 5320 a
see: celiprolol
rev 5320a
see: celiprolol
revarterenol
see: noradrenalin

reviron
see: methandriol
revivan
see: dopamine
rexigen
see: clobenzorex
rexort
see: citicoline
r fluprednylidene acetate
see: fluprednidene acetate
rg 833
see: betamethasone
rhefluin
see: amiloride plus hydrochlorothiazide
rhefluin mite
see: amiloride plus hydrochlorothiazide

rheodextran

rheomacrodex
see: dextran
rheopolyglucin
see: rheodextran
rheopolyglucine
see: rheodextran
rhinalar
see: flunisolide
rhinalator
see: amphetamine
rhinivict
see: beclometasone dipropionate
rhinocort
see: budesonide
rhinocort aqua
see: budesonide
rhinolar
see: fluocortin
ricortex
see: cortisone

ridazolol

rimexel
see: rimexolone

rimexolone

rimiterol

rimiterol hydrobromide
see: rimiterol
rinarol
see: buphenine
rinderon
see: betamethasone
rinderon a
see: betamethasone sodium phosphate
rinderon dp
see: betamethasone dipropionate
rinderon v
see: betamethasone valerate
ritalin
see: methylphenidate
ritalin hydrochloride
see: methylphenidate
ritalin la
see: methylphenidate
ritalin sr
see: methylphenidate
ritodrin
see: ritodrine

ritodrine

ritodrine hydrochloride
see: ritodrine
rivizor
see: vorozole
rm 101
see: perfluorobutyltetrahydrofuran
rm101
see: perfluorobutyltetrahydrofuran
rmi 16,289
see: enclomifene
rmi 16289
see: enclomifene
rmi 16,312
see: zuclomifene
rmi 16312
see: zuclomifene
rmi 81,968 a
see: medroxalol
rmi 81968 a
see: medroxalol
'rms'
see: morphine sulfate
ro 10 6338
see: bumetanide
ro 10-6338
see: bumetanide
ro10 6338
see: bumetanide
ro10-6338
see: bumetanide

ro 10 7614
see: diflucortolone valerate
ro 12 7024
see: domoprednate
ro 16 8714
see: 4 [3 [bis(beta hydroxyphenethyl)amino]butyl]benzamide
ro 16-8714
see: 4 [3 [bis(beta hydroxyphenethyl)amino]butyl]benzamide
ro 17 2218
see: 6 [2 (3,4 dihydroxyphenyl) 2 hydroxyethylamino] n [4 (trifluoromethyl)phenyl]heptanamide
ro 17 8648
see: 6 [2 (3,4 dihydroxyphenyl) 2 hydroxyethylamino] n [4 (trifluoromethyl)phenyl]heptanamide
ro 17 9651
see: 6 [2 (3,4 dihydroxyphenyl) 2 hydroxyethylamino] n [4 (trifluoromethyl)phenyl]heptanamide
ro 1 9569
see: tetrabenazine
ro 23 9982
see: cilazapril plus hydrochlorothiazide
ro 31 1118
see: flusoxolol
ro 31-1118
see: flusoxolol
ro31 1118
see: flusoxolol
ro31-1118
see: flusoxolol
ro 31 1411
see: flusoxolol
ro 31-1411
see: flusoxolol
ro31 1411
see: flusoxolol
ro31-1411
see: flusoxolol
ro 3 4787
see: bufuralol
ro 363
see: 1 (3,4 dihydroxyphenoxy) 3 (3,4 dimethoxyphenethylamino) 2 propanol
ro 4 5282
see: mefenorex
ro 4-5282
see: mefenorex
ro 6 62827
see: prasterone sulfate
ro 6 6827
see: prasterone sulfate
ro 6 6827-2
see: prasterone sulfate
ro 66827-2
see: prasterone sulfate
rodazol
see: aminoglutethimide
rogletimide
see: pyridoglutethimide
romecor
see: etamivan
rondimen
see: mefenorex
rontyl
see: hydroflumethiazide
ronyl
see: pemoline
rosilar
see: deflazacort
rosimon neu
see: morazone
rotalol
see: sotalol
roxanol
see: morphine sulfate
roxanol sr
see: morphine sulfate
roxicodone
see: oxycodone
roxycodone
see: oxycodone
rp 11614
see: canrenone
rp11614
see: canrenone
rp 2831
see: heptaminol
rp 8228
see: levofacetoperane
rp 8357
see: triamcinolone
rp8357
see: triamcinolone
(R,R) labetalol
see: dilevalol
rs 1320
see: flunisolide acetate
rs1320
see: flunisolide acetate
rs 1401 at
see: fluocinolone acetonide

Index

rs1401 at
see: fluocinolone acetonide
rs 21314
see: 6alpha,9alpha difluoro 11beta,17alpha dihydroxy 16beta methyl 17beta methylthiocarbonylandrosta 1,4 dien 3 one 17 acetate
rs 2177
see: flumetasone
rs2177
see: flumetasone
rs 2252
see: fluclorolone acetonide
rs 2362
see: procinonide
rs2362
see: procinonide
rs 2386
see: ciprocinonide
rs2386
see: ciprocinonide
rs 35909
see: ticabesone propionate
rs 35909 00 00 0
see: ticabesone propionate
rs 3999
see: flunisolide
rs3999
see: flunisolide
rs 40584
see: flumoxonide
rs40584
see: flumoxonide
rs 4691
see: cloprednol
rs 49947
see: gonadorelin[6 dextro [3 (2 naphthyl)alanine] 10 azaglycine]
rs 6245
see: tazolol
rs 85095
see: 6alpha,9alpha difluoro 11beta,17alpha dihydroxy 16beta methyl 17beta methylthiocarbonylandrosta 1,4 dien 3 one 17 propionate
rs 85446 007
see: timobesone acetate
rs 85446-007
see: timobesone acetate
rs 85446007
see: timobesone acetate
rs 94991
see: nafarelin
rs 94991 298
see: nafarelin acetate
rsr 13
see: efaproxiral
rsr13
see: efaproxiral
ru 1697
see: trenbolone acetate
ru1697
see: trenbolone acetate
ru 1881
see: metribolone
ru 22092
see: 6,7 dihydrocanrenone
ru 2323
see: gestrinone
ru2323
see: gestrinone
ru 26752
see: 7alpha propylspironolactone
ru 26988
see: 11beta,17beta dihydroxy 17 (1 propynyl)androsta 1,4,6 trien 3 one
ru 27333
see: trestolone
ru27333
see: trestolone
ru 28318
see: oxprenoate potassium
ru 28362
see: 11beta,17beta dihydroxy 6 methyl 17alpha (1 propynyl)androsta 1,4,6 trien 3 one
ru 39411
see: 11 [4 (2 dimethylaminoethoxy)phenyl]estradiol
ru 51599
see: niravoline
ru 58668
see: 11 [4 [[5 [(4,4,5,5,5 pentafluoropentyl)sulfonyl]pentyl]oxy]phenyl]estradiol
rudilin
see: buphenine
ruful
see: fluocinonide
rwj 17070
see: histrelin
rwj17070
see: histrelin
rx 6029 m
see: buprenorphine
rx 6029m
see: buprenorphine
rx6029m
see: buprenorphine

rydrin
see: buphenine
s 1320
see: budesonide
s 1520
see: indapamide
s1520
see: indapamide
s 1540
see: bitolterol
s 2395
see: tertatolol
s 2620
see: almitrine dimesilate
s2620
see: almitrine dimesilate
s 3460
see: alclometasone dipropionate
s 3500
see: butizide
s 5614
see: dexfenfluramine
s 596
see: arotinolol
s 62
see: chlorphentermine
s 73 4118
see: piretanide
s 734118
see: piretanide
s734118
see: piretanide
s 77 0777
see: prednicarbate
s 770777
see: prednicarbate
s77 0777
see: prednicarbate
s770777
see: prednicarbate
s 8666
see: 6,7 dichloro 2,3 dihydro 5 (n,n dimethylsulfamoyl)coumarilic acid
sagittol
see: propranolol
saheh
see: centchroman
saheli
see: centchroman
saizen
see: human growth hormone
salamol
see: salbutamol
salbuair
see: salbutamol
salbulin
see: salbutamol
salbumol fort
see: salbutamol
salbupart
see: salbutamol

salbutamol

salbutamol sulfate

salbutax
see: salbutamol sulfate
salbuvent
see: salbutamol

salcardolol

salena
see: flumetasone pivalate plus salicylic acid
salgem
see: salbutamol

sali aldopur

sali decoderm
see: fluprednidene acetate
salidur
see: furosemide plus triamterene
salinex
see: furosemide
sali puren
see: hydrochlorothiazide plus triamterene
sali spiroctan
see: butizide plus spironolactone

salmefamol

salmetedur
see: salmeterol xinafoate

salmeterol

salmeterol hydroxynaphthoate
see: salmeterol xinafoate

salmeterol xinafoate

saltos
see: salbutamol
saltucin
see: butizide
saluacard
see: nikethamide
saludactone
see: canrenoate potassium
salures
see: bendroflumethiazide
salures k
see: bendroflumethiazide
saluretic agent
see: diuretic agent
saluric
see: chlorothiazide
salurin
see: mersalyl
salurin (wadel)
see: trichlormethiazide
saluron
see: hydroflumethiazide
salvacard
see: nikethamide
salvacerin
see: nikethamide
salvasma
see: isoprenaline
salyrgan
see: mersalyl
salzen
see: human growth hormone
sanabolicum
see: nandrolone cyclohexylpropionate
sanamethasone
see: dexamethasone
sanasma
see: isoprenaline
sanasthmax
see: beclometasone dipropionate
sanasthmyl
see: beclometasone dipropionate
sandonorm
see: bopindolol

sandoz 204545

sandoz li 32468
see: spirendolol
sanedrin
see: ephedrine
sanedrine
see: ephedrine
sanorex
see: mazindol
sas 1060
see: spironolactone
sas1060
see: spironolactone
satalol
see: sotalol
satolol
see: sotalol
sauran
see: citicoline
sauteralgyl
see: pethidine

sauvagine

savacort
see: prednisolone acetate
saventrine
see: isoprenaline
saxizon
see: hydrocortisone sodium succinate
sb 05
see: gonadorelin[6 medphalan]
sb 223030
see: idoxifene
sb223030
see: idoxifene
sb 226552
see: cyclohexyl[4 [2 [2 hydroxy 3 (4 hydroxyphenoxy)propylamino]ethyl]phenoxymethyl]phosphinic acid
sb 7505
see: ibopamine
sc 11585
see: oxandrolone
sc 14266
see: canrenoate potassium
sc14266
see: canrenoate potassium
sc 25152
see: mexrenone
sc 26714
see: mexrenoate potassium
sc 33643
see: bemitradine
sc 5233
see: 6,7 dihydrocanrenone

sc 5705
see: 4 [4 methyl 2 [4 [2 (1 piperidinyl)ethoxy]phenyl] 7 pivaloyloxy 2h 1 benzopyran 3 ylphenyl] pivalate
sc5705
see: 4 [4 methyl 2 [4 [2 (1 piperidinyl)ethoxy]phenyl] 7 pivaloyloxy 2h 1 benzopyran 3 ylphenyl] pivalate
sc 66110
see: eplerenone
sc66110
see: eplerenone
sc 9376
see: canrenone
sc9376
see: canrenone
sc 9420
see: spironolactone
sc9420
see: spironolactone
scandine
see: ibopamine
sch 11460
see: betamethasone dipropionate
sch 15719w
see: labetalol
sch15719w
see: labetalol
sch 18020w
see: beclometasone dipropionate
sch 19927
see: dilevalol
sch 22219
see: alclometasone dipropionate
sch 32088
see: mometasone furoate
sch32088
see: mometasone furoate
sch 4358
see: meprednisone
sch 4831
see: betamethasone
schericur
see: hydrocortisone
scherisolon
see: prednisolone
scherofluran
see: fludrocortisone acetate
scherofluron
see: fludrocortisone acetate
scheroson
see: cortisone
scherosone
see: cortisone
scherosone f
see: hydrocortisone
schiwadex 40
see: dextran 40
schiwadex 60
see: dextran 60
scitropin
see: human growth hormone
s cortophin
see: corticotropin
scurenaline
see: adrenalin
s.d. 1601
see: moprolol
sd 1601
see: moprolol
sd 171 12
see: clobenzorex
sd 2124 01
see: procinolol
sd 2124-01
see: procinolol
sd2124 01
see: procinolol
sd2124-01
see: procinolol
sd 271 12
see: clobenzorex
se 1520
see: indapamide
se1520
see: indapamide
se 2395
see: tertatolol
se 2620
see: almitrine dimesilate
se2620
see: almitrine dimesilate
sectral
see: acebutolol
sedolin
see: amphetamine
segontin
see: prenylamine
segontin 60
see: prenylamine
seguril
see: furosemide
selacryn
see: tienilic acid

selecal
see: tilisolol
selecor
see: celiprolol
selectol
see: celiprolol
seledat
see: selegiline

selegiline

selegiline hydrochloride
see: selegiline
selokeen
see: metoprolol tartrate
seloken
see: metoprolol tartrate
seloken zoc
see: metoprolol tartrate
selokomb
see: hydrochlorothiazide plus metoprolol tartrate
selopres
see: hydrochlorothiazide plus metoprolol
selopress
see: hydrochlorothiazide plus metoprolol
selozide
see: hydrochlorothiazide plus metoprolol tartrate
selozok
see: metoprolol tartrate
semcox
see: hydromorphone
semilente iletin
see: insulin zinc suspension
semilente insulin
see: insulin zinc suspension
semitard
see: insulin zinc suspension
semoxydrine
see: methamphetamine
seragon
see: seric gonadotropin
ser ap es
see: hydralazine plus hydrochlorothiazide plus reserpine
serapes
see: hydralazine plus hydrochlorothiazide plus reserpine
seretide
see: fluticasone propionate plus salmeterol
serevent
see: salmeterol xinafoate
seric gonadotrophin
see: seric gonadotropin

seric gonadotropin

seric gonadotropins
see: seric gonadotropin
serilone
see: prednisolone
sermaka
see: fludroxycortide

sermorelin

serogan
see: seric gonadotropin
serophene
see: clomifene citrate
serostim
see: human growth hormone
serotim
see: human growth hormone
serotropin
see: seric gonadotropin
serpasil apresoline esidrex
see: hydralazine plus hydrochlorothiazide plus reserpine
sertum
see: soquinolol mucate
serum immunoreactive insulin
see: immunoreactive insulin
servicort topical
see: hydrocortisone acetate
servidone
see: chlortalidone
servier 2620
see: almitrine dimesilate
sevanil
see: etamivan
sevredol
see: morphine sulfate
sexovid
see: cyclofenil
sf
see: growth hormone
sh 440
see: methylprednisolone aceponate
sh 467
see: mespirenone
sh 470
see: drospirenone
sh470
see: drospirenone
sh 489
see: atamestane

sh 723
see: mesterolone
sh 863
see: clocortolone pivalate
sh863
see: clocortolone pivalate
shaeli
see: centchroman
sh d515
see: 15beta,16beta methylenemexrenone
she 222
see: mepindolol
s hemoglobin
see: hemoglobin S
sh k 203
see: fluocortin butyl
sh k203
see: fluocortin butyl
shatorn
see: buphenine
shl 183a
see: diflucortolone valerate
sickle cell haemoglobin
see: hemoglobin S
sickle cell hemoglobin
see: hemoglobin S
sickle hemoglobin
see: hemoglobin S
sicorten
see: halometasone
sidnocarb
see: sydnocarb
sidnophen
see: sydnofen
sigasalur
see: furosemide
sigmacort
see: hydrocortisone acetate
simaron
see: etamivan
simesalgina
see: pethidine
simpamina
see: amphetamine
simpamina d
see: dexamphetamine
simpamine
see: amphetamine
simpatedrin
see: amphetamine
simpatedrine
see: amphetamine
sim pelate
see: bamethan
simplene
see: adrenalin
sinalgin
see: methadone
sincomen
see: canrenoate potassium
sincortex
see: deoxycorticosterone acetate
sinesalin
see: bendroflumethiazide
sinkol
see: dextran
sinkron
see: citicoline
sintabolin
see: nandrolone phenpropionate
sinthiodal
see: oxycodone
sintoclar
see: citicoline
sionon
see: sorbitol
sisuril
see: hydroflumethiazide
sj 0011
see: human growth hormone
sj 0021
see: recombinant follitropin
sj0021
see: recombinant follitropin
sk 110
see: azosemide
sk and f 5137
see: dextromoramide
sk and f 8542
see: triamterene
sk and f 92657
see: prizidilol
skenan
see: morphine
skenan lp
see: morphine sulfate
skf 100168
see: ibopamine
skf 100168 a
see: ibopamine

skf 105494

skf105494
see: skf 105494

skf 105517
see: carvedilol
skf105517
see: carvedilol
skf 1085 a
see: epinine
skf 110679
see: histidyl dextro tryptophylalanyltryptophyl dextro phenylalanyllysinamide
skf 40383
see: carbuterol
skf 5137
see: dextromoramide
skf 62698
see: tienilic acid
skf 6611
see: norclostebol
skf 7692
see: benorterone
skf 82526
see: fenoldopam
skf 82526 j
see: fenoldopam mesilate
skf 8542
see: triamterene
skf8542
see: triamterene
skf 92657
see: prizidilol
skf 92657 a2
see: prizidilol
skf 95018
see: 6 [4 [3 [[3 [4 [2 (cyclopropylmethoxy)ethyl]phenoxy] 2 hydroxypropyl]amino]propionamido]phenyl] 4,5 dihydro 5 methyl 3(2h) pyridazinone
skf r 106114
see: fenoldopam 7,8 bis(n ethylcarbamate)
skf r 82526
see: fenoldopam
skf uk 52
see: oxprenolol
skinostelon
see: pregnenolone
sl 75177 10
see: cicloprolol
sl 75212
see: betaxolol
slankosan
see: mazindol
slimin
see: hydrochlorothiazide plus triamterene
slow lopresor
see: metoprolol tartrate
slow trasicor
see: oxprenolol
slow trasitensin
see: trasitensin
slow-trasitensin
see: trasitensin
slyn ll
see: phendimetrazine tartrate
sm 11044
see: 3 (3,4 dihydroxyphenyl) 2 [3 (4 fluorophenyl)propylamino] 3 hydroxypropionic acid pyrrolidine amide
sm 9500
see: somatrem
sm9500
see: somatrem
sn 203
see: clobetasone butyrate
sn 408
see: salmeterol xinafoate
sn 6187
see: butizide
snb 5001
see: recombinant erythropoietin
sodium caffeine benzoate
see: caffeine benzoate
sodium chlorothiazide
see: chlorothiazide

sofradex

solacthyl
see: corticotropin
soladren
see: adrenalin
solbutamol
see: salbutamol
soldactone
see: canrenoate potassium
soldesam
see: dexamethasone sodium phosphate
solgol
see: nadolol
solgol mite
see: nadolol
solodelf
see: triamcinolone acetonide
solomet
see: methylprednisolone
solone
see: prednisolone

Index

solucelestan
see: betamethasone sodium phosphate
solucort
see: prednisolone sodium phosphate
solu cortef
see: hydrocortisone sodium succinate
solucortef
see: hydrocortisone sodium succinate
solu cortef mix o vial
see: hydrocortisone
soludacortin
see: prednisolone sodium succinate
soludactone
see: canrenoate potassium
soludecadrol
see: dexamethasone sodium phosphate
solu decadron
see: dexamethasone sodium phosphate
soludecadron
see: dexamethasone sodium phosphate
solu decortin
see: methylprednisolone
solu decortin h
see: prednisolone sodium succinate
soludecortin h
see: prednisolone sodium succinate
soludeltacortef
see: prednisolone sodium succinate
solu glyc
see: hydrocortisone sodium succinate
soluglyc
see: hydrocortisone sodium succinate
solu medrol
see: methylprednisolone sodium succinate
solumedrol
see: methylprednisolone sodium succinate
solumedrone
see: methylprednisolone sodium succinate
solupred
see: prednisolone 3 sulfobenzoate
solupren
see: prednisolone
soluprene
see: prednisolone
solvasma
see: isoprenaline
soly glyc
see: hydrocortisone sodium succinate
som 1122
see: alpha [[[3 (1 benzimidazolyl) 1,1 dimethylpropyl]amino]methyl] 2 fluoro 4 hydroxybenzyl alcohol
somacton
see: growth hormone
somagard
see: deslorelin
somantin
see: growth hormone
somatobiss
see: growth hormone releasing factor
somatocrinin
see: growth hormone releasing factor
somatocrinin 44
see: growth hormone releasing factor
somatocrinin derivative
see: growth hormone releasing factor derivative
somatohorm
see: somatrem
somatoliberin
see: growth hormone releasing factor

somatomedin

somatomedin A

somatomedin B

somatomedin C

somatomedins
see: somatomedin
somatonorm
see: somatrem
somatorelin
see: growth hormone releasing factor
somatotrofin
see: growth hormone
somatotrope hormone
see: growth hormone
somatotrophic hormone
see: growth hormone
somatotrophin
see: growth hormone
somatotropic hormone
see: growth hormone
somatotropin
see: growth hormone
somatotropin analog
see: growth hormone derivative
somatotropin derivative
see: growth hormone derivative

Index

somatotropin,human
see: human growth hormone
somatotropin,methionyl
see: somatrem
somatotropin releasing factor
see: growth hormone releasing factor
somatotropin-releasing hormone
see: growth hormone releasing factor
somatotropins, recombinant
see: recombinant growth hormone

somatrem

somatropic hormone
see: growth hormone
somatropin
see: human growth hormone
somazina
see: citicoline
sometribove
see: somatrem
soprol
see: bisoprolol

soquinolol

soquinolol mucate

sorbelite
see: sorbitol
sorbit
see: sorbitol
sorbital
see: sorbitol
sorbite
see: sorbitol

sorbitol

sorbo
see: sorbitol
sorbol
see: sorbitol
sosegon
see: pentazocine
sosigon
see: pentazocine
sotabeta
see: sotalol
sotacol
see: sotalol
sotacor
see: sotalol
sotahexal
see: sotalol
sotalex
see: sotalol

sotalol

sotalol hydrochloride
see: sotalol
sotapor
see: sotalol
sota saar
see: sotalol
sotastad
see: sotalol

soterenol

soterenol hydrochloride
see: soterenol
soxysympamine
see: methamphetamine
sp 104
see: tetrahydrocannabinol
spasmo mucosolvan
see: ambroxol plus clenbuterol
spectramedryn
see: medrysone
spersadex
see: dexamethasone sodium phosphate
sphygmogenin
see: adrenalin
spiranyl durules
see: terbutaline sulfate

spirendolol

spiricort
see: prednisolone
spiridon
see: spironolactone
spirocort
see: budesonide
spiroctan
see: spironolactone
spiroctan m
see: spironolactone
spiroctazide
see: aldactazine
spirolactone
see: spironolactone

spirolang
see: spironolactone
spirone
see: spironolactone
spironolacton
see: spironolactone

spironolactone

spironolactone plus altizide
see: aldactazine
spironolactone plus butizide
see: butizide plus spironolactone
spironolactone with butizide
see: butizide plus spironolactone
spironone
see: spironolactone
spiropent
see: clenbuterol
spirorenone,1,2 dihydro
see: drospirenone
spirothiobarbiturate 03620
see: spironolactone
spirotone
see: spironolactone

spiroxasone

spirozide
see: aldactazine
spolotane
see: prednisolone
spoloven
see: dexamethasone
spoloven 17 valerate
see: dexamethasone 17 valerate
sq 11725
see: nadolol
sq 16374
see: metenolone enantate
sq 17409
see: drocinonide
sq 27239
see: tipredane
sq 9538
see: testolactone
squibb hc
see: hydrocortisone acetate
sr 20
see: methylphenidate
sr 57227
see: 4 amino 1 (6 chloro 2 pyridyl)piperidine
sr57227
see: 4 amino 1 (6 chloro 2 pyridyl)piperidine
sr 57227a
see: 4 amino 1 (6 chloro 2 pyridyl)piperidine
sr57227a
see: 4 amino 1 (6 chloro 2 pyridyl)piperidine
sr 58375a
see: n (1,2,3,4 tetrahydro 7 hydroxy 2 naphthyl)phenylethanolamine
sr 58539b
see: 3 chloro n (7 ethoxycarbonylmethoxy 1,2,3,4 tetrahydro 2 naphthyl)phenylethanolamine
sr 58572a
see: 3 chloro n (1,2,3,4 tetrahydro 7 hydroxy 2 naphthyl)phenylethanolamine
sr 58611
see: [[7 [[2 (3 chlorophenyl) 2 hydroxyethyl]amino] 5,6,7,8 tetrahydro 2 naphthyl]oxy]acetic acid ethyl ester
sr58611
see: [[7 [[2 (3 chlorophenyl) 2 hydroxyethyl]amino] 5,6,7,8 tetrahydro 2 naphthyl]oxy]acetic acid ethyl ester
sr 58611a
see: [[7 [[2 (3 chlorophenyl) 2 hydroxyethyl]amino] 5,6,7,8 tetrahydro 2 naphthyl]oxy]acetic acid ethyl ester
sr58611a
see: [[7 [[2 (3 chlorophenyl) 2 hydroxyethyl]amino] 5,6,7,8 tetrahydro 2 naphthyl]oxy]acetic acid ethyl ester
sr 59230
see: 1 (2 ethylphenoxy) 3 (1,2,3,4 tetrahydro 1 naphthylamino) 2 propanol oxalate
sr 59230a
see: 1 (2 ethylphenoxy) 3 (1,2,3,4 tetrahydro 1 naphthylamino) 2 propanol oxalate
sr 59483a
see: 1 (2 ethylphenoxy) 3 (1,2,3,4 tetrahydro 1 naphthylamino) 2 propanol oxalate
sr 720 22
see: metolazone
sr 72022
see: metolazone
st
see: growth hormone
st 104
see: prednylidene
st 1085
see: midodrine
st1085
see: midodrine

st 1396
see: celiprolol
st 1512
see: hexoprenaline
st1512
see: hexoprenaline
stanaprol
see: androstanolone
stanazolol
see: stanozolol
stanolone
see: androstanolone
stanolone derivative
see: androstanolone derivative
stanolone propionate
see: androstanolone propionate
stanoprol
see: androstanolone
stanorone
see: androstanolone
stanozol
see: stanozolol
stanozole
see: stanozolol

stanozolol

stapranolol
see: propranolol
starch,hydroxyethyl
see: hetastarch
stc 1106
see: fluprednidene acetate
stc1106
see: fluprednidene acetate
stellamine
see: nikethamide

stenbolone

stenbolone acetate

stenediol
see: methandriol
stenesium
see: methandriol
stenobolone
see: stenbolone
stenobolone acetate
see: stenbolone acetate
stenolon
see: metandienone
steranabol
see: clostebol acetate
steranabol depot
see: oxabolone cipionate
sterandryl
see: testosterone propionate
sterandryl amp
see: testosterone propionate
sterandryl retard
see: testosterone propionate
steraq
see: deoxycorticosterone acetate
sterax
see: desonide
sterilocaine
see: cocaine
stermonid
see: domoprednate
steroid,anabolic
see: anabolic agent
steroid aromatase inhibitor
see: aromatase inhibitor
sterolone
see: prednisolone
sterotest
see: testosterone propionate
sth
see: growth hormone
stiedex
see: desoximetasone
stillcardiol
see: pentetrazole
stiminol
see: nikethamide
stimovul
see: epimestrol
stimulan
see: amphetamine
stimulant
see: central stimulant agent
stimulant agent
see: central stimulant agent
stimulant drug
see: central stimulant agent
stimulants (historical)
see: central stimulant agent
stimulating agent
see: central stimulant agent
stimulative agent
see: central stimulant agent
stimulexin
see: doxapram

stimulin
see: nikethamide
storzolamide
see: acetazolamide
stp
see: 2,5 dimethoxy 4 methylamphetamine
strabolene
see: nandrolone phenpropionate
stresson
see: bunitrolol
strichnine
see: strychnine
stromba
see: stanozolol
strombaject
see: stanozolol
strychnidin 10 one
see: strychnine

strychnine

strychnine hydrochloride
see: strychnine
stryphnon
see: adrenalone
stryphnone
see: adrenalone
stupenal
see: oxycodone
stypnon
see: adrenalone
stypnone
see: adrenalone
styptirenal
see: adrenalin
su 10568
see: clortermine
su 4885
see: metyrapone
su4885
see: metyrapone
su 8341
see: cyclopenthiazide
su 8874
see: metyrapone
su8874
see: metyrapone
suacron
see: carazolol
suberoyl insulin
see: insulin derivative
substance m
see: hydrocortisone
subtardum
see: insulin zinc suspension
subutex
see: buprenorphine
succinylated gelatin
see: gelatin succinate
succinyl insulin
see: insulin derivative
sulfemoglobin
see: sulfhemoglobin

sulfhemoglobin

sulfohemoglobin
see: sulfhemoglobin
sultanol
see: salbutamol
sultanol n
see: salbutamol
sumial
see: propranolol
summair
see: broxaterol
superanabolon
see: nandrolone phenpropionate
superanabolone
see: nandrolone phenpropionate
superbolin
see: nandrolone phenpropionate
supercortisol
see: prednisolone
supercortizol
see: prednisolone
superfact
see: buserelin
super ov
see: follitropin
supertendin
see: dexamethasone acetate
supplosal
see: pethidine
supprelin
see: histrelin
supracapsulin
see: adrenalin
supranephrane
see: adrenalin
supranephrin
see: adrenalin
supranol
see: adrenalin
supra puren
see: spironolactone

suprapuren
see: spironolactone
suprarenaline
see: adrenalin
suprasteron
see: methyltestosterone
suprasteron amp
see: testosterone propionate
suprasterone
see: testosterone propionate
suprecur
see: buserelin acetate
suprefact
see: buserelin
suprel
see: adrenalin
supremon
see: buserelin acetate
suprifen
see: oxilofrine
suprifen psb
see: buphenine
suprilent
see: isoxsuprine
surenine
see: adrenalin
surenosterone
see: deoxycorticosterone acetate
surfagon
see: gonadorelin[1-9] ethylamide[6 dextro alanine]
surrenine
see: adrenalin
susphrine
see: adrenalin
sustained release trasitensin
see: trasitensin
sustanon
see: testosterone
suxizon
see: hydrocortisone sodium succinate

sydnocarb

sydnofen

sydnophen
see: sydnofen
symbicort
see: budesonide plus formoterol
symoron
see: methadone
sympametin
see: amphetamine
sympamin
see: dexamphetamine
sympamine
see: amphetamine
sympatedrine
see: amphetamine
sympathin
see: noradrenalin
sympathin e
see: noradrenalin
sympathin i
see: adrenalin
synaclyn
see: flunisolide
synacort
see: hydrocortisone
synacten
see: tetracosactide
synacthen
see: tetracosactide
synacthen 1-39 peptide
see: corticotropin derivative
synacthen depot
see: tetracosactide zinc phosphate
synacthene
see: tetracosactide
synacthen immediat
see: tetracosactide
synacthen retard
see: corticotropin
synacthine
see: tetracosactide
synadrin
see: prenylamine
synalar
see: fluocinolone acetonide
synalar forte
see: fluocinolone acetonide
synalar gamma
see: fluocinolone acetonide
synalar nasal
see: fluocinolone acetonide
synandone
see: fluocinolone acetonide
synandrets
see: methyltestosterone
synandrol
see: testosterone
synandrotabs
see: methyltestosterone

synarel
see: nafarelin acetate
synasteron
see: oxymetholone
synathen
see: tetracosactide
synchrodyn 1-17
see: alsactide
synchrodyn[1-17]
see: alsactide
syncort
see: deoxycorticosterone acetate
syncorta
see: deoxycorticosterone acetate
syncortyl
see: deoxycorticosterone acetate
syndren
see: methyltestosterone
syndrox
see: methamphetamine
synemol
see: fluocinolone acetonide
synerone
see: testosterone propionate
synlaudine
see: pethidine
synotic
see: fluocinolone acetonide
syntaris
see: flunisolide
syntecort
see: paramethasone acetate
syntestan
see: cloprednol
synthetic acth
see: tetracosactide

synthetic insulin

syracort
see: fluocortolone
t 0509
see: 3 hydroxydenopamine
t 1583
see: n (3,4,5 trimethoxyphenethyl)noradrenalin
t 712
see: amfepramone
ta 064
see: denopamine
ta 2005
see: 8 hydroxy 5 [1 hydroxy 2 [n [2 (4 methoxyphenyl) 1 methylethyl]amino]ethyl]carbostyril
ta2005
see: 8 hydroxy 5 [1 hydroxy 2 [n [2 (4 methoxyphenyl) 1 methylethyl]amino]ethyl]carbostyril

tabimorelin

tachytalol
see: sotalol
takamina
see: adrenalin
talatrol
see: trometamol

talinolol

talioin
see: pentazocine
taluvian
see: apomorphine
talwin
see: pentazocine
tamofen
see: tamoxifen citrate
tamokadin
see: tamoxifen citrate
tamoplac
see: tamoxifen
tamoplex
see: tamoxifen citrate
tamoxasta
see: tamoxifen

tamoxifen

tamoxifen,3 hydroxy
see: droloxifene
tamoxifen analog ii
see: 1,1 dichloro 2,3 diphenylcyclopropane

tamoxifen aziridine

tamoxifen citrate

tamoxifen derivative

tamoxifene
see: tamoxifen
tamoxifen,hydroxy
see: hydroxytamoxifen
tamoxifen,nor
see: nortamoxifen

Index

tamoxiphen derivative
see: tamoxifen derivative
tamoxiphen,monohydroxy
see: hydroxytamoxifen
tamoxyfen,4 hydroxy
see: 4 hydroxytamoxifen
tandix
see: indapamide
tap 144
see: leuprorelin
tap144
see: leuprorelin
tap 144 sr
see: leuprorelin
tap144 sr
see: leuprorelin
taracortelone
see: prednisolone
tareg d
see: hydrochlorothiazide plus valsartan
tarugan
see: morazone
tat 59
see: miproxifene phosphate
tauliz
see: piretanide

tazolol

TBPS
see: tert butylbicyclophosphorothioate
te 176
see: 4 cyclohexylamino 1 (1 naphthyloxy) 2 butanol
te176
see: 4 cyclohexylamino 1 (1 naphthyloxy) 2 butanol
tebodal
see: oxycodone
tedarol
see: triamcinolone diacetate
tekodin
see: oxycodone
teleost insulin
see: insulin
telipex
see: methyltestosterone
temetex
see: diflucortolone valerate
temetex c
see: diflucortolone valerate
temgesic
see: buprenorphine
temovate
see: clobetasol propionate
temserin
see: timolol maleate
tenamfetamine
see: 3,4 methylenedioxyamphetamine
teneretic
see: atenolol plus chlortalidone
tenif
see: atenolol plus nifedipine
tenoblock
see: atenolol
tenolol
see: atenolol
tenordate
see: atenolol plus nifedipine
tenorectic
see: atenolol plus chlortalidone
tenoret
see: atenolol plus chlortalidone
tenoretic
see: atenolol plus chlortalidone
tenoretic ge
see: atenolol plus chlortalidone
tenoretic mite
see: atenolol plus chlortalidone
tenormin
see: atenolol
tenormin mite
see: atenolol
tenovate
see: clobetasol propionate
tensamin
see: dopamine

tensigradyl

tensinor
see: atenolol
tenuate
see: amfepramone
tenuate dospan
see: amfepramone
teoptic
see: carteolol
tepanil
see: amfepramone
terbasmin
see: terbutaline sulfate
terbutalin
see: terbutaline

Index

terbutaline

terbutaline sulfate

terbutalin sulfate
see: terbutaline sulfate
terbutylamine
see: phentermine
teriam
see: triamterene
terion
see: fominoben
teronac
see: mazindol

terracortril

terra cortril
see: terracortril
terracortril gel
see: terracortril

tertatolol

tertatolol hydrochloride
see: tertatolol
tertensif
see: indapamide
tes
see: testolactone
teslac
see: testolactone
teslen
see: testosterone

tesmilifene

tesmilifene hydrochloride
see: tesmilifene
testa c
see: testosterone cipionate
testaform
see: testosterone propionate
testahomen
see: methyltestosterone
testamone
see: testosterone
testandrone
see: testosterone
testaqua
see: testosterone
testerone
see: testosterone
testex
see: testosterone propionate
testhormone
see: methyltestosterone
testim
see: testosterone
testin
see: methyltestosterone
testin tabletter
see: methyltestosterone
testipron
see: methyltestosterone
testobase
see: methyltestosterone
testoderm
see: testosterone
testoderm ciii
see: testosterone
testodet
see: testosterone propionate
testodrin
see: testosterone propionate
testodrin prolongatum
see: testosterone cipionate
testoform
see: methyltestosterone
testogel
see: testosterone
testogen
see: testosterone propionate
testogenina
see: methyltestosterone
testogenine
see: methyltestosterone
testoject 50
see: testosterone

testolactone

testolactone propionate
see: testolactone

testololactone

testoluton
see: testosterone
testoluton forte
see: testosterone
testonique
see: testosterone propionate

Index

testonorpon
see: methyltestosterone
testora
see: methyltestosterone
testoral
see: fluoxymesterone
testore
see: methyltestosterone
testorex
see: methyltestosterone
testormol
see: testosterone propionate
testormon
see: testosterone propionate
testosid
see: testosterone propionate
testosteron
see: testosterone

testosterone

1 testosterone

testosterone,11 oxo
see: 11 oxotestosterone
testosterone 17beta cypionate
see: testosterone cipionate
testosterone 17 undecylate
see: testosterone undecanoate

testosterone 4 butylcyclohexanecarboxylate

testosterone buciclate
see: testosterone 4 butylcyclohexanecarboxylate
testosterone,4 hydroxy
see: 4 hydroxytestosterone
testosterone chloride
see: testosterone

testosterone cipionate

testosterone congeners
see: testosterone derivative
testosterone conjugate
see: testosterone
testosterone cypionate
see: testosterone cipionate

testosterone derivative

testosterone enantate

testosterone enantate benziloylhydrazone

testosterone enanthane
see: testosterone enantate
testosterone enanthate
see: testosterone enantate

testosterone ester

testosterone ester mixture
see: testosterone ester

testosterone ether

testosterone heptanoate
see: testosterone enantate
testosterone heptonate
see: testosterone enantate
testosterone heptylate
see: testosterone enantate
testosterone oenanthate
see: testosterone enantate

testosterone phenylpropionate

testosterone propionate

testosteronepropionate
see: testosterone propionate

testosterone undecanoate

testosterone undecylate
see: testosterone undecanoate
testosteron propionate
see: testosterone propionate
testosviron depot
see: testosterone enantate
testoviron
see: methyltestosterone
testoviron amp
see: testosterone propionate
testoviron depot
see: testosterone enantate
testovis
see: methyltestosterone
testovis compresse
see: methyltestosterone

testoxyl
see: testosterone propionate
testoxyl perlinguale
see: methyltestosterone
testral
see: methyltestosterone
testred
see: methyltestosterone
testred cypionate
see: testosterone cipionate
testrex
see: testosterone propionate
testrina m
see: methyltestosterone
testrone
see: testosterone
testryl
see: testosterone

tetrabenazine

tetracor
see: pentetrazole
tetracosactid
see: tetracosactide

tetracosactide

1 24 tetracosactide
see: tetracosactide
tetracosactide retard
see: tetracosactide
tetracosactide zinc
see: tetracosactide zinc phosphate

tetracosactide zinc phosphate

tetracosactin
see: tetracosactide
tetracosactrin
see: tetracosactide
tetracosactrin zinc phosphate
see: tetracosactide zinc phosphate

3 [4 (1,2,3,4 tetrahydro 6 methoxy 2 phenyl 1 naphthyl)phenoxy] 1,2 propanediol

n (1,2,3,4 tetrahydro 7 hydroxy 2 naphthyl)phenylethanolamine

tetrahydrocannabinal
see: tetrahydrocannabinol
tetrahydrocannabinoic acid
see: tetrahydrocannabinolic acid

tetrahydrocannabinol

tetrahydro cannabinol
see: tetrahydrocannabinol
tetrahydrocannabinol 1 ene
see: dronabinol
7,8,9,10 tetrahydrocannabinol
see: tetrahydrocannabinol
tetrahydrocannabinol delta1
see: dronabinol

delta8 tetrahydrocannabinol

tetrahydrocannabinol delta9
see: dronabinol

delta9(11) tetrahydrocannabinol

tetrahydrocannabinol derivative

delta8 tetrahydrocannabinol derivative

tetrahydrocannabinolic acid

tetrahydrocannabinolic acid a
see: tetrahydrocannabinolic acid
tetrahydrocannabinolic acid b
see: tetrahydrocannabinolic acid
tetrahydrocannabinol isomer
see: tetrahydrocannabinol
tetrahydrocannabiol
see: tetrahydrocannabinol

tetrahydrocortisol

tetrahydrocortisone

tetrahydro hydrocortisone
see: tetrahydrocortisol
tetrahydrohydrocortisone
see: tetrahydrocortisol

Index

tetrahydrogestrinone

tetramethylhes
see: 2,3 bis(4 hydroxyphenyl) 2,3 dimethylbutane
tetramethylhexestrol
see: 2,3 bis(4 hydroxyphenyl) 2,3 dimethylbutane

tetramethylsuccinimide

tetrazol
see: pentetrazole
tetroquinol
see: tretoquinol
tevacor
see: oxprenolol
th 1165
see: fenoterol
th 1165 a
see: fenoterol
th 1165a
see: fenoterol
th 152
see: orciprenaline
thalitone
see: chlortalidone
tham
see: trometamol
tham solution
see: trometamol
thecodin
see: oxycodone
thein
see: caffeine
theoadrenalin
see: theodrenaline

theodrenaline

theodrenaline plus cafedrine
see: cafedrine plus theodrenaline
theophyllineethylamphetamine
see: fenetylline
theptine
see: amphetamine
therabolin
see: methandriol dipropionate
theranabol
see: oxymesterone
therobolin
see: methandriol dipropionate
thiabulazid
see: butizide
thiabutazide
see: butizide
thiadril
see: hydrochlorothiazide
thiamizide
see: tiamizide
thiaretic
see: hydrochlorothiazide
thiaver
see: epitizide
thiazide
see: thiazide diuretic agent
thiazide derivative
see: thiazide diuretic agent
thiazide diuretic
see: thiazide diuretic agent

thiazide diuretic agent

thiazidil
see: methyclothiazide
thienilic acid
see: tienilic acid
thienylic acid
see: tienilic acid
thiobulazid
see: butizide
thiovalone
see: tixocortol pivalate
thiuretic
see: hydrochlorothiazide
thixocortol
see: tixocortol
thixocortol pivalate
see: tixocortol pivalate
thomasin
see: etilefrine
thomasin retard
see: etilefrine

thrombocyte concentrate

thrometamol
see: trometamol
ths 101
see: dexamethasone 17,21 dipropionate
ths 201
see: halopredone acetate
thylakentrin
see: seric gonadotropin
thymergix
see: pyrovalerone

tiabutazide
see: butizide

tiamizide

tibicorten
see: triamcinolone acetonide
tibiocorten
see: triamcinolone acetonide
tibofem
see: tibolone

tibolone

ticabesone

ticabesone propionate

ticrynafen
see: tienilic acid

tienilic acid

tienoxolol

tilcant
see: bunitrolol

tilisolol

tilisolol hydrochloride
see: tilisolol
timabak
see: timolol maleate
timacor
see: timolol maleate

timobesone

timobesone acetate

timodyne
see: mefexamide
timolate
see: timolol maleate

timolol

timolol hemihydrate
see: timolol
timolol hydrogen maleate
see: timolol maleate

timolol maleate

timoptic
see: timolol maleate
timoptic xe
see: timolol maleate
timoptol
see: timolol maleate
timpilo
see: timolol maleate
tiovalon
see: tixocortol pivalate

tipredane

tixocortol

tixocortol 21 pivalate
see: tixocortol pivalate

tixocortol pivalate

tixocortone 21 pivalate
see: tixocortol pivalate
tixocortone trimethylacetate
see: tixocortol pivalate
tobanum
see: cloranolol
tobradex
see: dexamethasone plus tobramycin
tobramycin plus dexamethasone
see: dexamethasone plus tobramycin
tocodrin
see: buphenine
tokuderm
see: betamethasone valerate
tolamidol
see: tolamolol

tolamolol

tolamolol hydrochloride
see: tolamolol

Index

toliprolol

tolubuterol
see: tulobuterol
tonazol
see: nikethamide
tonedron
see: methamphetamine
tonogen
see: adrenalin
topicon
see: halopredone acetate
topicort
see: desoximetasone
topicorte
see: desoximetasone
topifug
see: desonide
topilar
see: fluclorolone acetonide
topisolone
see: desoximetasone
topodil
see: fluocortolone
toprol
see: metoprolol succinate
toprol xl
see: metoprolol succinate
topsym
see: fluocinonide
topsyn
see: fluocinonide
topsyne
see: fluocinonide
toradiur
see: torasemide

torasemide

torem
see: torasemide

toremifene

tornalate
see: bitolterol mesilate

torrat

torrem
see: torasemide
torsemide
see: torasemide
tostrelle
see: testosterone
tostrex
see: testosterone
tostrin
see: testosterone propionate
tostrina m
see: methyltestosterone
totocortin
see: dexamethasone sodium phosphate
toxin f2
see: zearalenone
tradon
see: pemoline
tramacin
see: triamcinolone acetonide
tramcinolone
see: triamcinolone
trandate
see: labetalol
tranquo alupent
see: orciprenaline
trans cannabidiol
see: cannabidiol
trans cisclomiphene
see: clomifene
trans clomifene
see: enclomifene
transclomifene
see: enclomifene
trans clomifene citrate
see: enclomifene citrate
trans clomiphene
see: enclomifene
transclomiphene
see: enclomifene
trans clomiphene citrate
see: enclomifene citrate
trans dehydroandrosterone
see: prasterone
transfusion substitute
see: plasma substitute
trans morphine
see: morphine
trans tamoxifen
see: tamoxifen
trans testosterone
see: testosterone
trans tetrahydrocannabinol
see: tetrahydrocannabinol
trasacor
see: oxprenolol

trasicor
see: oxprenolol
trasicor retard
see: oxprenolol
trasidex
see: cyclopenthiazide plus oxprenolol
trasidrex
see: cyclopenthiazide plus oxprenolol
trasipresol
see: dihydralazine plus oxprenolol
trasipressol
see: dihydralazine plus oxprenolol
trasitencin
see: trasitensin

trasitensin

trasitensin retard
see: trasitensin
trasitensin sr
see: trasitensin
travocort
see: diflucortolone valerate

traxanox

trecadrine

tredalat
see: acebutolol plus nifedipine
trelstar
see: triptorelin
trenamist
see: adrenalin
trenantone
see: leuprorelin
trenbalone acetate
see: trenbolone acetate

trenbolone

17alpha trenbolone

trenbolone acetate

trepress

trestolone

tretoguinol
see: tretoquinol

tretoquinol

tretoquinol derivative

tretoquinol hydrochloride
see: tretoquinol
treupel
see: gelonida
triacet
see: triamcinolone acetonide
triacetylinsulin
see: insulin derivative
triacortyl
see: triamcinolone
triadcortyl
see: mycolog
triam
see: triamcinolone acetonide
triamalone
see: triamcinolone acetonide
triamcimetil
see: dexamethasone
triamcinolide acetonide
see: triamcinolone acetonide
triamcinolon
see: triamcinolone
triamcinolon acetonide
see: triamcinolone acetonide

triamcinolone

triamcinolone 16,17 acetonide
see: triamcinolone acetonide
triamcinolone acetamide
see: triamcinolone acetonide

triamcinolone acetate

triamcinolone acetonamide
see: triamcinolone acetonide
triamcinolone acetonid
see: triamcinolone acetonide

triamcinolone acetonide

triamcinolone benetonide
see: triamcinolone acetonide

Index

triamcinolone diacetate

triamcinolone hexacetonide

triamcort
see: triamcinolone
triampterene
see: triamterene
triampur
see: hydrochlorothiazide plus triamterene
triamterence
see: triamterene

triamterene

triamterene plus bemetizide
see: diucomb
triamterene plus benzthiazide
see: benzthiazide plus triamterene
triamterene plus cyclothiazide
see: cycloteriam
triamterene plus furosemide
see: furosemide plus triamterene

triamterene plus xipamide

triamterene with furosemide
see: furosemide plus triamterene
triamterene with xipamide
see: triamterene plus xipamide
triamterens
see: triamterene
triamteril
see: triamterene
triamterine
see: triamterene
triamthiazid
see: hydrochlorothiazide plus triamterene
triancinolon
see: triamcinolone
tri anemul
see: triamcinolone acetonide
trianide
see: triamcinolone acetonide
triazide
see: trichlormethiazide

tribendilol

tricarbamylinsulin
see: insulin derivative
trichlordiuride
see: trichlormethiazide
trichlormethazide
see: trichlormethiazide

trichlormethiazide

1,3,8 trichloro 6 methyldibenzofuran

trichloromethiazide
see: trichlormethiazide
tricrynafen
see: tienilic acid
tridesilon
see: desonide
tridesonit
see: desonide
tridomose
see: gestrinone
trienbolone
see: trenbolone
trienbolone acetate
see: trenbolone acetate
trienolone
see: trenbolone
trienolone acetate
see: trenbolone acetate
triflumen
see: trichlormethiazide
trifluoromethylhydrothiazide
see: hydroflumethiazide
trigon depot
see: triamcinolone acetonide

11beta,17alpha,21 trihydroxy 3,20 dioxopregna 1,4 diene 16alpha carboxylic acid methyl ester

tri(hydroxymethyl)aminomethane
see: trometamol
trihydroxy methylaminomethane
see: trometamol
trihydroxymethyl amino methane
see: trometamol
trihydroxymethylaminomethane
see: trometamol
trihydroxypregnanedione
see: tetrahydrocortisone
trikort
see: triamcinolone acetonide
trimcaps
see: phendimetrazine tartrate

trimepranol
see: metipranolol
trimethochinol
see: tretoquinol
trimethokinol
see: tretoquinol
trimethoquinol
see: tretoquinol
trimethoquinol derivative
see: tretoquinol derivative
trimethoquinol hydrochloride
see: tretoquinol

n (3,4,5 trimethoxyphenethyl)noradrenalin

trimethylol
see: trometamol
trimethylolaminomethane
see: trometamol
trimethylxanthine
see: caffeine
1,3,7 trimethylxanthine
see: caffeine
trimetoquinol
see: tretoquinol
trimetoquinol derivative
see: tretoquinol derivative
trimexolone
see: rimexolone
trimolet
see: phenylpropanolamine
triniol
see: paramethasone acetate

triniton

triolandren
see: testosterone ether

trioxifene

trioxifene mesilate

trioxifene mesylate
see: trioxifene mesilate
trioxifene methanesulfonate
see: trioxifene mesilate

tripamide

triphenylethylene derivative
see: 1,1,2 triphenylethylene derivative

1,1,2 triphenylethylene derivative

triptorelin

triquinol
see: tretoquinol
trirexan
see: triamterene plus xipamide
tris
see: trometamol
trisamine
see: trometamol
tris amino
see: trometamol
trisaminol
see: trometamol
tris buffer
see: trometamol
tris chloride
see: trometamol
tris cl
see: trometamol
tris concentrate
see: trometamol
tris(heptafluoropropyl)amine
see: perfluorotripropylamine
tris hydrochloride
see: trometamol
tris hydroxymethylaminomethan
see: trometamol
trishydroxymethylamino methane
see: trometamol
trishydroxymethylaminomethane
see: trometamol
tris(hydroxymethyl)methylamine
see: trometamol
tris steril
see: trometamol
tris trometamol
see: trometamol
trisyn
see: fluocinolone acetonide
triteren
see: triamterene
trithiazid
see: hydrochlorothiazide plus triamterene

Index

trizma
see: trometamol
trometamine
see: trometamol

trometamol

trometamol edetate

tromethamine
see: trometamol
tromethamine e
see: trometamol edetate
tromethamol
see: trometamol
tromethane
see: trometamol
tromethanine
see: trometamol
trymex
see: triamcinolone acetonide
tryptal
see: gonadorelin[1-9] ethylamide[6 dextro tryptophan]
tryptex
see: gonadorelin[1-9] ethylamide[6 dextro tryptophan]
tryptorelin
see: triptorelin
ts 1020
see: hydrocortisone butyrate
ts 408
see: hydrocortisone 17 butyrate 21 propionate
tse 424
see: bazedoxifene
tse424
see: bazedoxifene
tsiklometiazid
see: cyclopenthiazide
tuloboterol
see: tulobuterol

tulobuterol

tulobuterol hydrochloride
see: tulobuterol
turbinaire
see: dexamethasone sodium phosphate
turfa
see: hydrochlorothiazide plus triamterene
turinabol
see: clostebol acetate
turobuterol
see: tulobuterol
tyb 5220
see: recombinant erythropoietin
tylinal
see: amfepramone
tylox
see: oxycodone
u 100
see: pig insulin
u 10997
see: mibolerone
u10997
see: mibolerone
u 11 100 a
see: nafoxidine
u 11100 a
see: nafoxidine
u 11100a
see: nafoxidine
u 19763
see: bolasterone
u1 tetrahydrocannabinol
see: dronabinol
u 23469
see: 3 [4 (1,2,3,4 tetrahydro 6 methoxy 2 phenyl 1 naphthyl)phenoxy] 1,2 propanediol
u 34865
see: diflorasone diacetate
u34865
see: diflorasone diacetate
u4 3,17 androstenedione
see: androstenedione
u 433
see: methoxyphenamine
u4 androsten 3,17 dione
see: androstenedione
u4 androstene 3,17 dione
see: androstenedione
u4 androstenedione
see: androstenedione
u 6013
see: isoflupredone acetate
u 67590a
see: methylprednisolone suleptanate
u 6817
see: norethandrolone
u 75799e
see: histidyl dextro tryptophylalanyltryptophyl dextro phenylalanyllysinamide
u9 tetrahydrocannabinol
see: dronabinol

Index

uk 11443
see: primidolol
uk 14,304
see: brimonidine
uk14,304
see: brimonidine
uk 14304
see: brimonidine
uk14304
see: brimonidine
uk 14304 18
see: brimonidine
uk1430418
see: brimonidine
uk 14304-18
see: brimonidine
uk14304-18
see: brimonidine
uk 6558 01
see: tolamolol
ulcosilvanil
see: acetazolamide
ulcosylvanil
see: acetazolamide

ulobetasol propionate

ultandren
see: fluoxymesterone
ultracorten
see: prednisone
ultracortene h
see: prednisolone sodium tetrahydrophthalate
ultracorten h
see: prednisolone sodium tetrahydrophthalate
ultracortenol
see: prednisolone pivalate
ultracortensol
see: prednisolone acetate
ultracortinol
see: prednisolone acetate
ultracur
see: fluocortolone
ultralan
see: fluocortolone caproate
ultralente
see: insulin zinc suspension
ultralente insulin
see: insulin zinc suspension
ultratard
see: insulin zinc suspension
ultratard hm
see: insulin zinc suspension
ultratard mc
see: insulin zinc suspension
ultravate
see: ulobetasol propionate

ultroser g

um 583
see: 7alpha (4 aminophenylthio)androstenedione
um 952
see: buprenorphine
um952
see: buprenorphine
umatrope
see: human growth hormone
umuline
see: neutral insulin
unat
see: torasemide
undecyloyl norandrostenolone
see: nandrolone undecanoate
undecyloylnorandrostenolone
see: nandrolone undecanoate
unephral
see: mercuderamide
unicard
see: dilevalol

uniderm

unidocan
see: deoxycorticosterone acetate
unilobin
see: lobeline
uniteston
see: testosterone propionate
unstable hemoglobin
see: hemoglobin
up 78842
see: tienoxolol
uprima
see: apomorphine
uractone
see: spironolactone
uragan
see: mersalyl
urbason
see: methylprednisolone
urbason retard
see: methylprednisolone acetate
urbason solubile
see: methylprednisolone sodium succinate

urea plus hydrocortisone
see: hydrocortisone plus urea
uregit
see: etacrynic acid
uregyt
see: etacrynic acid
uretren
see: triamterene
uricosid
see: probenecid
urocaudal
see: triamterene
urocid
see: probenecid
urodiazin
see: hydrochlorothiazide
urodiazine
see: hydrochlorothiazide
urofinil
see: chlortalidone
urofollitrophin
see: urofollitropin

urofollitropin

urozide
see: hydrochlorothiazide
urtilone
see: prednisone
usv 2555
see: indapamide
usv2555
see: indapamide
utemerine
see: ritodrine
uticort
see: betamethasone benzoate
utopar
see: ritodrine
vaderm
see: alclometasone dipropionate
val 1177
see: fenfluramine
val1177
see: fenfluramine
val 679
see: flunisolide
val679
see: flunisolide
valisone
see: betamethasone valerate
valnac
see: betamethasone valerate
valodex
see: tamoxifen citrate
vanabol
see: metandienone
vancenase
see: beclometasone dipropionate
vancenase aq
see: beclometasone dipropionate
vanceril
see: beclometasone dipropionate
vandid
see: etamivan
vanillic acid diethylamide
see: etamivan
vantol
see: bevantolol
vapedrine
see: amphetamine
vapo n iso
see: isoprenaline
variant,hemoglobin
see: hemoglobin variant
vasazol
see: pentetrazole
vasazol kwisda
see: nikethamide
vasculat
see: bamethan
vasculate
see: bamethan
vasculit
see: bamethan
vaseretic
see: enalapril plus hydrochlorothiazide
vasiten
see: buphenine
vasoconstrictine
see: adrenalin
vasocort
see: hydrocortisone
vasodilan
see: isoxsuprine
vasodilian
see: isoxsuprine
vasodrine
see: adrenalin
vasoplex
see: isoxsuprine
vasoretic
see: enalapril plus hydrochlorothiazide
vasosuprine
see: isoxsuprine

vasotonin
see: adrenalin
vasotonin forte seron
see: adrenalin
vasotran
see: isoxsuprine
vasoxine
see: methoxamine
vasoxine hydrochloride
see: methoxamine
vasoxyl
see: methoxamine
vasoxyl hydrochloride
see: methoxamine
vaspit
see: fluocortin butyl
vasylox
see: methoxamine
vasylox hydrochloride
see: methoxamine
vebenol
see: boldenone undecenoate
vectarion
see: almitrine dimesilate
velasulin
see: neutral insulin
velosulin
see: neutral insulin
vems
see: tretoquinol
venactone
see: canrenoic acid
venam
see: isoxsuprine
venetlin
see: salbutamol
venosan
see: pholedrine
ventilan
see: salbutamol
ventipulmin
see: clenbuterol
ventodisk
see: salbutamol
ventodisks
see: salbutamol
ventolase
see: clenbuterol
ventolin
see: salbutamol
ventolin aerosol
see: salbutamol
ventoline
see: salbutamol
ventolin nebules
see: salbutamol
ventolin tablets
see: salbutamol
ventramine
see: nikethamide
ventrazol
see: pentetrazole

veratide

veriderm medrol
see: methylprednisolone acetate
veritol
see: pholedrine
verobol
see: metandienone
verospiron
see: spironolactone
verospirone
see: spironolactone
veroxil
see: indapamide
vesix
see: furosemide
vetalog
see: triamcinolone acetonide
vetidrex
see: hydrochlorothiazide
vexol
see: rimexolone
viadur
see: leuprorelin
vialin
see: mephentermine
viani
see: fluticasone propionate plus salmeterol
viarex
see: beclometasone dipropionate
viarox
see: beclometasone dipropionate
vigil
see: modafinil
vilan
see: nicomorphine
vilescon
see: prolintane
villescon
see: prolintane
vioform millicorten
see: clioquinol plus dexamethasone

Index

vioform millicortenol
see: clioquinol plus dexamethasone
viozan
see: 4 hydroxy 7 [2 [2 [3 (2 phenylethoxy)propylsulfonyl]ethylamino]ethyl]benzothiazol 2(3h) one
virex oral
see: methyltestosterone
virilon
see: testosterone
virormolo
see: methyltestosterone
virormone
see: testosterone
virormone depot
see: testosterone enantate
virormone oral
see: methyltestosterone
virormone x
see: testosterone propionate
virosterone
see: testosterone
visacor
see: epanolol
visderm
see: amcinonide
visderm h
see: amcinonide

viskaldix

viskeen
see: pindolol
visken
see: pindolol
visken mite
see: pindolol
visken retard
see: pindolol
vistagan
see: levobunolol
vistimon
see: mesterolone
visumethazone
see: dexamethasone
vivarin
see: caffeine
vivazid
see: hydrochlorothiazide plus lisinopril
vobaderm
see: fluprednidene acetate
volex
see: hetastarch
volital
see: pemoline
volmac
see: salbutamol
volmax
see: salbutamol sulfate
volon
see: triamcinolone
volon a
see: triamcinolone acetonide
volon a 40
see: triamcinolone acetonide
volon a 80
see: triamcinolone acetonide
volon a tincture
see: triamcinolone acetonide
volonimat
see: triamcinolone acetonide
volume expander,plasma
see: plasma substitute
voranil
see: clortermine
voren
see: dexamethasone isonicotinate

vorozole

vortel
see: clorprenaline
vufb 6502
see: deacetylmetipranolol
w 2900
see: etozolin
w2900
see: etozolin
w 2946m
see: reproterol
w2946m
see: reproterol
w 6309
see: difluprednate
w6309
see: difluprednate
w 6412 a
see: bunolol
w 6412a
see: bunolol
w 7000a
see: levobunolol
w 752 a
see: human growth hormone
wandonorm
see: bopindolol

warduzuide
see: chlorothiazide
warner 6309
see: difluprednate
way 140424
see: bazedoxifene
way140424
see: bazedoxifene
we 704
see: soquinolol mucate
wellcortin
see: hydrocortisone acetate
westcort
see: hydrocortisone valerate
wg 253
see: rimiterol
wg253
see: rimiterol
wilpo
see: phentermine
win
see: methadone
win 14833
see: stanozolol
win 17757
see: danazol
win17757
see: danazol
win 20,228
see: pentazocine
win 20228
see: pentazocine
win 25978
see: amfonelic acid
win 27914
see: nivacortol
win 3046
see: isoetarine
win 32784
see: bitolterol mesilate
win 5162
see: isoprenaline
win 55212
see: 2,3 dihydro 5 methyl 3 (morpholinomethyl) 6 (1 naphthoyl)pyrrolo[1,2,3 de][1,4]benzoxazine
win 55212 2
see: 2,3 dihydro 5 methyl 3 (morpholinomethyl) 6 (1 naphthoyl)pyrrolo[1,2,3 de][1,4]benzoxazine
win 55212 3
see: 2,3 dihydro 5 methyl 3 (morpholinomethyl) 6 (1 naphthoyl)pyrrolo[1,2,3 de][1,4]benzoxazine
winobanin
see: danazol
winstrol
see: stanozolol
wintersteiner compound f
see: cortisone
wintonin
see: gepefrine tartrate
ws 7528
see: 3 methylnaringenin
ws7528
see: 3 methylnaringenin
wx 2426
see: chlorphentermine
wx 2462
see: chlorphentermine
wy 18481
see: gonadorelin[1-9] ethylamide[6 dextro alanine]
wy 3475
see: norboletone
wy3475
see: norboletone
wy 40972
see: lutrelin
wyamin
see: mephentermine
wyamine
see: mephentermine
wymesone
see: dexamethasone sodium phosphate
wymesone sodium
see: dexamethasone sodium phosphate
wysolone
see: prednisolone

xamoterol

xamoterol fumarate
see: xamoterol hydrogen fumarate
xamoterol hemifumarate
see: xamoterol hydrogen fumarate

xamoterol hydrogen fumarate

xamtol
see: xamoterol hydrogen fumarate
xenabol
see: 3beta androstanediol
xenalon
see: spironolactone

Index

xibenolol

xipamide

xipamide plus triamterene
see: triamterene plus xipamide
xopenex
see: levalbuterol
xuprin
see: isoxsuprine
xypamide
see: xipamide
xyvion
see: tibolone
y 12141
see: traxanox
yasmin
see: drospirenone plus ethinylestradiol
yb 2
see: indenolol
yetrazol
see: pentetrazole
ym 08316
see: formoterol fumarate
ym08316
see: formoterol fumarate
ym 09538
see: amosulalol
ym 17798
see: somatrem
ym17798
see: somatrem
ym 511
see: 4 [n (4 bromobenzyl) n (1,2,4 triazol 4 yl)amino]benzonitrile
ym 9538
see: amosulalol
yn 102
see: triamcinolone acetonide
yutopar
see: ritodrine
z 1170
see: broxaterol
28316z
see: indenolol
zambesil
see: chlortalidone
zami 1305
see: 1 tert butylamino 3 (3 methyl 2 nitrophenoxy) 2 propanol
zaroxolyn
see: metolazone
zd 1033
see: anastrozole
zd1033
see: anastrozole
zd 182780
see: fulvestrant
zd182780
see: fulvestrant
zd 2079
see: 4 [2 [(2 hydroxy 2 phenylethyl)amino]ethoxy]phenylacetic acid
zd 7114
see: 4 [2 [(2 hydroxy 3 phenoxypropyl)amino]ethoxy] n (2 methoxyethyl)phenoxyacetamide
zd 9238
see: fulvestrant
zd9238
see: fulvestrant
zearalanol
see: zeranol

zearalanone

zearalenon
see: zearalenone

zearalenone

zearalenone mycotoxin
see: zearalenone
zebeta
see: bisoprolol fumarate
zedrin
see: amphetamine
zedrine
see: amphetamine
zeisin
see: pirbuterol
zelapar
see: selegiline
zemide
see: tamoxifen citrate
zemide 20
see: tamoxifen citrate
zephrol
see: ephedrine

zeranol

zestoretic
see: hydrochlorothiazide plus lisinopril

Index

ziac
see: bisoprolol fumarate plus hydrochlorothiazide
zilmax
see: zilpaterol

zilpaterol

zilpaterol hydrochloride
see: zilpaterol
zinc insulin
see: insulin zinc suspension
zinc insulin crystalline
see: insulin zinc suspension
zinc insuline
see: insulin zinc suspension
zinc protamine insulin
see: isophane insulin

zindoxifene

zinterol

zipix
see: xipamide
zitazonium
see: tamoxifen citrate
zk 30595
see: drospirenone
zk30595
see: drospirenone
zk 32055
see: mexrenone
zk 90798
see: 4 ethyl 6,7 dimethoxy beta carboline 3 carboxylic acid methyl ester
zk 91587
see: 15beta,16beta methylenemexrenone
zk 91588
see: methylprednisolone aceponate
zk 94679
see: mespirenone
zk 97894
see: 17 hydroxy 15beta,16beta methylene 7alpha methylthio 3 oxo 17alpha pregna 1,4 diene 21 carboxylic acid gamma lactone
zm 182780
see: fulvestrant
zm182780
see: fulvestrant
zm 215001
see: 4 [2 [(2 hydroxy 3 phenoxypropyl)amino]ethoxy]phenoxyacetic acid
zok zid
see: hydrochlorothiazide plus metoprolol tartrate
zoladex
see: goserelin
zoladex depot
see: goserelin
zomacton
see: human growth hormone
zoolobelin
see: lobeline

zuclomifene

zuclomifene citrate

zu clomiphene
see: zuclomifene
zuclomiphene
see: zuclomifene

Index